This authoritative and comprehensive new publication looks in depth at a range of medical syndromes characterised by serious and unpredicted internal overheating of the body. These episodes may arise suddenly and unexpectedly in certain individuals, with life-threatening consequences, either as a result of heat stress, exceptional physical exertion or in response to certain common anaesthetics and some drugs, including ecstacy. The chapters focus on the full range of these syndromes, their metabolic and physiological basis, the important predisposing factors for the prediction of those at risk and the medical management of these conditions. The volume includes important contributions from authors of international repute and incorporates a wealth of information from the Leeds malignant hyperthermia investigation unit – the world's leading centre of research and investigation in this area.

This compilation provides an essential source of reference for those wishing to understand these disorders and a practical account of their medical management.

HYPERTHERMIC AND HYPERMETABOLIC DISORDERS

HYPERTHERMIC AND HYPERMETABOLIC DISORDERS

Exertional heat stroke, malignant hyperthermia and related syndromes

Edited by

PHILIP M. HOPKINS

*Senior lecturer in Anaesthesia, University of Leeds,
and Honorary Consultant Anaesthetist,
St James's University Hospital, Leeds*

and

F. RICHARD ELLIS

Professor of Anaesthesia, University of Leeds

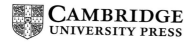 **CAMBRIDGE**
UNIVERSITY PRESS

Published by the Press Syndicate of the University of Cambridge
The Pitt Building, Trumpington Street, Cambridge CB2 1RP
40 West 20th Street, New York, NY 10011-4211, USA
10 Stamford Road, Oakleigh, Melbourne 3166, Australia

First published 1996

Printed in Great Britain at the University Press, Cambridge

A catalogue record for this book is available from the British Library

Library of Congress cataloguing in publication data

Hyperthermic and hypermetabolic disorders: exertional heat stroke,
   malignant hyperthermia, and related syndromes / edited by Philip M.
   Hopkins and F. R. Ellis.
      p.   cm.
      Includes index.
      ISBN 0 521 44381 4 (hardback)
   1. Fever.   2. Malignant hyperthermia.   3. Heatstroke.
   4. Neuroleptic malignant syndrome.   I. Hopkins, Philip M.
   II. Ellis, F. R. (Francis Richard)
      [DNLM: 1. Heat Stress Disorders.   2. Fever.   WD 610 H998 1996]
   RB129.H97   1996
   616′.047 – dc20
   DNLM/DLC
   for Library of Congress   96-13981   CIP

ISBN 0 521 44381 4 hardback

To Carmel (PMH) and to our patients

Contents

Contributors

P. J. Adnet
Service d'Accueil des Urgences, Hôpital B, CHU Lille, 59037 Lille Cédex, France

J. F. Antognini
Department of Anesthesiology, University of California School of Medicine, Davis, CA 95616, USA

C. G. Batty
Medical Branch, HQ 4 Division, Steeles Road, Aldershot, Hampshire, GU11 2DP, UK

P. E. Belchetz
General Infirmary at Leeds, Great George Street, Leeds LS1 3EX, UK

J. G. Dickinson
Duchess of Kent Military Hospital, Catterick Garrison, North Yorkshire, UK

J. Dinsmore
Department of Anaesthesia, St George's Hospital Medical School, Jenner Wing, Cranmer Terrace, London SW17 0RE, UK

F. R. Ellis
Malignant hyperthermia Investigation Unit, St James's University Hopsital, Leeds LS9 7TF, UK

J. E. Fletcher
Department of Anesthesiology, Hahnemann University, Broad and Vine, Philadelphia, PA 19102-1192, USA

W. A. Freeland
RGIT, 338 King Street, Aberdeen, AB2 3BJ, UK

G. A. Gronert
Department of Anesthesiology, University of California School of Medicine, Davis, CA 95616, USA

G. M. Hall
Department of Anaesthesia, St George's Hospital Medical School, Jenner Wing, Cranmer Terrace, London SW17 0RE, UK

P. J. Halsall
Malignant Hyperthermia Investigation Unit, St James's University Hospital, Leeds LS9 7TF, UK

P. Harnden
General Infirmary at Leeds, Great George Street, Leeds LS1 3EX, UK

J. A. Henry
Guy's Hospital, St Thomas Street, London SE1 9RT, UK

P. M. Hopkins
Malignant Hyperthermia Investigation Unit, St James's University Hospital, Leeds LS9 7TF, UK

J. P. Knochel
UT Southwestern Medical Centre and Department of Internal Medicine, Presbyterian Hospital of Dallas, Dallas, TX 75231, USA

R. M. Krivosic-Horber
Département d'Anesthésie-Réanimation, Hôpital B, CHU Lille, 59037 Lille Cédex, France

J.-F. Payen
Departement d'Anesthésie-Réanimation Chirurgicale, CHU Grenoble, F-38043 Grenoble Cédex G, France

H. Reyford
Département d'Anesthésie-Réanimation, Hôpital B, CHU Lille, 59037 Lille Cédex, France

H. Rosenberg
Department of Anesthesiology, Hahnemann University, Broad and Vine, Philadelphia, PA 19102-1192, USA

P. Stieglitz
Département d'Anesthésie-Réanimation Chirurgicale, CHU Grenoble, F-38043 Grenoble Cédex G, France

S. P. West
Northern Regional Genetics Service, 19/20 Claremont Place, Newcastle-upon-Tyne NE2 4AA, UK

Section 1

Exertional heat stroke

1

History and epidemiology: definitions and groups at risk

J. G. DICKINSON

History

'While he was out in the fields supervising the binding of the sheaves, he got sunstroke, took to his bed and died...' (Apocrypha). Such was the end of Manasses, husband of the beautiful Judith, heroine of the book named after her, in the sixth century BC. (She went on to use her feminine guile to behead the Commander in Chief of Nebuchadnezzar's army in Judea.) This may well be the earliest written description of heat stroke.

Mammals require homeothermia. If body temperature is to remain constant, heat gain must always be equal to heat loss. We can therefore assume that increased pressure on the system, heat stress, and occasional breakdown of control have been with us as long as humans have existed. Although detailed diagnostic data are not available, it seems reasonable to suppose, for example, that the deaths of 123 British prisoners in the notorious Black Hole of Calcutta on a single night in 1756 were the result of heat illness (Woodruff, 1954). In more recent times, a heat wave in Athens in 1987 killed nearly 1000 people, most of them elderly (Katsouyanni *et al.*, 1988). In the USA, Ellis (1972) has analysed the deaths in heat wave years using recorded International Coding of Disease (ICD) statistics and concludes that there are high rates in the elderly and to some extent among infants. He believes that there was considerable under reporting and that heat contributed considerably to deaths that were given codes other than that for heat illness. He also blamed inadequate power supplies leading to failure to meet the demands of air-conditioning.

Every year there are many cases of heat stroke in pilgrims making the Hadji to Mecca in Saudi Arabia. An interesting report by Yaqub *et al.* (1986) details the clinical picture and outcome of 30 cases of heat stroke during the pilgrimage in 1984. The authors describe 'strenuous exercise' as a contributing factor,

3

but give no details of the nature of the exercise. They also give a mean age of 58 years, and mention overcrowding and inadequate hygiene and sanitation which may perhaps be more important factors in the situation of the Hadji.

All, or most, of these descriptions probably relate to 'classical' heat stroke in which high environmental temperatures cause weakened individuals to lose the homeostatic battle. The destruction of the Roman Army in Saudi Arabia in 24 BC was an early example of a different form of heat illness in which the victims were young and vigorously active (Jarcho, 1967). There have been other military examples since. In civilian life, the recent blossoming of mass participation in marathons, half-marathons, fun runs and cycling events has produced many and sometimes tragic cases of heat illness. For such cases the terms 'exertional hyperpyrexia' and 'exertional heat stroke' have come to be used.

A further step in the definition of the problem is recognition that typical, even fatal, cases of heat stroke with marked elevation of core temperature can occur in fit people exercising in quite mild conditions of temperature and humidity. Table 1.1 summarises some of these cases of 'low temperature heat stroke'. If we use the term 'heat stroke' therefore, we must be careful to recognise that the 'heat' which produces it is endogenous rather than environmental. Environmental conditions may be such as to hinder the loss of endogenous heat, but it is the latter which is directly responsible for raising the body temperature and causing tissue damage.

Even the resting body produces heat, but muscular activity increases this heat production enormously, as shown in Table 1.2.

Definitions and descriptions

Terms such as heat stroke and heat illness have been used rather loosely so far in this chapter and, indeed, rigid definitions can be difficult or misleading. However, it is necessary to explain some of the terms commonly used and the ways in which they are applied.

Heat stroke

This is used to describe the situation in which core temperature rises to dangerous levels as a result of heat stress, leading to tissue damage. Exertional heat stroke, or exertional hyperpyrexia, applies to cases where physical activity is an important factor, even though high ambient temperature may also be partly responsible. Many authors have chosen an arbitrary core temperature to define heat stroke, commonly 40.6 °C (e.g. Anderson *et al.*, 1983) or 41.1 °C

Table 1.1. *Cases of heat illness below 21 °C*

References	Air Temp. (°C) (Method)[a]	Humidity %	Initial Body temp.(°C) (Method)[b]	Dress	Result
Carson & Webb (1973)	10.2 (DB)		40.4(R)	Full military kit	Recovered
Sutton (1984b)	12.0 (WBGT)		42.0(R)	Running kit	Recovered
Dickinson (1989)	12.0 (DB)	88	40.5(A)	Tropical combat kit	Died
Richards & Richards (1984)	15.0 (DB)	82	40.0(R)	Running kit	Recovered
Hanson & Zimmerman (1979)	16.0 (DB)	60	42.5	Running kit	Recovered
Carson & Webb (1973)	16.6 (DB)		39.4(R)	Full military kit	Recovered
Parnell & Restall (1986)	16.7 (DB)	87	40.0(R) 42.8(Oes)	Light clothing	Died
Whitworth & Wolfman (1983)	19.0 (DB)	30	40.0(R)	Running kit	Died
Sutton (1984b)	21.0 (DB)		41.5(R)	Running kit [c]	Recovered

Key to methods of temperature measurement:
[a]Air temperature: DB, dry bulb or not defined; WBGT, wet bulb globe temperature.
[b]Body temperature: R, rectal; A, Axillary; O, Oral; Oes, Oesophageal.
[c]female patient; all others male.

Table 1.2. *Approximate heat production for a 60 kg man*

Activity	Heat production in kJ/h
Resting	270
10 km run (slower athlete)	2000
10 km run (faster athlete)	6250
Marathon	4000

(Knochel, 1974). There are problems with this approach, however, and Shapiro & Seidman (1990) from Israel have counselled wisely against such a strict definition. Victims collapse with heat stroke away from hospital. If temperature is measured at all, it is oral or axillary, which does not necessarily reflect core temperature. It is often not possible to perform rectal or other core temperature measurements until arrival at hospital, by which time cooling measures have often quite rightly been undertaken. Also, in some fit, exercising people temperature may exceed 40 °C without producing significant symptoms (Gilat *et al.*, 1963).

Most authors so far have used rectal temperature as synonymous with core temperature which is certainly superior to oral or axillary temperatures taken in the usual way with a mercury thermometer. A small recent study (Ash *et al.*, 1992), however, compared rectal with oesophageal, skin and auditory canal temperatures in two subjects during heating and cooling in a water bath. The ear temperature was measured with an infrared thermopile radiometer that does not make direct contact with the tympanic membrane. The authors suggest that rectal readings lag behind both rises and falls in the ear and oesophageal temperatures. From the practical point of view, this may mean overcooling and unnecessary shivering if rectal temperatures are used to control cooling, and from the theoretical point of view it raises further doubt about the use of arbitrary rectal temperatures in the definition of heat illness. We should note, however, that the study was a small one and the results need confirmation.

The above factors indicate great difficulties with ICD Code 9920, heat stroke. Some clinicians will only include cases where rectal temperature has been measured at 41 °C or above and assign another diagnosis, such as heat syncope or heat exhaustion, to all other cases. Some will extrapolate to probable temperatures at the time of collapse, and others will make the diagnosis on clinical features other than core temperature. (These will be discussed in Chapter 2.) It should be noted that there is no specific code for exertional heat stroke and, indeed, in many cases it is difficult to decide if the main cause of illness was the ambient temperature or the exercise. Of course, it is the combination that leads to problems in the majority of cases.

Heat exhaustion

The condition in which the victim collapses from the effects of depletion of salt and water and resulting hypovolaemia is called heat exhaustion. Some of the apparent effects of hypovolaemia are probably connected with the shift of blood volume from the centre to the periphery when the blood vessels in the skin dilate to transfer heat to the environment. In unacclimatised people who replace fluid losses with water alone, salt depletion is the predominant factor, whereas acclimatised personnel who do not have access to water are likely to be mainly water depleted; however, a mixed picture is common. The clinical findings are those to be expected from dehydration, salt depletion and hypovolaemia. The core temperature may rise, but not to the same levels as in heat stroke, and tissue damage does not occur. There are three different ICD codes for heat exhaustion: 'anhidrotic' (water depleted), salt depleted and unspecified.

Relationship between heat stroke and heat exhaustion

Although standard teaching makes a plain distinction between these two conditions, there are overlaps from both the theoretical and the practical points of view. Clearly the processes in heat exhaustion may predispose to the development of heat stroke. For example, hypovolaemia and circulatory failure increase the difficulty in conducting endogenous heat to the surface and dissipating it. As regards cutaneous vascular tone, the body may be faced with a 'choice' as to whether to support the circulation at the expense of temperature homeostasis or vice versa. Some of these problems will be discussed in Chapter 2 as they relate to management, and the pathophysiology will be explored further in Chapter 3, but a few points must be made here to clarify the inter-relationship between the processes of hyperpyrexia (heat stroke) and salt and water depletion (heat exhaustion). In a recent study on artificially heated rats (de Garavilla *et al.*, 1990), it was shown that previous sodium restriction and water deprivation reduced by 25–50% the time taken for rectal temperature to reach 42.6 °C. In another study, Sawka *et al.* (1992) deliberately raised the core temperatures of military volunteers by exercising them to exhaustion in conditions designed to exceed their cooling capacity before and after dehydration. They found that subjects collapsed from 'exhaustion from heat strain' at lower core temperatures when they were dehydrated. This was a physiological study rather than a clinical one and the authors suggest that the clinical end state might have been described as heat exhaustion, but they also note that '...collapse was imminent due to either ataxia or syncope' at the time subjects could no longer continue. The presence of ataxia in particular could be construed as evidence that nervous tissue damage had already occurred and therefore of the presence of heat stroke.

The vastly experienced medical advisors to the City to Surf race complicate the terminology further by refusing to use the term 'exertional heat stroke', preferring 'exertion-induced heat exhaustion', the title of their excellent and practical recent review (Richards *et al.*, 1992). The clinical features and complications they list, however, are precisely those given for exertional heat stroke by other authors. They use a broad definition to include victims who collapse on strenuous exercise with a rectal temperature greater than 38 °C.

They believe that this definition, although it may include some very mild cases, ensures that all who are at risk are treated appropriately. Some patients they describe under this term had temperatures of 42 °C and over, so they have clearly included the whole spectrum from mild heat exhaustion to fatal heat stroke. Such 'lumping together' reflects the practical concerns of physicians dealing with prevention and management on a large scale and should therefore be taken seriously.

Though the two main clinical syndromes can often be distinguished, there is much to be said for the view of Lind (1983) that 'heat exhaustion and heat stroke represent different degrees of severity on a continuum of disordered thermoregulation'. For the purposes of description and analysis of cases of heat illness it would be preferable to report cases using three parameters: a scale of clinical dehydration and hypovolaemia, highest recorded core temperature and complications. If, together with these clinical features, the ambient conditions and the level of physical exertion were to be recorded, we would have a basis for epidemiological work, prospective studies and the comparison of results that is not possible using simple ICD codes.

Other forms of heat illness

These are heat cramps, heat syncope and heat oedema which all have separate ICD codes. They will not be further considered here as they have less relevance to exertional heat stroke, although there may be some confusion over differential diagnosis and ICD coding.

Risk factors: environment

In addition to the air temperature, several other factors affect comfort in high temperatures and the risk of heat illness. The evaporation of sweat is the most important way of losing heat from the body, and is impaired in humid conditions. For this reason, 'dry heat' is generally felt to be more tolerable than the 'wet heat' of humid conditions, but one danger of dry heat is that sweat may evaporate so rapidly and imperceptibly that subjects may not realise the degree to which they are liable to dehydration. Air movement is important as it aids the evaporation of sweat and the convection of heat from the body, and it is for this reason that fans make life more tolerable in hot conditions. Once air temperature reaches body temperature, however, fanning loses much of its efficiency and movement of hot air may actually have a heating effect. Solar radiation directly heats the body, so that shade is a source of comfort in heat. Clothing should be thin to allow heat to escape, light in colour to reflect radiant heat and loose to allow air to circulate beneath it.

The formula of Winslow *et al.* (1937), expresses these influences on the amount of heat stored by the body and therefore the tendency to a rise in core temperature:

$$S = M \pm R \pm Cd \pm Cv - E$$

where S is the amount of stored heat: M is the metabolic heat production (exercise); R is the heat gained or lost by radiation (sun); Cd is the heat gained or lost by conduction (negligible); Cv is the heat gained or lost by convection (wind, motion); E is the heat lost by evaporation (sweating).

Ambient temperature alone is not sufficient to quantify the risk of heat illness or to define comfortable conditions, and so various measurements have been devised to correct air temperature taking other factors into account.

Effective temperature (ET)

Landsberg (1972) defines this as 'a measure of sensation of temperature in which, for a given air temperature and humidity, the state of comfort is equal to that experienced from an environment at a lower temperature with saturated water (100%)'. It can be calculated from a series of curves obtained experimentally.

Corrected effective temperature (CET)

Further correction of ET for wind velocity and global radiation gives the CET (Gregorczuk, 1966; Landsberg, 1972). This was found by the Sydney group (Richards *et al.*, 1984) to be the environmental measure that correlated best with the number of heat casualties in the City to Surf race, enabling accurate predictions to be made.

Wet bulb globe temperature (WBGT)

This is rather easier to measure using commercial equipment and is widely used for controlling sporting events and military training. It is calculated as follows:

$$WGBT = 0.7 \times Twb + 0.2 \times Tg + 0.1 \times Tdb$$

where Twb is the wet bulb temperature; Tg is the black globe temperature; Tdb is the dry bulb temperature. Details of the use of these measurements in the prevention of heat illness will be examined in Chapter 2.

Risk factors: activities

Individual risk factors will be considered in Chapter 2, but clearly the groups at risk of exertional heat stroke are those whose occupation or leisure activities involve vigorous physical activity, especially, but not exclusively, in adverse ambient conditions or when wearing some form of clothing that impedes loss of heat. Fire-fighters, boilermen and foundry workers are typical examples of workers at risk in the course of their employment, and the Armed Services have a certain risk as we shall see, but we will begin by considering sporting activities.

Running

As a salutary warning, a doctor who is himself a marathon runner, quotes 'the spectacle of Gaby Anderson-Schiess, hyperthermic, dehydrated, uncoor-dinated and almost hemiparetic, weaving her way over the finish line in the first women's marathon in Los Angeles' (Sutton, 1984a). If trained athletes can be affected like that, he argues, how much more vulnerable are the thousands of less experienced people who take part in fun runs and other events? The first 'City to Surf' race in Sydney, Australia, took place in 1971 and, of 1600 competitors, 29 (1.8%) collapsed from heat effects (Richards & Richards, 1984). After producing regression curves relating the number of casualties to the CET and using these curves to predict the number of casu-alties in the 1983 and 1984 races with considerable accuracy, the same group was able to ensure that the necessary resources were available to deal with them (Richards *et al.*, 1984). By means of improved preparation, education of the competitors and management at the event, a marked reduction in the heat casualty figures was achieved: in 1971–77, 0.33% of starters suffered heat illness and 23.5% of these were admitted to hospital, whereas by 1978–84 the equivalent figures were 0.15% and 1.5%.

Although there is a good correlation of heat casualties with environmental temperature, cases occur in conditions that would not normally be regarded as risky. An example is the 26-year-old graduate student who became case number 4 in the paper of Hansen & Zimmerman (1979) and who appears in Table 1.1. In spite of being reasonably fit, he collapsed 200 m from the finishing line of a 10 km charity fun run. Recovering temporarily, he finished the race only to collapse again. In hospital he was unconscious with a rectal temperature of 42.5 °C. The ambient temperature during the run had been only 16 °C and the relative humidity 60%. He survived to run again.

It would be wrong to suppose that running is necessary for exertional heat stroke to occur. Pattison *et al.* (1988) describe the case of a 26-year-old woman who collapsed while walking in the Grand Canyon. Her rectal temperature was greater than 104 °F, she was unconscious and only barely survived acute renal failure. This case (among others, such as that of Sutton (1984b)) also explodes the popular myth that women are immune from heat illness.

Mountaineering

Climbers at high altitude carry heavy loads, wear warm clothing in anticipation of the temperature to drop at sunset and are exposed to strong solar radiation reflected from the snow and ice. Himalayan mountaineers have reported that daytime heat may be more troublesome than night-time cold. While there are few reports of confirmed cases of heat stroke in mountaineers, it is possible that such cases have been mistaken for acute mountain sickness, especially given the difficulty of measuring core temperature in a well-swaddled mountaineer in a small tent at night.

American football

In American College Football during 1964–73, matches or training led to an average of 3.9 deaths from heat stroke per year (Murphy, 1984). As a result of improved preventive measures, the equivalent figure for 1974–83 was 1.5 per year.

Other sports

It is hard to find significant case reports from other sports in the literature, but it is equally hard to believe that they do not exist. A letter to the *Australian Medical Journal* (Hansen & Brotherhood, 1988) expressed concern about untrained squash players on the basis of observations on higher level players, but does not quote any actual cases. The British paper that it quotes about deaths in squash actually attributes the majority of deaths to cardiac disease (Northcote *et al.*, 1984).

Military activities

It is no accident that much of the research on heat illness has been carried out by armed forces institutions, notably in Israel and the USA. When a death or severe disability results from heat illness in a serviceman, there is an outcry from the media about the dangers of military training. Yet servicemen must be trained to fight in many different environments and must be physically fit. They usually have to wear, at least, minimally protective clothing and carry their own equipment. There have been great strides in our understanding of how to prevent heat illness in the Services and these will be considered in Chapter 2. If scantily-dressed fun runners sometimes become tragic victims of heat illness in well-supervised events, it should not be surprising if precautions occasionally break down in the special circumstances of the Services. One problem is that a serviceman may be thought to be malingering when he is actually suffering heat effects; the converse is that many are so well motivated to succeed in spite of adversity that they will not allow themselves to give up or draw attention to their distress until it is too late. On top of this, it is not always possible to ensure that all physical activity, including personal fitness training, is supervised by medical or other trained personnel.

The clothing used to protect against nuclear, biological and chemical warfare presents a particular problem. To be impervious to vapours, the clothing inevitably prevents the evaporation of sweat. This may lead to adverse effects even in a person who is not engaged in strenuous physical acitivity. Mitchell (1991) reports an American helicopter pilot who was taking part in a study of heat stress effects during flights when wearing individual protection equipment (IPE). Following the second flight, his rectal temperature monitor showed 38.5 °C which was regarded as unsafe and, to his disappointment, he was withdrawn from the day's study. Five minutes later he became vague and collapsed and his temperature rose to just over 39 °C: he recovered over a ten minute period. The author discusses whether the correct diagnosis was heat syncope, heat exhaustion or heat stroke. He appears unwilling to accept heat stroke, presumably because the arbitrary 40 °C was not reached, but thought the rapid rise of temperature during the period before collapse meant that processes similar to those of heat stroke were at work.

As in the Gulf War, the threat of nerve gas attack requires large numbers of troops to take pretreatment, but this does not appear to affect heat tolerance. Atropine, however, which might be required in an actual chemical attack, inhibits sweating and certainly does increase the risk of heat illness.

British Ministry of Defence Statistics

The figures presented in this section are derived from the analysis of listings provided by the Medical Statistics Department of the Ministry of Defence for the years 1981–91. Only patients who have been admitted to hospital are recorded. Computerised records were used to list the details of hospital discharges assigned the ICD codes 9920 to 9929 which concern heat related

Table 1.3. *Tri-Service heat related admissions 1981–91 by diagnosis*

	ICD 9920 Heat Stroke	ICD 9921 Heat Syncope	ICD 9922 Heat Cramps	ICD 9923–5 Heat Exhaustion	ICD 9928–9 Other/ unspecified	All codes
Royal Navy	21	4	0	58	18	101
Army	153	93	6	983	61	1296
Royal Air Force	14	12	0	25	0	51
All	188	109	6	1066	79	1448
Percentage	13	7.5	0.4	73.6	5.5	100

illness. The NATO standard codes for 'Cause of Injury' were also listed. Individual case records were not examined.

There is clearly room for inaccuracy in this retrospective analysis. The difficulties in defining and distinguishing heat stroke and heat exhaustion have already been discussed and it is not possible to have confidence that all reporting clinicians have applied the same criteria. Doctors may have preferred to choose Codes 9928 (other heat effects) or 9929 (unspecified) rather than give a more specific name to the condition. A marked clustering of 12 such diagnoses in Royal Navy figures for 1988 is probably an example of some such process. As we have seen, there is no specific code for exertional heat stroke.

'Cause of Injury' codes might be expected to resolve the question of whether the exercise or the ambient temperature was mainly responsible for a given illness. The choice, however, remains subjective and the codes may not have been assigned by those qualified to make the decision. Some may have selected 'running' where others might have judged the environmental temperature to be of greater importance and chosen 'heat'. Such inaccuracies and uncertainties are inevitable unless a prospective study is carried out using strict criteria.

The following figures must be interpreted with all those reservations in mind; however, they do give a reasonable indication of the size of the problem in the Armed Forces. Table 1.3 summarises the hospital events for the 11 years. To the total of 1448 could be added three cases of heat fatigue, one of heat oedema and 32 cases in which heat related codes were given as secondary diagnoses. This gives a total of 1484, or an average of 135 admissions per year. On the basis of average numbers of cases in males and females per year and average proportions of each sex per Service, values for the average annual incidence per 100 000 have been calculated (Table 1.4).

The predominance of Army cases is to be expected in view of the greater

Table 1.4. *Average incidence per 100 000 per year by Service and sex*

	Total	Male	Female
Army	72	74	18
Royal Navy	14	14	5
Royal Air Force	5	5	9
All services	41	42	11

Table 1.5. *Length of time off duty (Army)*

	Less than 1 week	1–2 weeks	2–3 weeks	More than 3 weeks
Number	1073	77	72	74
Percentage	82.8	5.9	5.6	5.7

Table 1.6. *Heat related deaths 1981–91*

Army	Heat Stroke	7
	Heat exhaustion	2
	Heat syncope	2
	Other heat related	1
	Total	11
Royal Navy and Royal Air Force		No deaths

frequency of strenuous activities compared with the other two Services. Female numbers were small: Army 13; RN two; RAF six. The incidence of heat illness in females was lower than in males: 11 compared with 42.

To assess the severity of these illnesses, an analysis was made of the length of time required before the Army victims returned to duty. The results are given in Table 1.5. It will be seen that nearly 83% returned to duty in a week or less and, in fact, a large proportion had only one day off work. A further calculation gives an average 15.5 soldiers a year requiring more than one week off duty because of heat illness. At the other end of the scale, the longest time off duty was 153 days.

There were 11 deaths, the details of which are summarised in Table 1.6. Five of these resulted from heat illness occurring in the UK, three in Germany, one each in Cyprus and Belize and one in the 'Borneo, Brunei and Nepal' location. Cause of Illness coding gives 'excessive heat' in nine cases and a code which includes running and other forms of exercise for the remaining two. The

Table 1.7. *Incidence of heat illness in certain locations*

Location	Total cases	Average incidence per 100 000 per year
United Kingdom (including Northern Ireland)	584	66
Germany	203	36
Cyprus	57	193
Hong Kong	168	233
Gibraltar	5	93

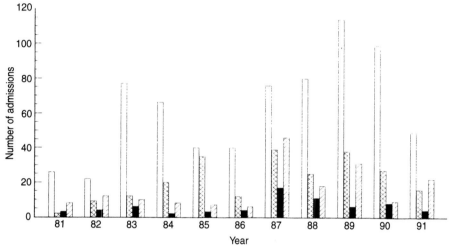

Figure 1.1. Admissions for heat illness: Army. Main locations by year. ▨▨ HK; ▭ Cyprus; ▨▨ BAOR; ■ UK.

significance of this is doubtful and it seems likely that exercise was involved in all cases.

Comparing the incidence of heat illness in the 11 years studied, it is evident that there are more cases in the second half of the period than in the first, and this is broadly true of all locations (Figure 1.1). Although possible explanations are that heat illness is increasing or that the weather is growing warmer, it seems most likely that awareness and reporting have increased, reflecting one of the limitations of a study of this nature.

It may come as a surprise to note that the UK is the location at which the majority of heat illness occurs in the Army. There are certain difficulties in comparing incidences in different locations because manpower deployment figures are not presented in precisely the same form as medical statistics. Also,

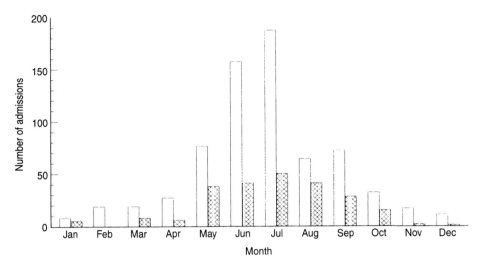

Figure 1.2. Admissions for heat illness: Army. UK and BAOR by month 1981–91. ▨ BAOR; ☐ UK.

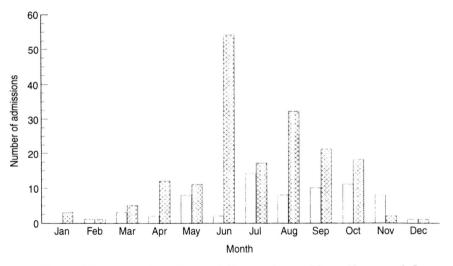

Figure 1.3. Admissions for heat illness: Army. Hong Kong and Cyprus by month, 1981–91. ▨ Hong Kong; ☐ Cyprus.

full manpower figures for 1990 are not available. Making some reasonable assumptions we can reach the incidences (per 100 000) shown in Table 1.7. These make it clear that Cyprus and Hong Kong have considerably greater incidences than the UK and Germany, as would be expected from their climates. Further analysis of troops in Hong Kong shows the Gurkhas to have a lower incidence (195 per 100 000) than British-based troops (460 per 100 000).

The factors involved in the Gulf War will be discussed in Chapter 2, but it may be noted here that there were only eight cases in the British forces during the conflict.

Figures 1.2 and 1.3 show the number of cases per month in the Army over the 11 year period in the major locations. As would be expected, most of the cases in the UK and Germany are spread over the warmer months, May to September. There is a rather wider spread in Cyprus and Hong Kong, where the hot weather lasts longer. No month, however, is free of cases of heat illness, confirming the importance of exercise and endogenous heat.

The recorded ICD codes show that heat exhaustion (74%) was by far the most common diagnosis in all three Services, with heat stroke much less common at 13% (Table 1.3).

Rather surprisingly, only five servicemen were discharged from the Army in the 11 years because of heat illness, and none was discharged from the Royal Navy and Royal Air Force. Three of the discharged soldiers were coded as having suffered heat exhaustion, one as heat syncope and the other as unspecified. Discharge does not necessarily imply persistent disability.

To summarise then, over the past 11 years the British Armed Forces have suffered about 135 heat casualties per year of sufficient seriousness to warrant hospital admission. Fewer than 20 of these have been serious enough to be off duty for more than a week, but there has been an average of one death per year. The Army sustains the bulk of the heat casualties. Heat illness occurs in service women, but less commonly than in men. Most events occur in the UK or Germany and in the warmer months, but the risk is greatest in hot climates such as Hong Kong and Cyprus and no time of year is without heat casualties. If recorded ICD codes are to be believed, only 13% of all cases of heat illness are of heat stroke, but difficulties in coding make this an unreliable figure.

References

Anderson, R. J., Reed, G. & Knochel, J. (1983). Heat stroke. *Advances in Internal Medicine*, **28**, 115–40.

Apocrypha, New English Bible. Judith 8, 3.

Ash, C. J., Cook, J. R., McMurry, T. A. & Auner, C. R. (1992). The use of rectal temperature to monitor heat stroke. *Missouri Medicine*, **89**, 283–7.

Carson, J. & Webb, J.F. (1973). Heat illness in England. *Journal of the Royal Army Medical Corps*, **119**, 145–53.

De Garavilla, L., Durkot, M. J., Ihley, T. M., Leva, N. & Francesconi, R. P. (1990). Adverse effects of dietary and furosemide-induced sodium depletion on thermoregulation. *Aviation, Space and Environmental Medicine*, **61**, 1012–17.

Dickinson, J. G. (1989). Heat-exercise hyperpyrexia. *Journal of the Royal Army Medical Corps*, **135**, 27–9.

Ellis, F. P. (1972). Mortality from heat illness and heat-aggravated illness in the United States. *Environmental Research*, **5**, 1–58.

Gilat, T., Shibolet, S. & Sohar, E. (1963). Mechanism of heat stroke. *Journal of Tropical Medicine and Hygiene*, **66**, 204–12.

Gregorczuk, M. (1966). Diagram biocyclometryczyny. *Przegl Geofiz*, **11**, 57–60.

Hansen, R. D. & Brotherhood, J. R. (1988). Prevention of heat induced illness in squash players. *Medical Journal of Australia*, **148**, 100.

Hanson, G. & Zimmerman S. W. (1979). Exertional heat stroke in novice runners. *Journal of the American Medical Association*, **242**, 154–7.

Jarcho, S. (1967). A Roman experience with heat stroke in 24 BC. *Bulletin of the New York Academy of Medicine*, **43**, 767.

Katsouyanni, K., Trichopoulos, D., Zavitsanos, X. & Touloumi, G. (1988). The 1987 Athens heat wave. *Lancet*, **2**, 573.

Knochel, J. P. (1974). Environmental heat illness; an eclectic review. *Archives of Internal Medicine*, **133**, 841–64.

Landsberg, H. E. (1972). A limited review of physical parameters: the assessment of human bioclimate. *Technical notes no. 331*, World Meteorological Organisation.

Lind, A. R. (1983). Pathophysiology of heat exhaustion and heat stroke. In *Heat Stroke and Temperature Regulation*, ed. M. Khogali, & J. R. S. Halse, pp. 179–88. Sydney, Academic Press.

Mitchell, G. W. (1991). Rapid onset of severe heat illness: a case report. *Aviation, Space and Environmental Medicine.* **62**, 779–82.

Murphy, R. J. (1984). Heat illness in the athlete. *American Journal of Sports Medicine*, **12**, 258–61.

Northcote, R. J., Evans, A. D. & Ballantyne, D. (1984). Sudden death in squash players. *Lancet*, **1**, 148–50.

Parnell, C. J. & Restall, J. (1986), Heat stroke: a fatal case. *Archives of Emergency Medicine*, **3**, 111–14.

Pattison, M. E., Logan, J. L., Lee, S. M. & Ogden, D. A. (1988). Exertional heat stroke and acute renal failure in a young woman. *American Journal of Kidney Diseases*, **9**, 184–7.

Richards, R. & Richards, D. (1984). Exertion-induced heat exhaustion and other medical aspects of the City-to-Surf fun runs, 1978–84. *Medical Journal of Australia*, **141**, 799–805.

Richards, R., Richards, D. & Sutton, J. (1992). Exertion-induced heat exhaustion. *Australian Family Physician*, **21**, 18–24.

Richards, R., Richards, D. & Whittaker, R. (1984). Method of predicting the number of casualties in the Sydney City-to-Surf fun runs. *Medical Journal of Australia*, **141**, 805–8.

Sawka, M. N., Young, A. J., Latzka, W. A., Neufer, P. D., Quigley, M. D. & Pandolf, K. B. (1992). Human tolerance to heat strain during exercise: influence of hydration. *Journal of Applied Physiology*, **73**, 368–75.

Shapiro, Y. & Seidman, D. S. (1990). Field and clinical observations of exertional heat stroke patients. Medicine and Science in Sports and Exercise, 22 (1), 6–14.

Sutton, J. R. (1984*a*). Not so fun run. *Medical Journal of Australia*, **141**, 782–83.

Sutton, J. R. (1984*b*). Heat Illness. In *Sports Medicine*, ed. R. H. Strauss, pp. 307–321. Philadelphia, Saunders.

Whitworth, J. A. G. & Wolfman, M. J. (1983). Fatal heat stroke in a long distance runner. *British Medical Journal*, **287**, 948.

Winslow, C. E. A., Herrington, L. P. & Gagge, A. P. (1937). Physiological reactions of the human body to various atmospheric humidities. *American Journal of Physiology*, **120**, 288–9.

Woodruff, P. (1954). *The Men Who Ruled India*. I. *The Founders*. London, Jonathan Cape.

Yaqub, B. A., Al-Harthi, S. S., Al-Orainey, I. O., Laajam, M. A. & Obeid, M. T. (1986). Heat stroke at the Mekkah pilgrimage: clinical characteristics and course of 30 patients. *Quarterly Journal of Medicine*, New Series, **59**, 229, 523–30.

2

Predisposing factors, clinical features, treatment and prevention

J. G. DICKINSON

Predisposing factors

The environmental conditions of temperature, humidity, air movement, insulation and clothing that may affect heat tolerance have already been discussed in Chapter 1, as well as different forms of exercise. We are now concerned primarily with the personal factors that cause one person to collapse, while others continue to exercise or compete under the same conditions. These are summarised in Table 2.1.

It is a general experience that obese people have more difficulty in coping with heat (and exercise) than thinner ones and a study of obese boys showed a greater rise in body temperature on standard exercise than occurred in others (Haymes *et al.*, 1975). Risk of exercise-induced heat illness rises with any pre-existing fever and it is generally unwise to undertake strenuous exercise while suffering from such illnesses. The detrimental effects of alcohol on performance in heat are a matter of common experience and a possible explanation lies in the diuresis and intracellular dehydration caused by alcohol. Tired, sleep-deprived people seem to be particularly at risk (Armstrong *et al.*, 1990).

Any influence that causes dehydration before exercise predisposes to heat illness. This includes diarrhoea, use of diuretics, diabetes insipidus and uncontrolled diabetes mellitus. Self-dehydration to avoid the need to pass urine during the exercise is particularly ill advised.

Similarly, any factor that interferes with heat loss will render the subject liable to heat stroke. Such factors include certain drugs and diseases of the skin. Patients with congenital anhidrosis, of which ectodermal dysplasia is the commonest form, are at great risk. In miliaria ('prickly heat') the sweat ducts are obstructed and sweating is inefficient. It is also thought that sweat gland function may be impaired as a result of a previous episode of heat stroke (Baba

Table 2.1. *Predisposing factors to heat intolerance*

Obesity
Current upper respiratory infection or febrile illness
Recent alcohol consumption
Sleep deprivation
Dehydrating illness, e.g. diarrhoea, vomiting
Failure to replace fluid losses
Skin diseases, e.g. anhidrosis, psoriasis, miliaria
Conditions increasing heat production, e.g. thyrotoxicosis
Lack of acclimatisation
Lack of physical fitness
Drugs
    Anticholinergics, e.g. atropine, 'Lomotil'
    Diuretics
    Phenothiazines
    Tricyclic antidepressants
    Antihistamines, cold remedies
    Anti-Parkinsonian drugs
    Beta-blockers
    Amphetamines, 'ecstasy'
Previous heat stroke

& Ruppert, 1968). Recently it has been shown that patients with psoriasis showed a sharper rise of temperature and a reduced sweat rate compared with normals in a heat exercise test and it is suggested that they have a reduced ability to dissipate heat (Leibowitz *et al.*, 1991). This may be true of patients with other widespread skin diseases.

Conditions that increase heat production, such as thyrotoxicosis, clearly predispose to heat stroke. Sympathomimetic and stimulant drugs such as amphetamines and alpha-adrenergic agonists have a similar effect.

Acclimatisation to heat involves a variety of physiological responses. The body adapts to produce a larger volume of more dilute sweat, and this has the important corollary that the acclimatised subject requires more fluid replacement than the unacclimatised. There are important cardiovascular adaptations also, involving expanded intravascular volume, increased maximum cardiac output, increased stroke volume and reduced maximal heart rate. These adaptations take at least three weeks to complete, so that a newcomer to a hot environment will be at special, but decreasing, risk during this period.

This raises the question of physical training and fitness, which, although it cannot substitute for heat acclimatisation, is still of some value. The cardiovascular adaptations of physical training are beneficial as the trained subject both produces less heat for a given amount of work and dissipates it more quickly as a result of his well-tuned cardiovascular system. Conversely, a person with cardiovascular disease who indulges in vigorous exercise runs many risks, including the danger of heat illness. Physiological aspects of physical training and acclimatisation are discussed in detail in Chapter 3.

Drugs may affect heat tolerance in a variety of ways. Anticholinergics such as atropine impede sweating: a small amount of atropine is present, for example, in the antidiarrhoeal preparation 'Lomotil'. Many drugs used in Parkinson's disease have anticholinergic effects. Phenothiazines and antihistamines (which may be present in cold remedies) also suppress sweating. Diuretics have already been mentioned and lead to depletion of water and salt. Tricyclic antidepressants increase motor activity and therefore heat production. Beta-blocking drugs may increase risk by reducing cardiovascular responses. Sympathomimetics and amphetamines (including 'ecstasy' and other drugs of abuse) increase psychomotor activity.

The question of whether previous heat stroke predisposes to further episodes is a difficult one. Israeli workers (Shapiro *et al.*, 1979) compared exercise responses in former patients with exertional heat stroke with normal controls and found impaired performance, higher rectal temperatures and higher pulse rates. A recent review of the whole subject of heat intolerance (Armstrong *et al.*, 1990) concludes that temporary or persistent heat intolerance occurs in only a small percentage of prior exertional heat stroke patients. Epstein (1990) concludes that recurrent heat stroke is more often due to pre-existing factors rather than induced by the first episode. Of these, anhidrosis and skin disease are important. Possible interrelations with malignant hyperthermia and the neuroleptic syndrome will be considered later in this book.

It is an open question whether susceptibility to exertional heat stroke is equal to the sum of all these known factors or whether there are additional factors or personal idiosyncrasies.

Symptoms and signs

Reports of cases of exertional heat stroke often mention collapse just before, at or after a finishing line, which probably represents the determination of athletes to finish in spite of the distress signals relayed from their bodies. In the early stages a runner, for example, might feel weak and dizzy and develop a headache. As the condition progresses, he may be nauseated and vomit, stagger and show abnormal behaviour. (Contrary to popular opinion, determination to keep going in such circumstances is not abnormal in a dedicated athlete, although one might call it an error of judgement!) He may become irritable (especially with officials who try to make him stop) and eventually will collapse, conscious or unconscious, on the ground. It is likely that these early features are a combination of hypovolaemia and the early effects on nervous tissue, especially brain oedema.

Examination at this stage will almost certainly reveal some dehydration, a fast pulse, perhaps low blood pressure, and a markedly raised core temperature. Oral or axillary temperatures may be normal or low, even low enough to suggest hypothermia (Sutton, 1984). In the past it has been said that a dry, hot skin is characteristic of heat stroke. This is not true in exertional cases, although failure of sweating may be found in classical heat stroke. In an analysis of casualties in the 'City to Surf' races moist, sweaty skin was found in over 90% of men and over 50% of women with rectal temperatures above 40 °C (Richards & Richards, 1984). Hot and dry, cold and clammy, and cold and dry skin may also be observed, probably depending on whether the predominant physiological responses at the time are primarily defending circulation or temperature and how successful they have been.

Pathogenesis is considered in Chapter 3, but Table 2.2 summarises the main processes that lead to symptoms, signs and complications in exertional heat stroke. It is obvious that the management of a severe heat stroke victim involves anticipating, detecting and treating many metabolic complications and multiple organ failure (Sprung *et al.*, 1980; Chao *et al.*, 1981; Anderson *et al.*, 1983; Jarmulowicz & Buchan, 1988).

Assessment

At any stage, a first aider, paramedic or doctor will find it helpful to assess and treat under four headings in the following order of priority:

> Airway and breathing
> Circulation: dehydration, hypovolaemia, shock
> Temperature: rectal if possible
> Complications.

The clinical picture on arrival at hospital will depend on many factors, including the length of time that has elapsed and the measures that have been used in first aid and during transport. At best, the patient will be conscious with a falling core temperature, adequate hydration and no complications. At the worst, the temperature may still be rising, the conscious state impaired, possibly deteriorating, and there will be evidence of dehydration, hypovolaemia or shock. Complications such as convulsions may already be evident.

A reasonable scheme for initial hospital assessment, therefore, is as follows:

Table 2.2. *Complications of heat stroke*

Organ	Pathology	Effects
Brain	Oedema	Convulsions
	Petechial haemorrhages	Coma
	Congestion	
Muscle	Rhabdomyolysis	Acute renal failure
		Hyperkalaemia
		Hyperuricaemia
		Hypocalcaemia
		Hyperphosphataemia
		Enzyme release, esp. CK
		Possibly DIC
	Lactic acidosis	
Blood	Disseminated intravascular coagulation (DIC)	Fragmentation of red blood cells
		Acute renal failure
		Thrombocytopenia
		Haemorrhage
		Thrombosis
		Haemolysis
Liver	Centrilobular necrosis	Liver cell failure
		Jaundice
		Haemorrhage
		Hypoglycaemia
		Enzyme release
Kidneys	Acute tubular necrosis	Acute renal failure
		Oliguria
		Acidosis
		Hyperkalaemia
Lungs	Respiratory alkalosis	Tetany
	Aspiration pneumonia	Hypoxia
	Haemorrhagic pneumonia	
Heart	Haemorrhagic myocarditis	Shock
Gastrointestinal tract	Non-specific	Nausea, vomiting, diarrhoea
	General bleeding diathesis	Haemorrhage

CK, creatine kinase.

Check airway, breathing and state of consciousness, correcting airway and breathing problems as a matter of urgency.

Seek evidence of shock or hypovolaemia and set up adequate intravenous infusion with crystalloids, colloids or both.

Check rectal temperature and institute or continue cooling methods as indicated.

Examine fully to exclude alternative diagnoses, establish baselines and detect early complications.

Arrange necessary laboratory and other tests.

With rather less urgency, it is necessary to elicit from the patient and witnesses the circumstances of the illness, the presence of any predisposing factors and details of any previous episodes. This information is important in giving advice for the future and in considering special investigations.

Investigation

Although mild cases can be managed with less information, the following observations and investigations are necessary for severe cases.

Bedside

Continuous monitoring of core temperature by rectal or tympanic membrane probe
Pulse, blood pressure and respiration
Urine output (catheterise if necessary) and fluid balance
Arterial oxygen saturation by pulse oximetry
Central venous pressure
12 lead electrocardiogram and continuous monitoring
Glasgow Coma Scale.

Laboratory

Haemoglobin, white count, platelets and blood film
Serum urea, creatinine and electrolytes
Serum calcium and phosphate
Blood glucose
Serum osmolarity
Liver function tests, including enzymes
Muscle enzymes, especially creatine kinase (CK)
Arterial blood gases and pH
Clotting factors, fibrinogen levels and fibrin degradation products
Urine for protein, casts, myoglobin and osmolarity.

Complications

Cardiovascular system

Two types of haemodynamic states are recognised in exertional heat stroke, although in the original description only one instance of the second type is described (O'Donnell & Clowes, 1972). In the first, increased cardiac output is associated with reduced peripheral vascular resistance, mild arterial hypotension and mildly raised central venous pressure. These would seem to be appropriate responses to the demands of heat and exercise. In the second type, cardiac output and blood pressure are markedly reduced, central venous pressure is considerably raised and there may be cyanosis. It would appear that, in these cases, compensation has been insufficient and cardiovascular collapse is imminent.

The elevation of central venous pressure is of some interest. It has been noted independently, and in one study from Mecca (Seraj *et al.*, 1991) it was considered to indicate that dehydration was not important in the pathogenesis of heat stroke and that cardiac overload might be a danger in management. The cases, however, were not exertional ones, and the fluid deficit may have been less of a problem.

Cardiac problems may arise as a result of hypovolaemia, but also from direct damage to the myocardium. Postmortem studies show subendocardial and other haemorrhages in the heart muscle, together with oedema and evidence of myofibrillar damage. A recent study of two patients in Israel (Zahger *et al.*, 1989) suggests that, although there is dysfunction of both ventricles, the right may be more severely affected and take longer to recover. If confirmed, this might provide a basis for the elevated central venous pressure in the presence of hypovolaemia. Some workers have suggested that pulmonary vascular resistance is increased, which could provide a mechanism for the greater effects on the right ventricle.

The electrocardiogram often shows conduction defects and non-specific changes in the T waves either initially or during cooling.

Central nervous system

Autopsy shows cerebral oedema, petechial haemorrhage and degeneration of nerve cells, especially in the cerebellum. Symptoms include irritability, aggressiveness, abnormal behaviour, ataxia, impaired consciousness and coma. Convulsions occur in as many as 60% of cases (Shapiro & Seidman, 1990). On examination, the pupils may be constricted or fixed and dilated, although not necessarily irreversibly. There may be papilloedema and other neurological features such as hemiparesis. These features are virtually identical with those of cerebral acute mountain sickness, another environmental condition in which autopsy shows oedema and haemorrhage. In this condition, also, there is impairment of nerve cell function (Dickinson, 1983), related, however, to hypoxia rather than hyperpyrexia.

Blood

Reduced coagulability of the blood is a feature of severe heat stroke. Contributing factors are hepatic damage, leading to the reduction of clotting factors, and disseminated intravascular coagulation (DIC) leading to consumption coagulopathy. Thrombocytopenia, occurring even in the absence of DIC, suggests that there may be a direct effect on the bone marrow, but this is not reflected in the white blood cell count, which is usually elevated.

Haemorrhage may occur into the skin, conjunctivae, gastrointestinal and renal tracts, myocardium and lungs. A haemorrhagic pneumonia is a common terminal event (Chao *et al.*, 1981).

The stimulus to DIC is not clear. It may be some product of rhabdomyolysis or of endothelial damage resulting from the hyperpyrexia or another, unknown, cause. DIC may be detected by the finding of hypofibrinogenaemia, raised fibrin degradation products in the blood, and fragmentation of red blood cells. As well as haemorrhage and sometimes thrombosis, its effects include haemolysis and acute renal failure.

Kidneys

It is common to find proteinuria and the presence of casts in the urine. Acute renal failure is said to occur in about 25% of cases of severe exertional heat stroke (Shapiro & Seidman, 1990) but less commonly in classical cases. Such figures, however, are likely to reflect the nature of the hospital reporting them and the severity of the condition of the patients that it receives. Hypovolaemia and shock may contribute and other important factors include DIC and tubular damage from myoglobinuria, hyperuricaemia and hypokalaemia. The female patient described by Pattison *et al.* (1988) had no evidence of DIC, but had severely depleted extracellular fluid volume, myoglobinuria and hyperuricaemia. The authors speculate along the lines of Knochel (1974) that serum potassium may have been low in the early stages, although it was raised on arrival at hospital.

Acid-base balance

When measuring blood gases and pH in hyperpyrexic patients it is important to apply a correction for temperature (Bradley *et al.*, 1956). Heat and exercise both stimulate respiration and the early stages of heat stroke are characterised by respiratory alkalosis (Sprung *et al.*, 1980). Lactic acidosis, however, may be the dominant effect as a result of factors such as hypovolaemia and tissue ischaemia. Renal failure may lead to further metabolic acidosis.

Muscle

Rhabdomyolysis is a condition in which disruption of skeletal muscle fibres causes pain and weakness in the muscles and an outpouring of myoglobin, uric acid, potassium and various enzymes into the blood. In the interpretation of results, however, it should be remembered that distance running is normally associated with the elevation of myoglobin, creatine kinase (CK), aspartate transaminase (AST) and lactic dehydrogenase (LDH), and these may remain elevated for hours or days after the exercise (Young, 1987). Severe rhabdomyolysis occurs in hyperpyrexia without exercise in malignant hyperthermia, and following exertion without heat stroke (Knochel, 1990). It is less common in classical heat stroke than in the exertional form. Marked rhabdomyolysis without heat stroke resulted in acute renal failure after a runner had competed in two 400 m sprint races in one day (Stevens *et al.*, 1988).

Runners may notice pain or cramps in muscles and the muscles may be found to be tender. It is usual to monitor CK and other enzymes after exertional heat stroke, but the significance of the initial findings is not clear. The development of a compartment syndrome may lead to a secondary rise in CK (Knochel, 1989). Brown (1992) describes a secondary rise in CK on the tenth day in hospital associated with pyrexia and shivering. This appeared to respond to intravenous methylprednisolone. There had been an unusual bacteraemic complication on the fifth day, however, and the exact significance of the enzyme rise, the symptoms and the effect of steroids must remain in doubt.

Whether the rhabdomyolysis is attributed to the exercise or the hyperpyrexia, the most feared complication is acute tubular necrosis and acute renal failure resulting from the toxic effect on the renal tubules of ferrihaemate derived from myoglobin. Uric acid deposition may also be a factor.

Electrolytes

Knochel (1974) has discussed at length the possibility of hypokalaemia in the early stages of heat stroke and its possible effects on muscle and kidney. By the time patients arrive at hospital, however, serum potassium is often normal or raised as a result of release from damaged muscle or from early renal failure. Serum calcium levels are commonly depressed as a result of deposition of calcium salts in damaged muscle, but tetany does not usually occur because acidosis is usually present by the time hypocalcaemia develops. Phosphate levels may be low, resulting from respiratory alkalosis, or increased because of release from muscle. Magnesium levels may also be low. The significance of such changes must be assessed in the light of the acid–base state and the overall picture and managed accordingly.

Liver and gastrointestinal tract

Nausea, vomiting and diarrhoea may occur early in the presentation of exertional heat stroke and gastrointestinal bleeding may be a late complication. The liver may show centrilobular necrosis at autopsy and hepatocellular failure may occur after two to three days. Jaundice may result from haemolysis, liver damage or both. Prothrombin time may be prolonged and this is one element in the bleeding diathesis. Hypoglycaemia occurs and may be a factor in the development of convulsions. Hypoglycaemia may result from liver damage or from exhaustion of the glycogen stores. Hassanein *et al.* (1992) have recommended that some patients with severe hepatic failure who have survived early neurological complications may require liver transplantation, and they report two such cases.

Treatment

Early diagnosis and treatment are of vital importance in ensuring a good outcome. Experience gained in the 'City to Surf' race (Richards *et al.*, 1992), shows that complications do not occur if casualties are treated within 15 minutes of collapse and if the temperature is below 38 °C within one hour of starting treatment. At all stages of treatment, protection of the airways takes precedence over all else and cooling measures should be carried out continuously and with adequate monitoring.

Both hospitals and first aid centres will achieve better results in saving lives and avoiding complications if they are set up to receive heat casualties. This involves the availability of personnel trained and drilled in the management of heat victims and the equipment that they use.

First aid care

This should be well understood by any person responsible for the organisation and health support of sporting events, military training and occupations at risk. Victims should be placed at rest in the shade and stripped of all unnecessary clothing. Core temperature should be measured as soon as possible. If the victim is able to take it, cool water should be administered by mouth. There are various ways of cooling the body in the field, the simplest and best being wetting the skin and remaining clothing and fanning. This can be carried out with an electric fan, by hand or using a natural breeze. A helicopter has been used as a rather extravagant fan in such circumstances and the US Navy has tried placing up to 12 victims at a time in an inflatable life raft and treating them with a fine spray of water. Partial immersion in any available body of water is an alternative, but care must be taken if consciousness is impaired. A saline infusion should be set up if possible and the legs may be raised if the blood pressure is low.

Some would advise that all victims should be transferred to hospital as soon as possible to be observed for the development of complications. Richards *et al.* (1992), however, feel that this is not necessary if there is no impairment of consciousness, no evidence of complications and if the temperature has fallen below 38 °C one hour after the prompt commencement of treatment.

During the transfer of patients to hospital, cooling and monitoring must be continued. Cooling can be maintained simply by keeping the body surface wet and allowing the draught from open windows to circulate around it. Small ice packs applied to the body also help. Rehydration should be continued as far as possible by mouth or intravenously.

Hospital care

On arrival at hospital, reassessment is carried out and the differential diagnoses must be considered. These will include septicaemia, malaria, meningitis and other febrile and infectious diseases. Any history of shivering before the collapse indicates a re-setting of the hypothalamic temperature control centre. This means a pyrexial process other than heat and exercise, which do not reset the centre, at least not until the cooling stage.

If further cooling is necessary, the wetting and fanning method is satisfactory. If wetting can be done by means of a fine spray, this is an advantage. Various arrangements of nets or hammocks and sprays are used in units that see many cases. Immersion in ice water, with or without massage, has been used in the past and still has some advocates (Costrini, 1990) who claim faster cooling and good results. The suspicion remains, however, that it may be counter-productive because it induces intense cutaneous vasoconstriction which interferes with the conduction of heat to the body surface. Immersion methods also cause difficulty in access to the patient. Knochel (1974) paints a grim picture of a convulsing, vomiting, incontinent patient being massaged in a bath of ice water. A reasonable compromise is to apply ice packs to forehead, axillae and groins while wetting and fanning the rest of the body.

Overcooling can lead to shivering which, of course, leads to further heat production. Below 38.5 °C cooling measures should be discontinued, although temperature monitoring should not. As stated in Chapter 1, there is a suggestion that the lag of rectal temperature behind other measures may give a falsely high reading in the cooling phase (Ash *et al.*, 1992). If shivering does occur, it can be inhibited by intravenous chlorpromazine, but this carries the danger of a fall in blood pressure and should be avoided if the blood pressure is already low.

No drug is effective in inducing cooling. Antipyretics cannot be expected to work as there is no re-setting of the thermoregulatory centre. Dantrolene is not generally effective in dogs (Amsterdam *et al.*, 1986) or humans (Bouchama *et al.*, 1991).

The volume and type of intravenous fluids to be used is a matter for judgement. On the one hand, cooling alone will shift blood from the dilated peripheral vessels to the centre, so that overenthusiastic fluid replacement may lead to circulatory overload. For this reason, some American authorities (Knochel, 1989) recommend avoiding infusion until the effect of cooling has been observed. As we have already seen, the Mecca group believes fluid deficit to be of little importance in their patients with non-exertional heat stroke. On the other hand, fluid replacement alone can reduce core temperature (Richards & Richards, 1984) and the Israeli practice (Shapiro & Seidman, 1990) is to begin with 2 L of saline or Ringer's lactate in the first hour followed by 1 L/h. On balance, it is reasonable to suppose that patients with exertional heat stroke are dehydrated, in some cases severely. The deficiency is more likely to be of water in the well-acclimatised patient and salt and water in the unacclimatised. Fluid should be given during cooling according to the initial assessment of the degree of dehydration and monitored by frequent measurements of serum electrolytes and osmolarity and of urine output and osmolarity. There may be other processes leading to cerebral or even pulmonary oedema, and because overload may make these complications worse, fluid administration should be monitored using a central venous pressure line or a Swan–Ganz catheter if possible. This becomes even more important in patients with shock, cardiac complications or pre-existing heart disease.

Although heat exposure may lead to hypokalaemia, replacement should not normally be instituted immediately as there is a danger of hyperkalaemia from muscle damage or renal failure. Replacement should be considered if levels remain low and if urinary output is good. If potassium levels rise dangerously, intravenous calcium and glucose and insulin infusions followed by ion exchange resins may be required. In acidosis, it is customary to rely on cooling and fluid replacement to restore the acid-base balance rather than using bicarbonate, but in the presence of rhabdomyolysis there is an argument for slight alkalinisation of the urine (see below).

It is reasonable to give oxygen by nasal catheter or mask in severe cases. If sedatives are necessary for agitated patients, small doses of diazepam may be used intravenously with caution.

Treatment of complications

Convulsions should be treated promptly as they generate more heat. If intravenous diazepam is insufficient for control, phenytoin infusion should be commenced with heightened awareness of the risk of arrhythmias. Hypoglycaemia, whether or not associated with convulsions, requires 50% glucose intravenously.

Rhabdomyolysis is not in itself amenable to treatment. Alkaline diuresis has been recommended as alkalinisation of the urine increases the solubility of ferrihaemate and reduces deposition in the renal tubules (Rainford & Bloodworth, 1990). There are some who do not believe that this is effective (Delaney, 1992) and it could be dangerous if the blood volume has not been corrected. If the serum uric acid level is high, it may be necessary to use allopurinol. It may sometimes be necessary to replace the calcium that has been deposited in damaged muscle. After some days, severe muscle pain and tenderness, together with a secondary rise of CK, may indicate the development of a compartment syndrome (Amundsen, 1989), that may require surgical decompression.

The management of shock may be difficult if it does not respond to cooling, fluid replacement, colloids and oxygen. Pressor agents are relatively contraindicated as they may constrict the skin and renal vessels. Arrhythmias should be treated promptly.

Acute renal failure must be treated in the usual way. Attempts may be made to avert renal failure in the early stages using low dose dopamine infusion which does not have significant pressor effects. Mannitol infusion and frusemide have also been used to stimulate diuresis, but it is important to ensure that volume replacement has been adequate before taking these steps. Rising potassium levels may require the use of ion exchange resins and glucose–insulin infusion. Peritoneal or haemodialysis may be life saving and should be undertaken early in rhabdomyolysis as these patients are in a highly catabolic state.

The most important treatment of DIC is to remove the cause. In heat stroke this means cooling and prevention of further muscle damage by decompression as necessary. Significant haemorrhage must be treated by blood transfusion. Infusion of platelets and fresh frozen plasma may be required. Neither heparin nor fibrinolytic therapy is appropriate.

Prognosis

The main determinants of prognosis are the speed and quality of treatment. Comparing published results over 70 years, Choo (1988) shows a reduction in mortality from over 60% to less than 10%, although exact comparability of the series is unlikely. Improved results are certainly the result of better understanding and earlier treatment. In classical heat stroke, mortality was only 15% when rapid cooling was achieved, but 33% when it was not (Vicario *et al.*, 1986). According to Choo (1988), the bad prognostic indicators are hyperkalaemia, hypotension, azotaemia, prolonged coma and prolonged temperature over 41 °C.

Although most victims who recover do so without residual effects, there have been reports of persistent cerebellar disease (Suri & Vijayan, 1978; Yaqub, 1987) and of peripheral neuropathy (Bouges *et al.*, 1987).

Prevention

Sir Roger Bannister wrote to *The Times* in 1989: 'The notion that courage and esprit de corps can somehow defeat the principles of physiology is not only wrong but dangerously wrong; lives can be quite needlessly lost and survivors may suffer permanent brain damage'. This in the context of exertional heat stroke and from the man who pushed the physiological limits of his day to their extreme with the first four minute mile.

Exertional heat stroke should be regarded as preventable on at least the second of two levels. The first level is prevention of the condition itself and this is unlikely ever to be fully achieved so long as humans pit themselves against one another and against the elements. The second level is prevention of fatalities and serious complications and this should be achievable in organised events, if not in personal activities. Prevention should be approached both at the personal and organisational level and its mainstay is education.

Sports events

Good advice for organisers and participants can be found, for example, in the *Position Stand on Prevention of Thermal Injuries during Distance Running* published by the American College of Sports Medicine in 1984. Although this is an excellent document, the advice to 'choose a comfortable speed' and 'run with a partner, each responsible for the other's wellbeing' is likely to be derided by serious competitors!

Many of the personal precautions are common sense measures to avoid the adverse effects of exercise generally; to increase one's level of physical fitness gradually, not to attempt strenuous activities without adequate and gradual training, to take an appropriate diet in the days before the event, to avoid alcohol for 24 hours before the event and to warm up and stretch the muscles immediately before exercise.

When an event is to take place in hot conditions, it is important to allow sufficient time to acclimatise to heat, which may mean three to four weeks. Even this precaution does not take account of unexpected heat waves in a normally temperate climate. Physical fitness does not substitute for heat acclimatisation. It is important not to fall into the error of training in the cool of the day for an event that is to take place (ill-advisedly) at noon. Adequate fluid should be taken before, during and after exercise. This needs to be done by an effort of will, as thirst is not a sufficient guide. Runners and tennis players, for example, may be unwilling to prehydrate themselves for fear of the need to empty their bladders during the event, which may be several hours long. Participants should be prepared to withdraw from an event if they feel they are not acclimatised, if they have an infection or are taking one of the medicines that affect heat tolerance. They should wear clothing appropriate to the conditions wherever possible, but this may be a problem, for example in a mountain race or an event that starts and ends on opposite sides of sunrise or sunset. They should make use of all available shade and consider wearing a hat or vest soaked in water to take advantage of the latent heat of evaporation in a way that does not draw on body fluids.

Organisers have great responsibilities. As well as providing competitor education, they should arrange strenuous events as far as possible to avoid hot and humid times of year or, failing this, in the early morning or evening. Routes should be designed to provide as much shade as possible. The risk of heat illness should be assessed using Wet Bulb Globe Temperature (WBGT) or Corrected Effective Temperature (CET) and the event should be cancelled or postponed if the WBGT is above 28 °C at the scheduled start time. Even below this, the WBGT should be published so that competitors are aware of the risk level. Adequate water should be provided at the start and finish and at frequent intervals, every 2–3 km, on the route. Sponges soaked in water provide both drinking water and 'substitute sweat' on heads and vests. There should be sufficient trained first aiders placed on the route, equipped with communications and backed up by medical personnel and cooling equipment, including plenty of water, ice and fans. Also available should be vehicles to

Table 2.3. *Check list for race organisers*

Before the race
    Choose a cool time of year
    Choose a cool time of day
    Competitor education: booklet, media
    Plan first aid and medical support
        Appoint a medical director to supervise:
            Training
            Equipment
            Radio communications
            Vehicles
            Routes for vehicles
            Alert hospitals
    Plan water stations: personnel,
      equipment

Race day
    Measure heat stress
    Be prepared to cancel or postpone (If
      this is necessary, you have not done
      your planning right!)
    Be prepared to disqualify competitors
      at special risk

---

move medical personnel to the scene and evacuate seriously affected victims. Local hospitals should be alerted well in advance and thought should be given to crowd-free routes for ambulances. These points are summarised in Table 2.3.

In the 'City to Surf' race, competitor education is given in local newspapers, in an *Instructions to Runners* booklet and through radio programmes (Richards & Richards, 1984). This also teaches competitors to recognise the early symptoms of heat stroke and advises them to withdraw from the race and seek help if they notice these symptoms. This good advice may well be ignored by highly motivated competitors, who may have been training for the event for months, but are still not prepared for the conditions. For this reason, organisers should be willing as far as possible to discourage or disqualify participants that they think are at risk.

Military activities

In a military context, it is not a matter of preparing for a single event, but an on-going process of educating all who supervise and participate in daily training and operational activities in the risks, prevention and management of

Table 2.4. *Interpretation of WBGT indices as guidance for commanders, organisers of sport and individuals (British Armed Services)*

WBGT Index °C	Acclimatised personnel	Unacclimatised personnel (less than one month)
Below 26 °C (White)	Work: normal Sport: normal	Work: normal Sport: normal
26 °C (Green)	Work: normal Sport: normal	72 h sedentary duty on arrival. Progressive increase to full activity by fourth week. Discretion to be exercised in any heavy exercise. 20 minutes' exercise maximum, followed by 20 minutes' rest in first 28 days. Supervised water consumption. Sport: discretion on sporting activities
29 °C (Green alpha)	Normal work but discretion in planning heavy exercise Periods of heavy exercise should not exceed 30 minutes with a rest period of one hour for cooling and rehydration Avoid standard Combat Fitness Tests Sport: may be undertaken with discretion. Regular rehydration	No strenuous activity Light exercise (walking) with adequate rest periods in the shade with rehydration Sport: organised sport with discretion
31 °C (Amber)	No strenuous exercise Limited activity for hardened acclimatised personnel (12 weeks or more training in the heat) Supervised rests and rehydration for 10 minutes every hour Sport: Organised sport with discretion and only after medical advice	All strenuous exercise is to cease. Sport: organised sport to cease. Voluntary sport discouraged but only to take place after medical advice
32 °C (Red)	All outdoor training, strenuous activity and non-essential duty should be halted for ALL personnel. Sport: no organised sport. Voluntary sport should only take place after medical advice	

WBGT, Web Bulb Globe Temperature.
Note: The effective level of WBGT is increased by 5°C when troops are wearing IPE (clothing protective against nuclear, chemical and biological attack).

heat illness. Although preventive activities must be targeted at hot parts of the world, it must never be forgotten that exertional heat stroke occurs in temperate countries and under moderate conditions. Table 2.4 shows the way in which the WBGT is used to regulate work and sport according to ambient conditions in British service personnel in Cyprus. Much the same system is used in Hong Kong and elsewhere (Henderson *et al.*, 1986).

Table 2.4 also shows the use of coloured 'flags' to indicate the level of risk. The levels and the colours have been standardised in UK military practice following a recent Defence Council Instruction. Practice in the US armed forces is similar (Barthel, 1990). It should be noted, however, that other organisations use different levels and different 'flags'. For example, the Position Stand of the American College of Sports Medicine (1984) gives lower levels and has a different colour flagging system.

'Water discipline' no longer means learning to do without it! There has been much progress in the areas of water requirements and work/rest periods and in the procedures for use of clothing protective against nuclear, biological and chemical warfare. Commanders have been provided with detailed tables of water requirements and work and rest periods in different conditions and different forms of dress. American military practice is again parallel (Barthel, 1990). Also there have been changes in the level of Individual Protective Equipment (IPE) worn at different levels of threat to take account of the additional heat stress involved while, at the same time, ensuring that complete protection is available at short notice if required. The system for drinking while wearing a respirator has been improved. It must be emphasised that servicemen must train regularly using this equipment and an American study showed that panic while wearing it was more of a problem than heat illness (Carter & Cammermayer, 1985). Such panic can readily be avoided by training.

Before deploying to the Gulf in 1990 and 1991, all British service personnel were given a leaflet entitled 'It's Your Health – look after it'. Among other things, it listed the signs and symptoms of heat illness and first aid measures, recommended work/rest periods in different forms of dress and summarised the heat stress guidelines based on WBGT. Although water for washing was sometimes in short supply, vast quantities of bottled drinking water were made available. In spite of the sometimes hot conditions and the extensive wearing of IPE, heat illness was not an important problem in Operation Granby and Operation Desert Storm. If the conflict had extended into still hotter parts of the year, however, the risks would certainly have been greater.

Occupational risk

In industry, while the risk of exertional heat stroke is always present in certain workers, heat stress for them is rather more predictable than in sport or in the armed services, and prevention should be easier. A heat wave, however, could endanger workers who are not normally in risky occupations. An interesting study (Livingstone *et al.*, 1989) showed that immersion of the hands in cold water for five minutes per hour during rest periods helped considerably to reduce heat stress.

Advice for the future

Finally, it is necessary to discuss the further investigation of victims of exertional heat stroke and the advice that they should receive. The limited data available to help us in this area are reviewed by Armstrong *et al.* (1990) and Epstein (1990). In their study of ten victims, Armstrong *et al.* found that nine out of ten had regained heat tolerance at about two months, but one did not show normal responses until nearly a year after the original episode. To study all victims in a heat laboratory would be a large undertaking and some would need to be studied several times. A further difficulty is that the subjects need to achieve a reasonable degree of physical fitness and be given an opportunity to acclimatise to heat before meaningful results can be obtained.

As we have seen, very few victims will have persistent heat intolerance and soldiers, in particular, feel aggrieved if their activities are curtailed and their careers jeopardised as a result of one episode of heat stroke. On the other hand, military authorities are vulnerable to criticism if they permit a former victim to take part in strenuous activities that result in a severe or fatal further episode.

A sensible policy is to advise all victims against strenuous activities for a period of three months, after which exercise may be gradually introduced under supervision. Exceptions to this policy would be those who have had previous episodes, those who have succumbed in mild conditions and those who have collapsed when all, or most, of an accompanying group have had no difficulty. If obvious risk factors such as obesity, alcohol and systemic or skin disease have been excluded, such people should be referred to a heat laboratory for testing three months after the episode.

References

American College of Sports Medicine. (1984). Position Stand on Prevention of Thermal Injuries During Distance Running. Reprinted by permission of the *Medical Journal of Australia* **141**, 876–9.

Amsterdam, J. T., Syverud, S. A., Barker, W. J., Bills, G. R., Goltra, D. D., Armao, J. C. & Hedges, J. R. (1986). Dantrolene sodium for treatment of heat stroke victims: lack of efficacy in a canine model. *American Journal of Emergency Medicine*, **4**, 399–405.

Amundson, D. E. (1989). The spectrum of heat related injury with compartment syndrome. *Military Medicine*, **154**, 450–2.

Anderson, R. J., Reed, G. & Knochel, J. P. (1983). Heatstroke. *Advances in Internal Medicine*, **28**, 115–40.

Armstrong, L. E. J., de Luca, J. P. & Hubbard, R. W. (1990). Time course of recovery and heat acclimation ability of prior exertional heatstroke patients. *Medicine and Science in Sports and Exercise*, **22**, 36–48.

Ash, C. J., Cook, J. R., McMurry, T. A. & Auner, C. R. (1992). The use of rectal temperature to monitor heat stroke. *Missouri Medicine*, **89**, 283–7.

Baba, N. & Ruppert, R. D. (1968). Alteration of eccrine sweat glands in fatal heat stroke. *Archives of Pathology*, **85**, 669–74.

Barthel, H. J. (1990). Exertion-induced heat stroke in a military setting. *Military Medicine*, **155**, 116–19.

Bouchama, A., Cafege, A., Devol, E. B., Labdi, O., El-Assil, K. & Seraj, M. (1991). Ineffectiveness of dantrolene sodium in the treatment of heatstroke. *Critical Care Medicine*, **19**, 176–80.

Bouges, F., Vijayan, G. & Jaufeerally, F. (1987). Peripheral neuropathy after heatstroke. *Lancet*, **1**, 224.

Bradley, A. F., Stupfel, M. & Severinghaus, J. W. (1956). Effect of temperature on PCO_2 and PO_2 of blood *in vitro*. *Journal of Applied Physiology*, **9**, 201–4.

Brown, J. (1992). A complicated case of exertional heat stroke in a military setting with persistent elevation of creatine phosphokinase. *Military Medicine*, **157**, 101–3.

Carter, B. J. & Cammermayer, M. (1985). Emergence of real casualties during simulated chemical warfare under high heat conditions. *Military Medicine*, **150**, 657–65.

Chao, T. C., Siniah, R. & Pakiam, J. E. (1981). Acute heat stroke deaths. *Pathology*, **13**, 145–56.

Choo, M. H. H. (1988). Clinical presentation of heat disorders. In *Heat Disorders*, ed. P. P. B. Yeo & M. K. Lin, pp. 6–15. Singapore, Headquarters Medical Services.

Costrini, A. (1990). Emergency treatment of exertional heatstroke and comparison of whole body cooling techniques. *Medicine and Science in Sports and Exercise*, **22**, 15–18.

Delaney, K. A. (1992). Heat stroke: underlying processes and lifesaving management. *Postgraduate Medicine*, **91**, 379–88.

Dickinson, J. G. (1983). High altitude cerebral oedema: cerebral acute mountain sickness. *Seminars in Respiratory Medicine*, **3**, 151–8.

Epstein, E. (1990). Heat intolerance: predisposing factor or residual injury? *Medicine and Science in Sports and Exercise*, **22**, 29–35.

Hassanein, T., Razack, A., Gavaler, J. S. & van Thiel, D. H. (1992). Heat stroke: its clinical and pathological presentation, with particular attention to the liver.

40   *J. G. Dickinson*

American Journal of Gastroenterology, **87**, 1382–6.

Haymes, E. M., McCormick, R. J. & Buskirk, E. R. (1975). Heat tolerance of exercising lean and obese pubertal boys. *Journal of Applied Physiology*, **39**, 457–61.

Henderson, A., Simon, J. W., Melia, W. M., Navein, J. F. & Mackay, B. G. (1986). Heat illness: a report of 45 cases from Hong Kong, *Journal of the Royal Army Medical Corps*, **132**, 76–84.

Jarmulowicz, M. R. & Buchanan, J. D. (1988). Exertional hyperpyrexia: case report and review of pathophysiological mechanisms. *Journal of the Royal Naval Medical Services*, **74**, 33–8.

Knochel, J. P. (1974). Environmental heat illness: an eclectic review. *Archives of Internal Medicine*, **133**, 841–64.

Knochel, J. P. (1989). Heat stroke and related heat stress disorders. *Disease a Month*, **35**, 301–77.

Knochel, J. P. (1990). Catastrophic medical events with exhaustive exercise: white collar rhabdomyolysis. *Kidney International*, **38**, 709–19.

Leibowitz, E., Seidman, D.S., Laor, A., Shapiro, Y. & Epstein, Y. (1991). Are psoriatic patients at risk of heat intolerance? *British Journal of Dermatology*, **124**, 439–42.

Livingstone, S. D., Nolan, R. W. & Cattroll, S. W. (1989). Heat loss caused by immersing hands in water. *Aviation, Space and Environmental Medicine*, **60**, 1166–71.

O'Donnell T. F. & Clowes, G. H. A. (1972). The circulatory abnormalities of heat stroke. *New England Journal of Medicine*, **287**, 734–7.

Pattison, M. E., Logan, J. L., Lee, S. M. & Ogden, D. A. (1988). Exertional heat stroke and acute renal failure in a young woman. *American Journal of Kidney Diseases*, **9**, 184–7.

Rainford, D. J. & Bloodworth, L. L. (1990). Pigment nephropathy. In *Acute Renal Failure*, ed. D. Rainford & P. Sweny, pp. 129–44. London, Farrand Press.

Richards, R. & Richards, D. (1984). Exertion-induced heat exhaustion and other medical aspects of the City to Surf fun runs, 1978–84. *Medical Journal of Australia*, **141**, 799–805.

Richards, R., Richards, D. & Sutton, J. R. (1992). Exertion induced heat exhaustion. *Australian Family Physician*, **21**, 18–24.

Seraj, M. A., Channa, A.B., Al Harti, S. S., Khan, F.M., Zafrullah, A. & Samarkandi, A. H. (1991). Are heat stroke patients fluid depleted? Importance of monitoring central venous pressure as a simple guideline for fluid therapy. *Resuscitation*, **21**, 33–9.

Shapiro, Y., Magazink, A., Udassin, R., Ben Baruch, G., Shvartz, E. & Shoenfield, Y. (1979). Heat intolerance in former heatstroke patients. *Annals of Internal Medicine*, **90**, 913–16.

Shapiro, Y. & Seidman, D. S. (1990). Field and clinical observations of exertional heat stroke patients. *Medicine and Science in Sports and Exercise*, **22**, 6–14.

Sprung, C. L., Portocarrero, C. J., Fernaine, A. V. & Weinberg, P. F. (1980). The metabolic and respiratory alterations of heat stroke. *Archives of Internal Medicine*, **140**, 665–9.

Stevens, P. E., Pusey, C. D. & Rainford, D. J. (1988). Sprinting can seriously damage your health. *British Medical Journal*, **297**, 1518.

Suri, M. L. & Vijayan, G. P. (1978). Neurological sequelae of heat hyperpyrexia. *Journal of the Association of Physicians of India*, **26**, 203–7.

Sutton, J. R. (1984). Heat illness. In *Sports Medicine*, ed. R. H. Strauss, pp.307–321. Philadelphia, Saunders.

Vicario, S. J., Okabajue, R. & Haltom, T. (1986). Rapid cooling in classic heatstroke: effect on mortality rates. *American Journal of Emergency Medicine*, **4**, 394–8.

Yaqub, B. A. (1987). Neurological manifestations at the Mecca Pilgrimage. *Neurology*, **37**, 1004–6.

Young, A. (1987). Sports medicine. In *Oxford Textbook of Medicine*, 2nd edn, vol.2, ed. D. J. Weatherall, J. G. G. Ledingham & D. A. Warrell, pp.26.1–8. Oxford, Oxford University Press.

Zahger, D., Moses, A. & Weiss, A. T. (1989). Evidence of prolonged myocardial dysfunction in heat stroke. *Chest*, **95**, 1089–91.

3

Pathophysiology of heat stroke

J. P. KNOCHEL

Introduction

Exertional heat stroke is characterised by a body temperature above 40.5 °C, central nervous system dysfunction and in about 50% of cases, anhidrosis. It occurs in individuals, almost always men, who are performing hard physical work at a rate such that the heat produced by metabolism cannot be adequately dissipated to the environment.

The aetiology of exertional heat stroke appears to be clearly evident in most cases (Knochel & Reed, 1994). Thus, intense, sustained physical activity is performed at such a level that the resulting metabolic heat production and its storage in the body exceeds the capacity for heat dissipation. It is also clearly evident that a host of contributory risk factors play a role (Chapters 1 and 2). These include the status of heat acclimatisation, heat and humidity, time of day, clothing, salt and water balance, the status of physical fitness, associated illnesses, medications or illicit drugs and male gender. Additional factors include the adequacy of rest, performing exercise under conditions of fasting and especially in military situations and fever from immunisations.

Failure of thermoregulation has been cited as a cause of heat stroke for many years. This implies failure of the hypothalamic centres that regulate cutaneous blood flow and sweat gland activity in response to an elevation of blood temperature. Sweat gland fatigue is another theoretical factor that has not attracted a great deal of interest from contemporary research scientists. The secretion of sweat depends on plasma flow to the secretory coil of the gland. A decline or cessation of sweating, a classical sign of heat stroke that usually occurs immediately before collapse, was originally interpreted to reflect circulatory failure. Failure of thermoregulation and sweat gland fatigue are generally more important considerations in cases of Classical Heat Stroke which usually occur in infants, the elderly or the chronically ill independently of physical exertion. In contrast to patients with classical heat stroke, victims of exertional heat stroke most often show persistent sweating at the height of their illness clearly indicating the 'sweat gland fatigue' probably plays little if any role in the pathogenesis of their illness. Many cases of exertional heat stroke occur in men who use poor judgement, who go too far and too fast for the prevailing conditions of heat and humidity.

The entire concept of 'sweat gland fatigue' may be erroneous. Older studies showed that prolonged cholinergic stimulation of perspiration resulted in a progressive fall in sweat rate. More recent evidence (Sawka & Wenger, 1988) indicates that the superficial layer of the corneum absorbs water, swells and eventually mechanically occludes the pore of the sweat gland. Either immediate removal of sweat as it is secreted or adhesive tape stripping of the superficial skin layer facilitates unimpaired sweating without evidence of 'fatigue'. Anhidrosis observed for weeks or months after recovery from frank heat stroke may reflect injury-mediated damage to the sweat gland or frank necrosis (Knochel & Reed, 1994). In such cases, histological examination of skin and sweat glands would be of great interest.

A number of isolated episodes of exertional heat stroke have occurred in temperate climates (Bailey, 1975). In nearly all instances, the victim was competing in an athletic event such as mountain climbing, cross-country skiing, long-distance running or American football. In the latter instance, collapse is often provoked by repetitive wind sprints at the end of a heavy practice session in large men who may have lost up to 10 kg of body fluids. Some believe that the coup de grace is a surge of effort towards the end of a competitive race which may not only increase heat production acutely, but also cause vasoconstriction of skin blood vessels because of noradrenaline (norepinephrine) release which reduces the ability of the body to lose heat (Kim *et al.*, 1979).

Idiosyncracy must be invoked to account for certain cases. Some patients without discernible risk factors unexpectedly collapse. Some of these victims had negotiated identical amounts of heat stress on previous occasions without difficulty.

This chapter will review certain elements of the pathophysiology of exertional heat stroke, some of its complications and, where appropriate, emphasise issues that in the author's view, deserve further research.

Acclimatisation to heat and its hazards

Acclimatisation to heat is a complex process requiring profound physiological, physical, endocrine and biochemical adaptations in many organs or systems. Physical fitness per se is a critically important component (Knochel & Reed, 1994).

The hallmark of the heat acclimatised state is a lesser rise of core temperature for a given unit of work than that which occurred in the untrained, unacclimatised state. Once acclimatised, a person can perform physical work in the heat that would have been impossible or even life-threatening in the untrained, unacclimatised state.

The major adaptations in acclimatisation are cardiovascular, endocrine, exocrine, haematological, renal, metabolic and immunological. Acclimatisation is induced by performing sufficient work in the heat to cause repeated elevations of core temperature. The degree of acclimatisation obtained, at least up to a point, will vary with the intensity and duration of the heat load. A trained, acclimatised person will demonstrate a reduced resting heart rate, a higher stroke output and the capacity to increase cardiac output to higher levels for any given level of work than before. The heart undergoes eccentric hypertrophy. Training itself improves vascular tone and improves autonomic regulation of the heart and peripheral vascular system. Thus, a trained, acclimatised person is much less likely to develop postural hypotension or fainting while working in the heat.

Muscular work, especially in the heat, results in a major translocation of blood flow to skeletal muscle (Kjellmer, 1965). The resulting fall in effective arterial volume activates the renin–angiotensin system, which in turn stimulates the production of aldosterone. Aldosterone in this setting has two critical effects (Knochel & Reed, 1994). First, it promotes net salt conservation by the kidney leading to an increased extracellular volume, which in turn reduces the fall in effective arterial volume during exercise. Second, aldosterone causes a reduction in sweat sodium concentration, thereby helping to conserve arterial volume during exercise. The quantity of sweat that can be produced during heat stress also increases significantly, an additional hallmark of the heat acclimatised state. Training and acclimatisation cause a net gain of total body water, part being intracellular reflecting a net gain of muscle (lean) mass (Nadel, 1984). The extracellular volume measured by radiosulphate dilution may increase 20%. Although the haematocrit falls modestly in a trained, acclimatised man, the so called 'anaemia of training', there also occurs an increase in red cell mass. Thus, plasma volume expansion exceeds the gain of red cell mass. These changes improve tissue perfusion and fuel delivery during work, which in turn serves to enhance the delivery of heated blood from the working muscle to the body surface (Knochel, 1990). The delivery of oxygen to working organs, especially muscle, improves not only by increased perfusion, but also by increased capillary density per muscle fibre (Brodal *et al.*,

Table 3.1. *Local adaptations in skeletal muscle to training that improve oxidative metabolism and reduce heat production*

1.	Increased capillarity
2.	Increased capillary filtration coefficient
3.	Decreased diffusion distance from capillary to mitochondria
4.	$\uparrow O_2$ extraction
5.	$\uparrow$Concentration of myoglobin
6.	$\uparrow$Mitochondrial mass
7.	$\uparrow$Production of antioxidants
8.	$\uparrow$Ion transport enzyme density

1977) and increased concentration of myoglobin in the muscle cell (Table 3.1). Of no less importance, there occurs a major increase in mitochondrial density and oxidative enzymes in the muscle. All of these factors increase metabolic efficiency herein defined as an increased capacity to produce ATP per mole of glucose or fatty acids oxidised to carbon dioxide and water (Knochel, 1990). The result is not only less heat production per unit of mechanical work, but also an improvement in factors allowing removal of heat.

Trained, acclimatised men show an increase of glomerular filtration rate that may rise 20% higher than the baseline (Knochel *et al.*, 1974). While part of this represents the effect of volume expansion, the results of renal studies suggest that renal hypertrophy may also play a role. A higher glomerular filtration rate could well provide protection against acute renal failure that may otherwise occur with extreme exertion in the heat.

The immunological effects of heat acclimatisation and training are currently under intense investigation. Hard work in the heat is associated with the appearance of endotoxins in the blood which in turn lead to the formation of tumour necrosis factor and other cytokines (Bouchama *et al.*, 1991a). Antibodies against these potentially harmful factors are found in heat acclimatised persons. During hard work, shunting of blood away from the visceral circulation to skeletal muscle and skin theoretically causes bowel ischaemia which permits absorption of bacterial endotoxins in the blood. This in turn leads to a cascade of cytokine formation, typified by tumour necrosis factor. Interventions that reduce, eliminate or block endotoxins and their related activation of cytokines have been shown to reduce mortality in experimental hyperthermia. These include administration of endotoxin antibodies, immunisation against endotoxin and prophylactic sterilisation of the bowel with antibiotics before inducing hyperthermia. Hyperthermia in germ-free animals is less harmful than in animals possessing a normal intestinal flora. Endotoxin absorption from the bowel during heat stress could explain certain serious complications of exertional heat stroke (Fong *et al.*, 1990). These include the extremely catabolic state of severe cases, capillary hyperpermeability, endothelial injury, disseminated intravascular coagulation (DIC), acute respiratory distress syndrome and the multiple organ failure syndrome.

Rhabdomyolysis: a complication of training in the heat and its possible cardiovascular consequences

An intact cardiovascular system is perhaps the single most important requirement to work safely under conditions of heat stress. Thus, cardiovascular disease, hypertension and medications used to treat these disorders are common and well-known risk factors for both exertional and classical forms of heat stroke. It is not widely appreciated that demands on cardiovascular performance imposed by hard work and environmental heat stress could be substantially increased by the coexistence of exertion-induced injury of skeletal muscle. Haller and his coworkers have made several important observations in this regard on patients with skeletal muscle disease (Haller *et al.*, 1983). Compared with control subjects, cardiac output is grossly exaggerated but total oxygen consumption is disproportionately low for any given level of work in patients with McArdle's disease. These patients may develop severe rhabdomyolysis with exercise. McArdle's disease is characterised by the inability to utilise skeletal muscle glycogen because of the absence of myophosphorylase. Thus, under conditions of hard work, glycogen can not be hydrolysed and therefore is not available to produce energy. When these patients exercise, their cardiac output is disproportionately increased in an apparent attempt to provide the skeletal muscle with more substrate for energy production and, as a result, myocardial work is considerably greater. Of interest, if one infuses glucose into a patient with McArdle's disease while they are working, their hyperdynamic cardiac output immediately falls to a normal level and oxygen consumption for the level of cardiac output rises. The same response is also seen in other myopathic illnesses (Haller *et al.*, 1983). Now consider what happens to a young military recruit in basic training in the summer time. Characteristically, after several days of training, his muscles become stiff and sore, they may cramp and his creatine kinase (CK) may rise to levels indicating frank rhabdomyolysis. Serum CK may reach levels of 50 000 IU/L in these men (Demos *et al.*, 1974). Other men without muscular symptoms may show CK elevations to 10 000 IU/L. Laboratory findings indicating rhabdomyolysis consist of creatinuria, hypocalcaemia secondary to calcium precipitation in injured muscle, hyperphosphataemia, hyperuricaemia and hyperuricosuria secondary to the release of purine from the injured muscle

(Knochel *et al.*, 1974). Although the exact studies performed by Haller and his associates (1983) have not been carried out on men training in hot weather, it seems possible that muscle cells injured by training could exert demands on the heart in the same way as occurs in myopathic patients. In addition to the exercise itself, muscle injury in a person training in the heat could also occur by means of potassium deficiency (Knochel *et al.*, 1972).

There are three mechanisms whereby intensive training in the heat may cause potassium deficiency. First, it is well known that men training in the heat may secrete ten or more litres of sweat each day (Knochel, 1989). Potassium concentration in sweat secreted at high rates may average 9 mEq/L (Emrich *et al.*, 1970; Verde *et al.*, 1982). Thus, if a trainee consumes a normal diet of 100 mEq K^+ per day, most of this will be lost in sweat. The second mechanism to explain K^+ loss is physiological hyperaldosteronism. The training induced complex of hyperreninaemia, sustained production of aldosterone, extracellular volume expansion and excretion of sodium into the urine, particularly at night, could mediate K^+ losses by Na^+–K^+ exchange in the renal tubule (Knochel *et al.*, 1972). Normal subjects made K^+ deficient reduce urinary K^+ excretion to values below 20 mEq/day. Men training in the heat excreted an average of 67 mEq/day despite K^+ depletion, a finding that suggests renal K^+ wasting. The third mechanism to explain a decrease in the total body K^+ could also occur by muscle injury itself (Knochel, 1982). One would not expect a seriously injured or necrotic cell to maintain its high concentration of K^+ ions. Consequent to cell injury, one anticipates loss of K^+ into the urine along with an appropriate quantity of nitrogen. By definition, loss of K^+ by this means does not cause K^+ deficiency. Rather, it resembles the reduction of total body K^+ that would occur if a leg were amputated. The average maximum K^+ deficit measured by total body isotope dilution in these men was 517 mEq (Knochel *et al.*, 1972). Our studies did not allow determination of the precise fraction of the total deficit that occurred by sweating, urinary losses or tissue loss consequent to cellular injury. That these men were actually K^+ deficient was supported by our finding that there was a reduction of total body K^+ by 10.6 mEq/kg of lean body mass.

When a muscle cell contracts in response to an electrical stimulus, potassium ions are released into the interstitial fluid surrounding the cell (Kjellmer, 1965; Knochel & Schlein, 1972). Local hyperkalaemia induces arteriolar vasodilatation which is thought to be at least partially responsible for increasing muscle blood flow during exercise. The increased flow not only subserves delivery of oxygen, fatty acids and glucose, but also facilitates the removal of metabolites such as carbon dioxide and lactate and the removal of heat generated during contraction. Experimental potassium deficiency blocks the release of potassium during electrical stimulation and muscle blood flow does not increase despite forceful contractions (Knochel & Schlein, 1972). The muscle becomes necrotic following work. Besides disturbances of blood flow, K^+ deficiency causes additional metabolic abnormalities of the muscle that also could contribute to rhabdomyolysis. Synthesis and storage of glycogen fall sharply in K^+ deficient animals and humans (Knochel, 1987). In addition, the usual stimulation of glycogen synthesis produced by exercise is not seen in K^+ deficient animals. Thus, K^+ deficiency establishes a situation somewhat similar to McArdle's disease, as glycogen is not available as a fuel in either instance.

Potassium deficiency can cause rhabdomyolysis in humans and can be reproduced in dogs (Knochel & Schlein, 1972); therefore it seems possible that muscle cell injury in young men during sustained training in the heat could be at least partially ascribed to this mechanism. It is also possible that such a myopathy might increase cardiovascular work requirements during exercise, similar to patients with McArdle's disease, which might in turn lower the threshold for the development of exertional heat stroke. In contrast to basic military training conducted in hot weather, men training in cool weather do not become potassium deficient and show little, if any, evidence of muscle injury (Knochel *et al.*, 1972).

Besides basic military training, other situations potentially capable of inducing the foregoing sequence of events includes football players undergoing twice daily sessions in late summer, and men performing sustained, prolonged physical labour day after day.

Do some victims of exertional heat stroke have malignant hyperthermia?

Malignant hyperthermia

This is a disease in which susceptible individuals become acutely hypermetabolic, rigid and hyperthermic, usually following administration of suxamethonium, or during anaesthaesia with volatile anaesthetics (e.g halothane, enflurane or isoflurane). (Malignant hyperthermia is discussed in detail in Section 2). The disease is familial and has been ascribed to deranged calcium homeostasis in skeletal muscle (Hopkins *et al.*, 1991). Dantrolene reverses the abnormality. A similar condition is found in pigs. Susceptible pigs may develop typical attacks of malignant hyperthermia when exposed to heat or alternatively during periods of extreme fright or physical stress. It has been postulated because of the similarities of malignant hyperthermia in pigs and humans that exertional heat stroke may, at least in some instances, be a manifestation of malignant hyperthermia. This postulation has not been proven. First of all, typical malignant hyperthermia induced during anaesthesia has been described in two professional American football players (Wingard & Gatz, 1978). If heat stress and physical effort could induce an attack of malignant hyperthermia, it seems that it would have occurred earlier in these men because they were both large lineman who, like all football players, had certainly become hyperthermic on many occasions as a result of training exercises, especially wind sprints. Neither man had a history of heat intolerance. Second, the clinical patterns of exertional heat stroke and malignant hyperthermia are quite different. At the onset of an attack induced by anaesthesia, patients with malignant hyperthermia display acute hypercarbia, hypoxia and muscle rigidity. In contrast, patients with exertional heat stroke show respiratory alkalosis, often combined with lactic acidosis related to preceding exercise, and a normal or elevated blood oxygen level. Muscular rigidity is not a feature of exertional heat stroke (unless they develop convulsive seizures during cooling). Spontaneous cooling is not likely to occur in malignant hyperthermia but if sweating is present, patients with exertional heat stroke generally do so. Several reports have described positive contracture tests in young men who had survived exertional heat stroke and in members of their families (Hackl *et al.*, 1991; Hopkins *et al.*, 1991). In patients who have recovered from exertional heat stroke, however, positive halothane or ryanodine-induced contractures do not prove the existence of malignant hyperthermia because these tests are not specific (Chapter 6). Some observers have advocated the use of dantrolene to reduce body temperature in patients with heat stroke because of the notion that exertional heat stroke may be a clinical manifestation of malignant hyperthermia. There is no evidence that dantrolene is useful in this condition (Bouchama *et al.*, 1991*b*). At least for the present, there is no acceptable alternative treatment for exertional heat stroke other than direct cooling and other supportive measures. In fact, because of the potentially harmful cardiovascular, pulmonary and hepatic effects of dantrolene, the drug could be dangerous.

Why is exertional heat stroke rare in women?

The fact that exertional heat stroke characteristically affects men was never a point of concern until it was realised that despite increasing participation in military training and competitive sports, women are much less prone to this disease (Chapter 1). One case was described by Pattison and his coworkers (1988) in a young woman who developed a typical case of exertional heat stroke while hiking down a mountain. As in the case of men, she developed frank rhabdomyolysis with renal failure but fortunately survived. Also of interest, independently of exertional heat stroke, exertional rhabdomyolysis is also extremely rare in women. Studies examining the release of CK as an index of muscle injury show that for any comparable level of exercise, muscle injury is invariably worse in men.

Many studies have been conducted comparing thermoregulation in women and men and these have been reviewed recently (Stephenson & Kolka, 1988). In general, when women undergo incremental elevations of core temperature by passive heating, the thermoregulatory set point, i.e the specific temperature at which sweating and cutaneous blood flow increase, is lower than that observed in men. Thus, if a woman's set point at which thermoregulatory reflexes are activated is lower than that for a man, one can infer that women should become less febrile or store less heat than men for a comparable degree of physical work or passive heating. This possibly explains why women must exercise at a higher comparable level of oxygen consumption than men to elevate their core temperature to the same level (Stephenson & Kolka, 1988).

In ovulatory women, the set point for activating sweating and cutaneous blood flow is lower in the follicular phase (days 0–15 of the cycle) than in the luteal phase (15–28 of the cycle). In quantitative terms, the difference between the thermoregulatory set point in the follicular and luteal phases, as well as the differences between women and men is about 0.5 °C. The difference in heat storage incident to exercise is about the same as that produced by passive heating. Another group of investigators (Tankersley *et al.*, 1992) examined thermoregulation during exercise in the heat in postmenopausal women before and after 14–23 days of therapy with conjugated oestrogens (premarin) or an oestrogen patch. Measurements were obtained after a 40 minute period of supine rest at a dry bulb temperature of 25 °C, wet bulb 17.5 °C and again after exercise in a dry bulb temperature of 36 °C, wet bulb 27.5 °C. Each woman exercised for a period of 60 minutes in the semi-recumbent position at an average level of 40% of their maximal oxygen uptake. After oestrogen replacement therapy in physiological doses, the women showed a lower thermoregulatory set point and their rectal and oesophageal temperature elevations were less by an average value of 0.6 °C.

Despite the foregoing information, there is no proof that gender or oestrogen protects women against exertional heat stroke. The possibility still exists that men are capable of generating more heat than women because of their proportionately larger muscle mass, and thus larger potential for work-related heat production. Obviously, the fact that women are less likely to develop exertional heat stroke, despite taking part in competitive sports, remains an interesting observation that deserves further study.

Core temperature versus brain temperature

The levels of core temperature at which exertional heat stroke occurs are widely variable. Some patients are found to have temperatures of 40.6 °C or less shortly after collapse, and others may have temperatures estimated to be 46.7 °C. It is well known that competitive events or military drills in the heat may cause frank hyperthermia in normal men who show no apparent harmful effects. One such athlete was described with a rectal temperature of 41.9 °C during a marathon (Maron *et al.*, 1977). Although there is no definitive answer, brain temperature per se could be a more logical determinant of exertional heat stroke. At least part of the human anatomy may have undergone a number of interesting evolutions in order to keep the brain cool while working in the heat.

Although most forms of highly competitive physical sports impose risks for developing exertional heat stroke, some sports with comparable levels of heat production carry less risk. One of these is competitive cycling. Although cyclists have indeed developed heat exhaustion and collapse, frank heat stroke and its complications are unusual (Moore *et al.*, 1995). It has been postulated that rapid air movement may reduce the risk by promoting more rapid heat loss. In addition, facial exposure to air may promote more efficient cooling of the brain. Venous drainage from the central portion of the face, oral and nasal passages flows beneath the surface of the brain en route to the heart (Cabanac, 1986), theoretically maintaining a lower brain temperature. A substantial portion of venous blood flowing from the face enters the cavernous sinus. The internal carotid artery is contained within the cavernous sinus, thus serving as a countercurrent heat exchanger.

Other anatomical facial characteristics may play a role in brain cooling. It has been proposed that the broad nose and mouth of persons of equatorial origin facilitate more efficient cooling of venous blood flowing beneath the brain, and hence the brain itself. This may represent an evolutionary phenomenon in these individuals to prevent overheating of the brain during hard work in the heat. In contrast, the narrow face and small nasal passages of those living in cold climates in the North or at high altitudes may theoretically subserve the purpose of reducing heat loss by this means.

Major complications of exertional heat stroke

Cardiovascular shock

Patients with acute exertional heat stroke commonly present in a state of shock. In most cases, the reduction in blood pressure results from translocation of blood from the central circulation to the skin and muscle, accounting for the common finding of flushed skin. Such patients always demonstrate frank hyperthermia and a rapid pulse. Others who have sustained sizeable deficits of salt and water as a result of perspiration may present in typical hypovolaemic shock. At least one-half of the victims of exertional heat stroke are still perspiring when first seen; because of this the effect of continued sweating is deceptive as vaporisation may cool the skin despite core hyperthermia. For this reason, it is critically important to measure rectal or core temperature. If the state of shock is the result of translocation of blood, in nearly all cases blood pressure spontaneously rises as cooling measures take effect which cause a shift of blood from the skin vessels back to the central circulation. For this reason, the most important initial treatment for shock is aggressive cooling. Infusion of saline in sufficient quantities to restore blood pressure to normal before cooling should be avoided as it may be followed by pulmonary oedema as body temperature is lowered. Under such circumstances, cooling results in translocation of blood to a normal or expanded central circulation which results in pulmonary congestion.

Myocardial injury in exertional heat stroke

Many patients with acute heat stroke show electrocardiographic abnormalities that may include an assortment of both atrial and ventricular arrhythmias, conduction defects or bundle branch block. Most of these resolve completely after cooling. In rare instances, frank transmural myocardial infarction has occurred and in cases subjected to autopsy, the coronary arteries have been normal (Knochel *et al.*, 1961). The cause of myocardial infarction under these conditions is unknown, but it seems possible that hypotension, decreased myocardial perfusion, high concentrations of catecholamines, and ischaemic cellular injury could easily permit calcium to enter the intracellular space in sufficient concentration to activate proteolytic enzymes and thus explain the myocardial necrosis. Similar results have been obtained in experimental animals by infusing poisonous concentrations of adrenaline (epinephrine) in conjunction with calcium salts, so-called 'infarctoid cardiomyopathy' (Selye & Bajusz, 1959). Similar findings occur in fatal cases of exertional heat stroke that show focal haemorrhagic infarctions in the left ventricle especially near the interventricular septum. A multitude of other potentially injurious factors are detectable in the plasma of patients with heat stroke which include free radicals, reactive oxygen species, cytokines, endothelin-1 and nitric oxide. Early in hyperthermia, splanchnic vasoconstriction apparently occurs in response to endothelin-1 (Bouchama *et al.*, 1994). This serves to increase intestinal permeability to bacterial endotoxins. Later in hyperthermia, nitric oxide release mediates an increased flow in the mesenteric circulation (Hall *et al.*, 1994), which could have a paradoxically harmful effect of increasing endotoxin delivery to the systemic circulation

Acid–base derangements and changes of plasma composition in early exertional heat stroke

Most patients with acute exertional heat stroke will have lactic acidosis at the time of onset. While part of this may be explained by shock, it should be remembered that lactic acidosis, even of pronounced degree, may be a normal result of severe exertion. Normal persons may show a reduction of blood bicarbonate to 5 mEq/L, an elevation of lactate to values as high as 25 mmol/L and a reduction of arterial pH to 6.8 units simply as a result of repetitive, exhaustive exercise (Osnes & Hermansen, 1972). Under these conditions, the acute metabolic acidosis clears as rapidly as blood is returned to the liver where lactate is converted back to glucose via the Cori cycle. Similarly, in patients with heat stroke, restoration of a normal circulatory volume generally leads to rapid clearing of lactic acidosis. In those who have presented in clinical shock, however, restoration of blood volume may allow reperfusion of skeletal muscle that is followed by a lactic acid washout resulting in a delayed appearance or even a reappearance of lactic acidosis. In these cases, simple correction of hypovolaemia will generally lead to rapid resolution of the lactic acidosis. Most patients also show acute respiratory alkalosis at the time of admission characterised by values for arterial carbon dioxide tension far below those usually seen in uncomplicated metabolic acidosis. In normal persons, simple exposure to heat and the elevation of body temperature is nearly always associated with hyperventilation, reduction of carbon dioxide tension and elevation of pH. This response accounts for 'heat paraesthesias' or 'heat-induced tetany' (Knochel & Reed, 1994).

Characteristic electrolyte disorders are also seen in the early phases of acute exertional heat stroke. Hypokalaemia is observed in at least one-half of these patients and has several explanations. Thus, the high levels of adrenaline (epinephrine) that occur with exertional heat stroke can drive potassium into cells because of its beta-agonist effect. Simple thermogenic hyperventilation with respiratory alkalosis can also cause acute hypokalaemia, an effect that now appears to be catecholamine dependent (Krapf *et al.*, 1995). Finally, it is possible that some of these individuals may be potassium deficient as a result of the losses incurred by sweating and renal wasting because of aldosterone (Knochel *et al.*, 1972). In most of these cases, the hypokalaemia spontaneously disappears within a few hours. Acute hypophosphataemia is also seen in many of these patients during the acute stage and apparently also results from cellular uptake of phosphate consequent to the effect of catecholamines and acute respiratory alkalosis (Knochel & Caskey, 1977). These events are generally not seen until the metabolic acidosis has been corrected. Presumably, the superimposition of respiratory alkalosis reduces intracellular carbon dioxide tension, intracellular pH rises, phosphofructokinase is activated by the elevation of pH, the rate of glucose phosphorylation increases and consumes the available stores of inorganic phosphorus thus explaining the acute hypophosphataemia. Serum phosphorus levels may fall well below 1 mg/dL (0.3 mmol/L). This situation does not require treatment because it resolves spontaneously.

Delayed acid–base and plasma composition changes and their relation to rhabdomyolysis

After the initial hours of exertional heat stroke, the acid–base disorder may spontaneously convert from a mixture of lactic acidosis and respiratory alkalosis to one of predominant metabolic acidosis. The changes in plasma composition now reflect tissue destruction. Essentially all of these patients have rhabdomyolysis. Skeletal muscle contains about 60 mmol of sulphate/kg, 60 mmol of phosphate/kg and smaller quantities of organic acids (adenylate, creatinine) that if released can cause profound metabolic acidosis (Knochel, 1988). Release of the contents from 1 kg of injured muscle is tantamount to infusing 120 mEq of sulphuric acid and 108 mEq of phosphoric acid. Since each mEq of fixed mineral acid that moves into the extracellular fluid titrates 1 mEq of bicarbonate, severe metabolic acidosis can appear at this time. Hyperphosphataemia is characteristically seen because of the cellular phosphate leak, resulting in calcium phosphate complex formation and hypocalcaemia. Injured muscle also takes up calcium ions from the circulation where it precipitates as $CaCO_3$ and calcium phosphate, both reactions themselves resulting in the liberation of hydrogen ions. Calcium accumulation in muscle explains the profound degrees of hypocalcaemia seen in these patients. Although tetany may occur, it is exceptionally rare, possibly because muscle injury destroys the usual excitation–contraction coupling response seen in normal muscle. Patients with severe rhabdomyolysis have had serum calcium values as low as 2.3 mg/dL (0.65 mmol/L) without tetany. Hypocalcaemia of this magnitude is also capable of depressing cardiac output (Henrich *et al.*, 1984).

All of these processes are grossly exaggerated if the patient has acute renal failure and is unable to excrete acid into the urine. The destruction of tissue also liberates large quantities of nitrogenous products that appear as urea. Rhabdomyolysis is also characterised by disproportionate elevations of creatinine in the serum compared with urea (usually 0.1 or less) reflecting release of muscle creatine phosphate which is spontaneously dehydrated to creatinine. Muscle enzymes display sharp elevations, including CK and aldolase. Young men with exertional heat stroke may show CK elevations as high as 2–3 million IU/L which reflect massive muscle destruction (Knochel, 1990).

Pronounced hyperuricaemia may occur in rhabdomyolysis (Knochel *et al.*, 1974). Levels exceeding 40 mg/dL have been observed. Uric acid is derived from purines released from the injured muscle. Not only is hyperuricaemia related to overproduction, but also renal uric acid excretion is reduced by the elevation of blood lactate.

Hyperkalaemia appears within hours following rhabdomyolysis and peaks between the sixth and 48th hour after injury. Severe muscular weakness may progress to paralysis that may involve the respiratory muscles. The concentration of potassium inside the normal skeletal muscle cell is approximately 150 mEq/L. The high concentration gradient between the intracellular and extracellular compartments is maintained for the most part by the Na^+-K^+Mg-dependent ATPase pump. One cycle of this pump transports 3 Na^+ ions from the interior of the cell in exchange for 2K^+ ions in the opposite direction. There is a greater net traffic of sodium ions moving out than potassium ions moving in, and the interior of the cell becomes negatively charged thus attracting potassium ions and generating the high intracellular–extracellular ratio. Adequate supplies of ATP to energise this pump requires a constant source of metabolic energy. Ischaemia, hyperthermia, hypoxia and reduced perfusion with the blood delivering chemical substrates leads to failure of the pump, a reduction of membrane potential and diffusion of potassium ions into the extracellular fluid. This results in acute hyperkalaemia. Hyperkalaemia is perhaps the most dangerous early complication of severe exertional heat stroke with rhabdomyolysis because of its side-effects of cardiotoxicity. The side-effects include atrial asystole, conduction disturbances, both atrial and ventricular arrhythmias, ventricular fibrillation and cardiac arrest. Functionally, progressive hyperkalemia causes a reduction of cardiac output. Even modest degrees of hyperkalaemia may become potentially fatal in the presence of severe hypocalcaemia because of the electrical opposition of calcium and potassium ions on membrane phenomena. I have personally observed fatal hyperkalaemia with a serum potassium of only 6.2 mEq/L in a young football player with exertional heat stroke whose serum calcium was 4.8 mg/dL (1.36 mmol/L). This emphasises two critically important points. First, one must not rely on serum potassium measurements alone to assess the import-ance or severity of hyperkalaemia. The electrocardiogram remains the single most powerful tool to determine when hyperkalaemia must be treated. Sec-ond, in the presence of frank, ominous hyperkalaemia, intravenous calcium chloride is the drug of choice as it will be effective immediately in reversing the electrical cardiotoxicity. Infusing calcium does not reduce potassium levels. In contrast to calcium infusions, glucose and insulin and various β-adrenergic agonists will reduce potassium levels but may require hours to become effec-tive. In addition, patients with exertional heat stroke who have diffuse muscle injury and possibly hepatic ischaemia, appear to respond poorly to insulin-glucose or β_2 receptor agonist infusions. Potassium exchange resins (disodium polystyrene sulphonate) may require up to 24 hours to become effective. Patients with severe hyperkalaemia usually have acute renal failure. Because continued infusions of calcium salts are themselves potentially dangerous, severe cases of hyperkalaemia often require haemodialysis for control. So-dium bicarbonate for treatment of hyperkalaemia has become somewhat controversial. Theoretically, alkalinisation of extracellular fluid results in shifts of potassium ions into cells, especially of the liver and skeletal muscle; however, employing $NaHCO_3$ for this purpose generates CO_2 which diffuses into cells and lowers intracellular pH. At least in patients with chronic renal failure, infusions of $NaHCO_3$ exert no effect on serum potassium independent-ly of dilution (Zager, 1989). In addition, infusions of $NaHCO_3$ can lower ionised calcium concentration which in turn could aggravate hyperkalaemia. The use of bicarbonate to treat hyperkalaemia needs to be re-evaluated.

Other complications of exertional heat stroke

Acute renal failure

The incidence of acute renal failure in exertional heat stroke is about 30%. Clinical factors favouring its appearance include renal hypoperfusion because of volume depletion and shock, high circulating levels of noradrenaline (norepinephrine), and myoglobinuria. It is likely that cytokines formed in response to absorbed intestinal endotoxins or those generated primarily by tissue damage (Zager *et al.*, 1995) injure proximal tubular cells and vascular endothelium. Usually, acute renal failure is multifactorial in these patients (Knochel, 1994). Myoglobin is readily filtered by the glomerulus. A portion of the filtered myoglobin is taken up by the proximal tubular cell by pinocytosis. It then is thought to enter lysosomes where the acid pH serves to split the pigment into ferrihaemate and globin. The ferrihaemate, being an organic acid, is released and actively transported by the tubular cell to the peritubular blood, a process that reduces cellular stores of ATP. Low levels of ATP, superoxide free radicals (their formation favoured by iron released from ferrihaemate), and undoubtedly other factors, lead to cellular injury (Zager, 1996). Myoglobin not taken up by proximal tubular cells passes down the tubule; as myoglobin cannot be reabsorbed, its concentration rises in the distal nephron because of the renal concentrating mechanism. This, and the presence of a low tubular fluid pH result in gel formation of the pigment and tubular obstruction. Obstruction at this site increases the availability of myoglobin for absorption in the proximal tubule. Thus, the classic findings of acute renal failure in patients with exertional heat stroke, rhabdomyolysis and myoglobinuria consist of injured or necrotic proximal tubular epithelia and distal tubular obstruction with pigment-laden casts. Myoglobin may also bind nitric oxide, thus forestalling any vasodilatory effects of this substance (Zager, 1989, 1996; Zager *et al.*, 1995). Theoretically, if given very early, infusion of mannitol accelerates the rate of flow of proximal and distal tubular fluid, thus flushing myoglobin from the kidney. Alkalinisation of the urine theoretically reduces gel formation of myoglobin and thereby promotes its excretion. Classic urinary findings in patients with exertional heat stroke and rhabdomyolysis include a positive dipstick test for haem pigment and pigmented casts in the urinary sediment. Renal glycosuria is often seen because of proximal tubular injury. Oliguria is the rule in patients with this complication.

Haemorrhagic complications of exertional heat stroke

Exertional heat stroke is nearly always associated with haemorrhagic complications and in some cases these have been fatal (Knochel & Reed, 1994). Petechial haemorrhages and ecchymoses are common early clinical manifestations and possibly represent capillary damage as a result of hyperthermia itself. Nearly all patients with exertional heat stroke show laboratory findings of DIC. These consist of thrombocytopenia, hypofibrinogenaemia, prolongation of prothrombin and partial thromboplastin times, and accumulation of fibrin degradation products in the blood. Chemical evidence of mild and apparently harmless DIC can be demonstrated in normal persons performing only moderate exercise in hot weather. In patients with heat stroke, however, this complication may be severe. It tends to become most pronounced after the first 24 hours of injury. Administration of platelets and fresh frozen plasma may be helpful. While heparin was once advocated as a treatment for this condition, it has lost favour because of its potential haemorrhagic side effects. DIC usually begins to clear spontaneously by the fourth to seventh hospital days. Some patients with exertional heat stroke show haemorrhage as a result of fibrinolysis. This is apparently a rare event. Others, because of hepatocellular injury, show reduced prothrombin activity independently of DIC. During the recovery phase of heat stroke, polymorphonuclear cells may show hypersegmentation. Eosinophilia has also been observed. There is evidence that hyperthermia and endotoxin-mediated cytokines may explain the DIC in this condition (see later).

Endotoxins and cytokines

Although primary thermogenic tissue injury is of unquestionable importance, current evidence strongly suggests that much of the widespread damage of exertional heat stroke results from secondary causes, especially endotoxins and cytokines. More and more evidence centres on the importance of the simple concept that gut ischaemia occurs in persons performing hard work in the heat as a result of blood translocation to the skin and skeletal muscles (Rowell, 1986). Apparently, anything causing ischaemia in the intestinal circulation, including heat stress, facilitates absorption of bacterial endotoxins (Gathiram *et al.*, 1988). Thereupon, endotoxin leads to production of endogenous mediators of a syndrome closely resembling septic shock (Parillo *et al.*, 1990). These mediators, known to appear in the blood of patients with acute heat stroke (Bouchama *et al.*, 1991*a*), include tumour necrosis factor, interleukins 1, 2, 6 and 8, platelet activating factor, vasoactive amines, arachidonate metabolites and probably others. Their targets are the cardiovascular system, skeletal muscle, kidney, lung, central nervous system, liver and the coagulation system. Their effects include complex organ dysfunction or destruction that are typical of exertional heat stroke. These include myocardial injury, vascular injury including the capillary leak syndrome, diverse and widespread central nervous system injury, hepatic injury, acute renal failure, adult respiratory distress syndrome, rhabdomyolysis and DIC.

The immune response to endotoxaemia appears to play a major role in the process of heat acclimatisation, and protection against heat stroke (Gathiram *et al.*, 1987). Studies are needed to evaluate the possible salutory effects of immune therapy (specific antibodies against endotoxin and its derived cytokines) for patients with severe exertional heat stroke. Other issues concern the importance of reperfusion injury in patients with exertional heat stroke. Products of lysed leucocytes or other cells from crushed limbs have been implicated in widespread injury that appears after restoration of the circulation (Klausher *et al.*, 1988). Patients with exertional heat stroke and severe rhabdomyolysis display virtually identical complications.

Whether exertional heat stroke-associated injury occurs by hyperthermia per se or by secondary mechanisms is of considerable interest. Thermal injury to protein structures elicits synthesis of heat shock proteins in nearly every cell. These proteins, and the genetic mechanism regulating their synthesis, have been widely studied. After sublethal heating, they appear within hours and hypothetically provide resistance to further thermogenic cellular injury by protecting the cytoskeleton, augmenting intracellular antioxidants or preserving enzymes within the cell. The protein has been named a 'chaperone' because it appears to transport or target other thermolabile proteins to specific organelles such as mitochondria or microsomes. It seems likely that these substances and a host of other factors (Knochel *et al.*, 1985; Sen, 1995) play an important role in defence against thermogenic cell injury and are important in heat acclimatisation. It is possible that they play a role in the protection induced by previous heat stress against endotoxin (Ryan *et al.*, 1992). If certain individuals are unable to synthesise these proteins normally and whether such a defect could be responsible for heat stress injury are unanswered questions at this time but certainly need to be studied.

Any physician managing patients with exertional heat stroke must cool and resuscitate their patients as rapidly as possible. They also need to be acutely aware of the complex and often devastating complications of this illness which are as equally severe as those encountered in major trauma, burns or sepsis.

References

Bailey, J. C. (1975). Heat stroke during temperate climatic conditions: case reports. *Military Medicine*, **140**, 1–30.

Bouchama, A., Parhar, R. S., El-Yazigi, A., Sheth, K & Al-Sedairy, S. (1991*a*). Endotoxemia and release of tumour necrosis factor and interleukin 1 alpha in acute heat stroke. *Journal of Applied Physiology*, **70**, 2640–4.

Bouchama, A., Cafege A., Devol, E. B., Labdi, O., El-Assil, K. & Seraj, M. (1991*a*). Ineffectiveness of dantrolene sodium in the treatment of heat stroke. *Critical Care Medicine*, **19**, 176–80.

Bouchama, A., Hammami, M. M., Ilaq, A. & Al-Sedairy, S. (1994). Marked elevation of plasma level of endothelin-like immunoreactivity in patients with heat stroke. *American Journal of Respiratory and Critical Care Medicine*, **149**, 445 (abstract).

Brodal, P., Ingjer, F. & Hermansen, L. (1977). Capillary supply of skeletal muscle fibres in untrained and endurance-trained men. *American Journal of Physiology*, **232**, H705–H712.

Cabanac, M. (1986). Keeping a cool head. *News in Physiological Sciences*, **1**, 1–44.

Demos, M. A., Gitin, E. L. & Kagen, L. J. (1974). Exercise myoglobinemia and acute exertional rhabdomyolysis. *Archives of Internal Medicine*, **134**, 669–73.

Emrich, H. M., Stoll, E. & Rossi, E. (1970). Aldosteronwirkung auf die natrium-chlorid und kaliumausscheidung im schweib von pankreasfibrose-patienten und gesunden: *Klinische Wochenschrift*, **48**, 966–72.

Fong, Y., Marano, M. A., Moldawer, L. L., Wei, H., Calvano, S. E., Kenney, J. S.,

Allison, A. C., Cerami, A., Shires, G. T. & Lowry, S. F. (1990). The acute splanchnic and peripheral tissue metabolic response to endotoxin in humans. *Journal of Clinical Investigation*, **85**, 1896–904.

Gathiram, P., Wells, M. T., Brock-Utne, J. G. & Gaffin, S. L. (1987). Antilipopolysaccharide improves survival in primates subjected to heat stroke. *Circulatory Shock*, **23**, 157–64.

Gathiram, P., Wells, M. T., Raidoo, D., Brock-Utne, J. G. & Gaffin, S. L. (1988). Portal and systemic plasma lipopolysaccharide concentrations in heat-stressed primates. *Circulatory Shock*, **25**, 223–30.

Hackl, W., Winkler, M., Mauritz, W., Sporn P. & Steinbreithner, K. (1991). Muscle biopsy for diagnosis of malignant hyperthermia susceptibility in two patients with severe exercise-induced myolysis. *British Journal of Anaesthesia*, **66**, 138–40.

Hall, D. M., Buettner, G. R., Matthes, R. D. & Gisolfi, C. V. (1994). Hyperthermia stimulates nitric oxide formation: electron paramagnetic resonance detection of NO heme in blood. *Journal of Applied Physiology*, **77**, 548–53.

Haller, R. G., Lewis, S. E., Cook, J. D. & Blomqvist, C. G. (1983). Hyperkinetic circulation during exercise in neuromuscular disease. *Neurology*, **33**, 1283–7.

Henrich, W. L., Hunt, J. M. & Nixon, J. V. (1984). Increased ionized calcium and left ventricular contractility during hemodialysis. *New England Journal of Medicine*, **310**, 19–23.

Hopkins, P. M., Ellis, F. R. & Halsall, P. J. (1991). Evidence for related myopathies in exertional heat stroke and malignant hyperthermia. *Lancet*, **338**, 91–1492.

Kim, Y.D., Lake, C. R., Lees, D. E., Schuette, W. H., Bull, J. M., Weise, V. & Kopin, I. J. (1979). Hemodynamic and plasma catecholamine responses to hyperthermic cancer therapy in humans. *American Journal of Physiology*, **237**, H570–H574.

Kjellmer, I. (1965). Potassium ion as a vasodilator during muscular exercise. *Acta Physiologica Scandinavica*, **63**, 460–8.

Klausner, J. M., Paterson, I. S., Valeri, C. R., Shepro, D. & Hechtman, H. B. (1988). Limb ischemia induced increase in permeability is mediated by leukocytes and leukotrienes. *Annals of Surgery*, **208**, 755–60.

Knochel, J. P. (1982). Neuromuscular manifestations of electrolyte disorders. *American Journal of Medicine*, **72**, 521–35.

Knochel, J. P. (1987). Metabolism and potassium. In *Potassium Transport: Physiology and Pathophysiology. Current Topics in Membranes and Transport*, ed G. Giebisch, pp. 383–400. Orlando, Academic Press.

Knochel, J. P. (1988). Biochemical, electrolyte and acid–based disturbances in acute renal failure. In *Acute Renal Failure*, ed. B. M. Brenner & J. M. Lazarus. pp. 667–793. New York, Churchill Livingstone.

Knochel, J. P. (1989). Heat stroke and related heat stress disorders. *Disease-a-Month*, **35**, 306–77.

Knochel, J. P. (1990). Catastrophic medical events with exhaustive exercise: 'White collar rhabdomyolysis'. *Kidney International*, **38**, 709–19.

Knochel, J. P. (1994). Pigment nephropathy. In *Primer on Kidney Disease, National Kidney Foundation*, ed. A. Greenberg, Chapter 6. *Academic Press*, San Diego.

Knochel, J. P., Blachley, J. D., Johnson, J. H. & Carter, N. W. (1985). Muscle cell hyperpolarization and reduced exercise hyperkalemia in physically conditioned dogs. *Journal of Clinical Investigation*, **75**, 740–5.

Knochel, J. P., Beisel, W. R., Herndon, E. G. Jr., Gerard, E. S. & Barry, K. G. (1961). The renal, cardiovascular, haematological and serum electrolyte abnormalities of heat stroke. *American Journal of Medicine*, **30**, 299–309.

Knochel, J. P. & Caskey, J. H. (1977). The mechanism of hypophosphatemia in acute heat stroke. *Journal of the American Medical Association*, **238**, 425–6.

Knochel, J. P., Dotin, L. N. & Hamburger, R. J. (1972). Pathophysiology of intense physical conditioning in a hot climate. *Journal of Clinical Investigation*, **51** 242–55.

Knochel, J. P., Dotin, L. N. & Hamburger, R. J. (1974). Heat stress, exercises and muscle injury: effects on urate metabolism and renal function. *Annals of Internal Medicine*, **8**, 321–8.

Knochel, J. P. & Reed, G. (1994). Disorders of heat regulation. In *Clinical Disorders of Fluid and Electrolyte Metabolism*, ed. M. H. Maxwell, C. R. Keelman & R. G. Narins, Chapter 47. New York, McGraw-Hill.

Knochel, J. P. & Schlein, E. M. (1972). On the mechanism of rhabdomyolysis in potassium depletion. *Journal of Clinical Investigation*, **51**, 1750–8.

Krapf, R., Caduff, P., Wagdi, P., Staubli, M. & Hulter, H. N. (1995). Plasma potassium response to acute respiratory alkalosis. *Kidney International*, **47**, 217–24.

Maron, M. B., Wagner, J. A. & Horvath, S. H. (1977). Thermoregulatory responses during competitive running. *Journal of Applied Physiology*, **42**, 909–14.

Moore, G. E., Holbein, M. E. B. & Knochel, J. P. (1995). Exercise-associated collapse in cyclists is unrelated to endotoxemia. *Medicine and Science in Sports and Exercise*, **27**, 1238–42.

Nadel, E. R. (1984). Body fluids and electrolyte balance during exercise. Competing demands with temperature regulation. In *Thermal Physiology*, ed. J. R. S. Hales, pp. 365–76. New York, Raven Press.

Osnes, J. B. & Hermansen, L. (1972). Acid–base balance after maximal exercise of short duration. *Journal of Applied Physiology*, **32**, 59–63.

Parrillo, J. E., Parker, M. M., Natanson, C., Suffredini, A. F., Danner, R. L., Cunnion, R. E. & Ognibene, F. P. (1990). Septic shock in humans. *Annals of Internal Medicine*, **113**, 227–42.

Pattison, M. E., Logan, J. L., Lee, S. M. & Ogden, D. A. (1988). Exertional heat stroke and acute renal failure in a young woman. *American Journal of Kidney Disease*, **11**, 184–7.

Rowell, L. B. (1986). Circulatory adjustments to dynamic exercise and heat stress: competing controls. In *Human Circulation: Regulation During Physical Stress*, ed. L. B. Rowell, pp. 363–406. New York, Oxford University Press.

Ryan, A. J., Flanagan, S. W., Moseley, P.L. & Gisolfi, C. V. (1992). Acute heat stress protects rats against endotoxin shock. *Journal of Applied Physiology*, **73**, 1517–22.

Sawka, M. N. & Wenger, C. B. (1988). Physiological responses to acute exercise-heat stress. In *Human Performance Physiology and Environmental Medicine at Terrestrial Extremes*, ed. K. B. Pandoff, M. N. Sawka, R. R. Gonzales (Eds.), Benchmark Press, Indianapolis, Chapter 3.

Selye, H. & Bajusz, E. (1959). Conditioning by corticoids for the production of cardiac lesions with noradrenaline. *Acta Endocrinologica*, **30**, 183–193.

Sen, C. K. (1995). Oxidants and antioxidants in exercise. *Journal of Applied Physiology*, **79**, 675–86.

Stephenson, L. A., Kolka, M. A. (1988). Effect of gender, circadian period and sleep loss on thermal responses during exercise. In: *Human Performance Physiology and Environmental Medicine at Terrestrial Extremes*. ed. Pandolf, K. B., Sawka, M. N. & Gonzalez, R. R. Benchmark Press, Indianapolis, 267–304.

Tankersley, C. G., Nicholas, W. C., Deaver, D. R., Mikita D. & Kenney, W. L. (1992). Estrogen replacement in middle-aged women: Thermoregulatory responses to exercise in the heat. *Journal of Applied Physiology*, **73**, 1238–45.

Verde, T., Shephard, R. J., Corey, P. & Moore, R. (1982). Sweat composition in exercise and in heat. *Journal of Applied Physiology.* **53**, 1540–45.

Wingard, D. W. & Gatz, E. E. (1978). Some observations on stress susceptible patients. In *Second International Symposium on Malignant Hyperthermia*, Aldrete, J. A. & Britt, B. A. (eds). Grune & Stratton, New York, 363–72.

Zager, R. A. (1989). Studies of mechanisms and protective maneuvers in myoglobinuric acute renal failure. *Laboratory Investigation*, **60**, 619–29.

Zager, R. A., Burkhart, K. M., Conrad, D. S. & Gmur, D. J. (1995). Iron, heme oxygenase, and glutathoine: Effects on myohemoglobinuric proximal tubular injury. *Kidney International*, **48**, 1624–34.

Zager, R. A. (1996). Rhabdomyolysis and myohemoglobinuric acute renal failure. *Kidney International* (in press).

4

Investigation of heat stroke victims
1: The human physiology laboratory

C. G. BATTY and W. A. FREELAND

Introduction

Heat intolerance has been defined as an inability to adapt to exercise in a hot environment (Senay & Kok, 1976; Strydom, 1980; Epstein *et al.*, 1983). For those who have sustained a heat injury on more than one occasion, formal assessment in a hot environment should be considered.

In planning the assessment, the variables to be considered are physical fitness and the effect of working in the heat. Fitness is measured because it has been demonstrated that physical training and work in a hot environment improves heat tolerance (Gisolfi & Robinson, 1969).

Assessment

Clinical

A number of soldiers have been referred to the Centre for Human Sciences (CHE) DERA Farnborough, formerly the Army Personnel Research Establishment (APRE), for formal assessment and heat challenge testing under controlled conditions. These men have all sustained a heat injury requiring inpatient medical attention on at least two occasions during their military training in the UK. They had no past history of heat intolerance despite working in hot climates previously. Clinical examination and hospital investigations were normal apart from subject D whose muscle enzymes had been found to be abnormal. As an adjunct to their investigation, a work in heat test was sought.

Following a further clinical examination, on arrival at CHE, fully informed consent was obtained before subjecting the individual to exercise in the physiology laboratory and in the hot chamber.

Heat challenge

Hot chamber

A thermal challenge has been developed to satisfy the military requirements of assessing acclimatisation to heat. This takes the form of a one hour work-in-Heat Test (Turk, 1974). This was adapted for the assessment of the soldiers' heat intolerance. Dreosti (1935) clearly showed that all men were not the same in their reaction to heat and that a heat intolerant group existed who needed more treatment than others to reach a safe level of thermal tolerance.

The soldiers referred to CHE underwent a heat challenge in the Establishment's climatic (hot) chamber. This facility is capable of a maximum temperature of $+70\,°C$ and a relative humidity of between 20 and 80%. A solar load of up to 1100 watts/m^2 could be applied if required (Amor, 1983). The Wet Bulb Globe Treatment (WBGT) was calculated using a Grant Instruments Meter.

The test performed by the soldiers involved them stepping on and off a 12 inch step at a rate of 12 steps per minute for one hour (Turk, 1974). The rate was kept constant by the subjects stepping to the beat of an electronic metronome. The WBGT was kept in the range of $29.7–35.5\,°C$. The subjects were tested on two occasions on two consecutive days. Dress during the test consisted of shorts, with or without T shirt and training shoes (Figure 4.1).

Measurements

The clothed body weight, before and after exposure to heat, was measured using a weight capture unit incorporating a 200 kg Kelgray Platform (Berry, 1990). The weight of the clothes worn was recorded before and after exposure to estimate sweat loss. Core temperature was measured every five minutes using negative temperature coefficient aural thermistors. Heart rate was observed continuously on a Simonson and Weal Electrocardiographic (ECG) monitor and recorded every five minutes.

Procedure

The same procedure was followed for each soldier.

1. The subject arrived in the preparation room where he was given a plastic bag into which he placed the clothing and footwear to be worn in the chamber. These were weighed. He was allowed to drink fruit squash and then instructed to empty his bladder after which no further fluids were permitted. The clothing to be worn was donned and the aural thermistors inserted. (Rectal,

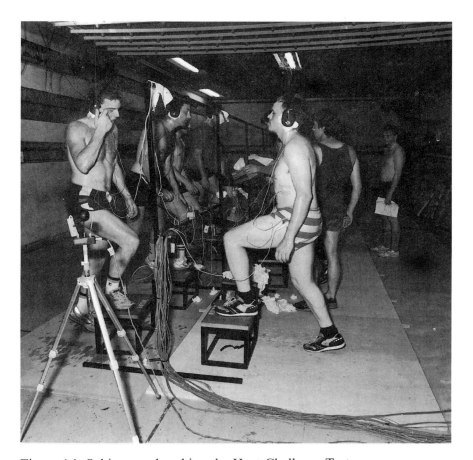

Figure 4.1. Subjects undertaking the Heat Challenge Test.

instead of aural, thermistors could have been used to measure the core temperature.) Three ECG electrodes were applied to the anterior chest wall. Thereafter he was weighed. Following a 30 minute period of equilibration, initial core temperatures were measured using a Grant Meter. The heart rate was also noted.

2. The subject entered the chamber, stood by the stool and the leads were connected to the data logger which was controlled by a computer and programmed to print, plot and store the data. The one hour Work-in-Heat test then commenced.

3. At the end of the period the subject was allowed to rest in the chamber before being taken out to be reweighed prior to being de-instrumented. Clothing and footwear were collected and reweighed. Thereafter he was allowed to rehydrate and shower.

Table 4.1. *Results of the hot chamber work assessment*

Subject	Core Temperature (°C)			Mean Skin Temperature (°C)			Heart rate (/min)			Sweat Loss	
	Initial	Maximum final	δ	Initial	Maximum	δ	Initial	Maximum	δ	Total (g)	g/kg body wt
A	37.1	37.92	0.82	35.27	37.10	1.83	108	140	32	1410	17.06
B	37.19	38.46	1.27	34.82	37.63	2.81	124	160	36	1290	16.97
C	36.99	37.63	0.64	34.98	37.28	2.20	107	155	45	990	17.0
D	37.0	38.6	1.6	Not recorded			140	187	47	1000	13.25

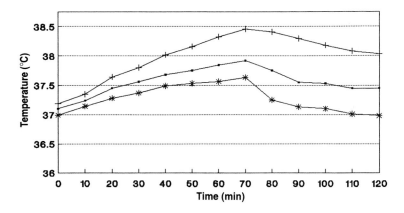

Figure 4.2. Core Temperature Heat Challenge Test. Wet Bulb Globe Temperature (WGBT) 29.7–31.92 °C. ■, Subject A; +, subject B; *, subject C.

Withdrawal criteria

The withdrawal criteria for all subjects were a core temperature of 38.5 °C and a heart rate of more than 180 beats/min as laid down by the Establishment's independent Ethics Committee. This is at variance with the original Work-in-Heat Test protocol (Turk, 1974). As can be seen by the results that follow, only one soldier had to be withdrawn on account of the core temperature criterion.

Results

A selection of the results for the thermal challenge is shown in Table 4.1 and Figures 4.2 and 4.3.

Subject B, although within the normal range for height and weight as defined in the 1983 Metropolitan Life Insurance Company Tables, was found to be physically unfit (VO_2 max = 42.4 ml/kg min) according to the criteria for passing the military basic fitness test (see later). Despite approaching the limit of 38.5 °C he completed the Work-in-Heat test, tolerating the heat stress well.

Subjects A and C demonstrated that they had a degree of thermal tolerance. Similar results were obtained on the second day of assessment.

Figure 4.3 shows subject D who was relatively unfit (VO_2 max = 46.05 ml/kg/ min) and was unable to maintain his core temperature within accepted limits. After 25 minutes the exercise was stopped as his core temperature rose to 38.6 °C. He was allowed to rest in the hot environment while his core temperature continued to be measured. Following an initial fall, it began

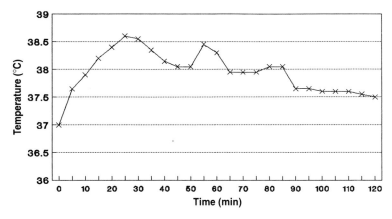

Figure 4.3. Core temperature Heat Challenge Test in subject D. Details as for Figure 4.2.

to rise again thus necessitating his removal to the cool preparation room which resulted in further recovery followed by a slight rise again. This again demonstrated his failure to thermoregulate. Once he was allowed to rehydrate, his recovery progressed without incident. His heart rate also rose above the threshold for withdrawal. He was seen to be sweating well and indeed he lost 13.25 g/kg body weight of sweat. Similar results were obtained when the heat challenge was repeated on the second day under comparable conditions. He was referred back to his Consultant Physician at the Queen Elizabeth Military Hospital, Woolwich, to ascertain the cause of his abnormal muscle enzyme levels found during his hospital based investigations.

From there he was referred for further investigation to the Malignant Hyperthermia Unit at St James's University Hospital, Leeds. Further investigations proved abnormal (Hopkins *et al.*, 1991) and are discussed in Chapter 6.

Sweat rates

There is considerable variation in the rate of sweating in normal men, even when all the conditions are controlled. During muscular exertion in a hot environment, sweat secretion reaches values as high as 1600 ml/h (Ganong, 1979), and in a dry atmosphere most of this sweat is vaporised. No standard can easily be laid down below which sweating is defective. From the results shown in Table 4.1, all subjects including subject D were found to be sweating well.

Mean skin temperature

All subjects showed a good rise in the mean skin temperature denoting increased peripheral blood flow. This vasodilatation aids the thermoregulation of the individual, provided a condition of low humidity is present to allow for adequate evaporation of sweat.

Physical assessment

Most subjects were reported to have collapsed or suffered a heat injury during some form of physical activity, e.g. military training, and so an assessment of physical fitness in terms of maximal oxygen uptake (VO_2 max) was undertaken.

As part of this assessment of physical fitness, basic lung function was measured using a bellows-type spirometer. The normal range of the ratio FEV_1 to FVC is 70–80% (Åstrand & Rodahl, 1977). Lung function tests are essentially measures of physiological changes and it is known that some individuals with a relatively poor FEV_1 may still be able to undertake comparatively strenuous work. A further indication of disability may be gained from exercise tolerance testing.

From the results in Table 4.2, only soldier A was outside the normal range as defined by Åstrand & Rodahl (1977). As has been demonstrated, however, this did not affect his overall physical fitness or work in heat.

Physical fitness assessment

The VO_2 max indicates the body's ability to conduct maximally and transport oxygen to the working muscles during exercise. It serves as an index of the functional capacity of the circulation and of cardiovascular fitness (Mitchell *et al.*, 1958; Saltin *et al.*, 1968; Mitchell & Blomqvist, 1971). The assessment can be carried out in any of three ways:
1. Direct measurement of VO_2 by measurement of expired gases during maximal exercise.
2. Prediction of VO_2 max from the workload achieved at maximal activity.
3. Prediction of VO_2 max from workload and heart rate during submaximal activity, e.g. The standard Åstrand Rhyming Test (Åstrand & Rodahl, 1988).

The common methods used in the measurement of cardiovascular fitness are a motorised treadmill (Taylor *et al.*, 1955) or, in its absence, the cycle ergometer method.

Saltin and Åstrand (1967) found that the mean value for the VO_2 max for

Table 4.2. *Pulmonary function test results*

Subject	Age (years)	Height (m)	Weight (kg)	FEV$_1$ (L)		FVC (L)		FEV$_1$/FVC	
				Actual	Predicted	Actual	Predicted	Actual %	Predicted
A	20	1.85	82.65	4.05	5.4	5.96	6.3	67.95	85.71
B	24	1.80	76.0	4.25	4.9	5.19	5.72	81.89	85.66
C	18	1.52	58.25	4.1	3.6	4.57	3.94	89.72	91.37
D	23	1.70	75.5	4.68	4.4	5.25	5.08	84.2	86.60

young untrained males was in the order of 48.7 $\pm$ 5.1 ml/kg/min. Other previously published studies for groups of British soldiers found their mean VO_2 max to be 53.1 mlk/g/min (Myles & Toft, 1982; Patton & Duggan, 1987).

The cycle ergometer has the advantage of more precise quantification of the work performed. A disadvantage may be that low exercise tolerance may result from unfamiliarity with bicycle pedalling and a lack of motivation. Treadmill exercising reduced this difficulty as everyone is familiar with walking and running.

During the treadmill assessment, measurements are taken of heart rate, respiratory rate, minute ventilation, tidal volume, oxygen consumption and carbon dioxide production. A close watch is kept of the ECG monitor for arrhythmias and possible ischaemia.

The assessment should be discontinued for the following reasons:

1. Exhaustion of the subject.
2. Attainment of 85% of the maximum predicted heart rate in those individuals aged older than 40 years (Åstrand,1960).
3. Arrhythmias, especially increasing premature ventricular contractions.
4. Chest pain.

Prior to any activity, a resting ECG is taken to act as a baseline reference while excluding ischaemic changes and arrhythmias. The ECG leads remain attached for the duration of the exercise test for continuous monitoring. Full resuscitation facilities with medical cover must also be available throughout.

As in all exercise, it is important that the subject is fully warmed up by the use of stretching exercises and a two minute session on the treadmill or on the bicycle. This latter exercise also serves to familiarise the subject with the equipment.

Motor-driven treadmill

Two forms of assessment can be performed using this method. In both, the treadmill is run at a constant velocity of 12 km/h; its gradient is increased incrementally from 0 to 5% and thereafter by steps of 2.5%.

1. *Continuous.* The subject exercises until the point of exhaustion is reached. The increase in gradient occurs every three minutes with the expired air being collected into Douglas bags during the last minute of each level for analysis. There are no rest periods during this test, thereby ensuring that a continuous run to exhaustion is achieved, or to the point where one or more of the withdrawal criteria is reached.

   The advantage of this method is that the period spent in testing the subject

Table 4.3. *Results VO$_2$ max*

Subject	Workload		VO$_2$ max
	Kmh	Gradient (%)	ml/kg/min
A	12	10	53.62
B	12	0	42.17
C	12	7.5	54.69
D	12	5	42.70

is short to allow greater throughput if large numbers of subjects are to be tested. Cumulative fatigue, however, results in a lower plateau of oxygen uptake and hence a lower VO$_2$ max value than if the test was performed using the interrupted method.

2. *Interrupted.* Subjects run for three minutes at each stage of the test and during the last minute of each run the expired air is collected for analysis. In between the runs, the individual rests before recommencing at a steeper gradient. This continues until the individual is unable to complete a run. Heart rate is monitored continuously. The test is stopped at the point of the subject's exhaustion or if one of the criteria, see above, is met (Åstrand, 1952; Boreha *et al.*, 1990).

The subjects at CHE underwent the interrupted treadmill test in accordance with the protocol and withdrawal criteria already described. Their results are shown in Table 4.3.

It can be predicted from these results that two subjects would fail the standard basic military fitness test (1.5 mile squadded warm up in 14 minutes followed immediately by 1.5 mile best individual effort run in 10.5 minutes for all soldiers under 30 years of age). The VO$_2$ max required to pass this test has been estimated at 49 ml/kg/min (Duggan & Patton, 1986; Duggan, 1988).

Cycle ergometer

The NATO cycle ergometer test has been well validated as a reliable predictor of aerobic power (Myles & Toft, 1982; Patton *et al.*, 1982; Hogdon & Beckett, 1983; Pederson & Neilson, 1983; NATO, 1986).

This exercise test involves the subject pedalling at a rate of 75 revolutions per minute (rpm) which is displayed on a LED screen. An initial load of 37.5 watts is applied. Thereafter the work load increases in stepped increments every minute by 37.5 watts until the subject is unable to continue or maintain the pedalling rate. The time taken to reach exhaustion or failure to maintain the pedalling rate is recorded. The VO$_2$ max is calculated using the equation:

$$VO_2 = 1.247 + \frac{0.301t}{\text{Body weight}}$$

where t = maximum cycling time in minutes and the body weight is measured in kilograms (NATO, 1986).

Conclusion

It is recommended that individuals with a history of exertional heat intolerance be investigated to assess their ability to thermoregulate adequately in the heat. Other factors, including anhidrosis, concurrent medical conditions and poor physical fitness, should be excluded. A technique for studying heat intolerance in the laboratory has been described. The value of the heat challenge may lie in its ability to act as a filter in determining the appropriate referral for further specialist investigation. Those individuals who demonstrate poor thermoregulation under laboratory conditions should be considered for further investigation to exclude a genetic predisposition similar to malignant hyperthermia.

References

Amor, A. F. (1983) *The APRE Hot Chamber Radiant Heat Facility*. MOD APRE Memorandum 83M522.

Åstrand, I. (1960). Aerobic work capacity in men and women with special reference to age. *Acta Physiologica Scandinavica*, **49**, 169.

Åstrand, P.-O. (1952). Experimental studies of physical working capacity in relation to sex and age. Munksgaard, Copenhagen.

Åstrand, P.-O. & Rodahl, K. (1977). *Textbook of Work Physiology*. New York, McGraw Hill.

Åstrand, P.-O & Rodahl, K. (1988). Evaluation of physical performance on the basis of tests. In *Textbook of Work Physiology, Physiological Basis of Exercise*, pp. 354–390. New York, McGraw Hill.

Berry, M. J. (1990). *Weight Capture Unit Incorporating A 200 Kg Kelgray Platform*. MOD APRE Working Paper 21/90.

Boreha, C. A. G., Paliczka, V. J. & Nichols, A. K. (1990). A comparison of the PWC170 and 20-MST tests of aerobic fitness in adolescent school children. *Journal of Sports Medicine and Physical Fitness*. **30**, 19–23.

Dreosti, A. O. (1935). The results of some investigations into the medical aspect of deep mining in the Witwatersrand. *Journal of the Chemical and Metallurgical Mining Society of South Africa*, 102–129.

Duggan, A. (1988). *Energy cost of basic fitness test performance in boots and running shoes*. MOD APRE Memorandum 88M503.

Duggan, A. & Patton, J. F. (1986). *Oxygen cost of performing a running test in boots: assessments on treadmill and road*. MOD APRE Memorandum 86M511.

Epstein, Y., Shapiro, Y. & Brill, S. (1983). Role of surface area to mass ratio and work efficiency in heat tolerance. *Journal of Applied Physiology*, **54**, 831–6.

Ganong, W. F. (1979). *Review of Medical Physiology*, 9th edn. Los Altos CA, Lange Medical Publications.

Gisolfi, C. & Robinson, S. (1969). Relations between physical training, acclimatisation and heat intolerance. *Journal of Applied Physiology*, **26**, 530–4.

Hogdon, J. A. & Beckett, M. A. (1983). Another validation of the RSG's maximal work capacity test. *Proceedings of the 5th meeting of NATO RSG 4*, Brussels DS/A/DR(83)320.

Hopkins, P. M., Ellis, F. R. & Halsall, P. J. (1991). Evidence for related myopathies in exertional heat stroke and malignant hyperthermia. *Lancet*, **338**, 1491–2.

Mitchell, J. H & Blomqvist, G. (1971). Maximal oxygen uptake. *New England Journal of Medicine*, **284**, 1018–22.

Mitchell, J. H., Sproule, B. J. & Chapman, C. B. (1958). The physiological meaning of the maximal oxygen intake test. *Journal of Clinical Investigation*, **38**, 538–47.

Myles, W. S. & Toft, R. J. (1982). A cycle ergometer test of maximal aerobic power. *European Journal of Applied Physiology*, **49**, 121–9.

NATO Research Study Group (1986). In *Physical Fitness*. Final Report of RSG 4, Brussels.

Patton, J. F. & Duggan, A. (1987). Upper and lower body anaerobic power: comparison between biathletes and control subjects. *International Journal of Sports Medicine*, **8**, 94–8.

Patton, J. F., Vogel, J. A. & Mello, R. P. (1982). Evaluation of a maximal predictive cycle ergometer test of aerobic power. *European Journal of Applied Physiology*, **49**, 131–40.

Pederson, A. & Neilson, J. E. (1983). Evaluation of the RSG 4 test in relation to tests measuring oxygen uptake and other test methods to determine VO_2 max. *Proceedings of the 5th meeting of NATO RSG4*, Brussels DS/A/DR(83)320.

Saltin, B. & Åstrand, P.-O. (1967). Maximal oxygen uptake in athletes. *Journal of Applied Physiology*, **23**, 353–8.

Saltin, B., Blomqvist, G., Mitchell, J. H. *et al.* (1968). Response to exercise after bed rest and after training; a longitudinal study of adaptive changes in oxygen transport and body composition. *Circulation*, **38**, 1–78.

Senay, L. C. & Kok, R. (1976). Body fluid responses of heat tolerant and intolerant men to work in a hot wet environment. *Journal of Applied Physiology*, **40**, 55–9.

Strydom, N. B. (1980). Heat intolerance: its detection and elimination in the mining industry. *South African Journal of Science*, **76**, 154–6.

Taylor, H. L., Buskirk, E. & Henschel, A. (1955). Maximal oxygen uptake as an objective measure of cardiorespiratory performance. *Journal of Applied Physiology*, **8**, 73–80.

Turk, J. (1974). *A reliable test of heat acclimatization for the Army*. MOD APRE Report 7/74 (R).

5

Investigation of heat stroke victims
2: Nuclear magnetic resonance spectroscopy

J.-F. PAYEN and P. STIEGLITZ

Introduction

Body temperature is determined by the balance between heat accumulation generated by physical activity or gained from the environment, and heat dissipation. Heat storage is thus the result of either excessive heat accumulation or the reduced ability to dissipate body heat. It is well recognised that there is an inherent competition between the maintenance of blood pressure, muscle vasodilation supplying substrates for energy metabolism and the thermoregulatory system (sweating and skin vasodilation) during exercise in the heat (Jessen, 1987). Exertional heat stroke then occurs when this physiological challenge to homeostasis fails to be maintained.

The exact origin of exertional heat stroke is still unclear, especially the role of skeletal muscle as a potential factor in triggering exertional heat stroke. It is beyond doubt that thermal load mostly derives from exercising muscles because of the low efficiency of muscle in converting chemical energy to external work. Previous studies have described the consequences of hyperthermia on contractile activity (Segal et al., 1986), the cost of generating force (Rome & Kushmerick, 1983) and on metabolism (Edwards et al., 1972; Kozlowski et al., 1985). Few studies, however, have investigated whether primary muscle impairment may compromise thermal homeostasis. It has been suggested that heat increases the permeability of the cell to sodium ions and enhances the intracellular acidosis, thus reducing the metabolic efficiency of the cell (Hubbard, 1990). Thus, a pre-existing impairment of muscle energy metabolism prior to heat exposure could result in a higher cellular sensitivity to hyperthermia.

The possibility of a predisposing muscle factor in the aetiology of exertional heat stroke raises two points. First, it is well known that exertional heat stroke principally occurs in young men extremely motivated to perform strenuous prolonged exercise in a hot environment because of peer pressure, discipline or athletic competition. Individual factors, as well as environmental conditions predisposing to exertional heat stroke have been listed recently (Richards & Richards, 1987; Epstein, 1990; Dickinson, 1993; Chapters 1 and 2). Several measures applied to the whole population have been thus edicted to prevent exertional heat stroke (Kielblock, 1987). The notion of muscle impairment prior to exertional heat stroke would inevitably question the validity of such a strategy. Second, the relationship between exertional heat stroke and malignant hyperthermia which shares many symptoms with exertional heat stroke is unclear. Increased sensitivity to halothane and/or caffeine using the *in vitro* contracture test have been reported in some patients with exertional heat stroke (Hopkins *et al.*, 1991; Hackl *et al.*, 1991; Denborough, 1982) which could suggest an underlying skeletal muscle abnormality in post-exertional heat stroke patients. Is there a common inherited defect or a non-specific phenotypic response (Bourdon & Canini, 1995)? A range of tests, including heat and exercise tolerance as well as tests of skeletal muscle, are needed to clarify these points.

Phosphorus nuclear magnetic resonance (^{31}P-NMR) spectroscopy seems to be highly relevant for studying muscle energy metabolism in humans because of three major advantages: (1) it enables biochemical identification of high-energy phosphate compounds and their follow-up during exercise, (2) it provides reliable determination of intracellular pH and (3) it is non-invasive. Numerous ^{31}P-NMR studies of various myopathies have been carried out. The interest for using ^{31}P-NMR to investigate victims of exertional heat stroke would be on the basis of non-invasive detection of persistent impairment of exercise-induced muscle energy.

This chapter includes an explanation of the principles of NMR and muscle bioenergetics as well as the results from investigations of patients with exertional heat stroke. It should be emphasised that few ^{31}P-NMR studies of post-exertional heat stroke patients have been conducted. More are needed as the implication of skeletal muscle as a primary factor in exertional heat stroke is of epidemiological, scientific and clinical importance.

Theoretical basis and clinical applications of ^{31}P-NMR spectroscopy

Principles of nuclear magnetic resonance

An NMR spectrometer consists of a radio transmitter capable of sending high frequency radio waves into a strong and homogeneous magnetic field. The interaction of the radio frequency waves with atomic nuclei in the magnetic field generates signals that can then be used to obtain a frequency spectrum.

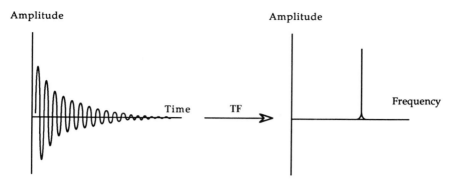

Figure 5.1. Free induction decay (FID) (left) is transformed using Fourier analysis (TF) into a frequency spectrum (right).

Although NMR is a nuclear phenomenon, the generation of measurable signals does not involve the use of ionising radiation.

The generation of an NMR signal is possible because there are some atomic nuclei rotating around their axes (i.e. ^{1}H, ^{31}P, ^{13}C and ^{19}F). These nuclei behave like a magnet as their spinning motion creates a magnetic momentum (spins). The application of an external magnetic field B_0 leads to alignment of these spins either along or against B_0. These two orientations in the magnetic field represent different quantum energy states. By means of radio frequency pulses (lasting from microseconds to milliseconds), the frequency of which is adjusted so as to match the energy differences between the two quantum states, it is possible to perturb the state of the spin system. In response to the radio frequency pulses, a nuclear signal is generated, which decays exponentially. This is called the free induction signal (FID). The characteristic decay time is called the transverse relaxation time (T2). Following the perturbation, the spin system returns towards its equilibrium state also in an exponential fashion. The characteristic time associated with this evolution is termed the longitudinal relaxation time (T1). Using Fourier transformation, the nuclear signal may be separated into its frequency component, thus generating an NMR spectrum (Figure 5.1). Several FIDs are often needed to improve the signal-to-noise ratio of the spectrum.

On the basis of these principles, two major NMR applications have been developed: NMR imaging and NMR spectroscopy. NMR imaging produces two or three-dimensional representations of the proton density in tissues. NMR spectroscopy relies on the fact that the magnetic field sensed by a nucleus is due not only to the external field but also to the electronic surroundings, i.e. the chemical environment. This method requires the use of large field strengths. For an extensive review of the basic principles of NMR spectroscopy, the reader is referred to the work of Gadian (1982).

What can be measured with ^{31}*P-NMR spectroscopy?*

NMR spectra may contain several peaks, each one corresponding to the resonance frequency of a given nucleus in a particular electronic environment. The amplitude of each peak is proportional to the number of nuclei resonating at that particular frequency. The minor differences in resonance frequency between peaks are expressed in parts per million (ppm) relative to the resonance frequency of a reference substance, and they are called chemical shifts.

Figure 5.2 shows typical ^{31}P-NMR spectra from human gastrocnemius muscle at rest, during exercise and during post-exercise recovery. Phosphorus is an attractive nucleus because it forms part of several molecules participating in the transfer of energy within the cell, i.e. ATP, ADP, AMP, phosphocreatine (PCr) and inorganic phosphate (P_i). Moreover, phosphorus is naturally abundant in muscle tissue and of good NMR sensitivity. These spectra are obtained in a magnetic field of 2.35 Tesla (1 Tesla = unit of magnetic field equal to 10 000 gauss) by applying a radio frequency pulse of 40.6 MHz which is the resonance frequency of phosphorus.

The ^{31}P-NMR spectroscopy also provides a reliable method of measuring the intracellular pH (pH_i) by determining the separation or chemical shift δ between P_i and PCr peaks (Moon & Richards, 1973). Indeed, the P_i frequency relative to that of PCr is slightly different according to its mono (HPO_4^{2-}) or diprotonated ($H_2PO_4^-$) forms. The pH_i is measured as follows (Taylor *et al.*, 1983):

$$pH_i = 6.75 + \log [(\delta - 3.27)/(5.69 - \delta)] \tag{1}$$

with an accuracy within 0.1 pH unit.

The area can be theoretically used to quantify the concentration of the studied compound as this area is the sum of the resonating nuclei. If this assertion is correct for *in vitro* NMR studies, one main reason impedes the ability to obtain absolute concentrations during *in vivo* NMR studies: the peaks lines are broader *in vivo* than *in vitro* because of magnetic susceptible variations within the tissue, resulting in an overlap between the peaks. The signal-to-noise ratio is proportional to the square root of the acquisition number, and so the measurement of compounds at low tissue concentration will require an acquisition time that is incompatible with the observation of biological phenomena. For these technical considerations, it is generally admitted that a compound gives a visible *in vivo* NMR signal when its tissue concentration is more than 0.5 mmol (Gadian, 1982). In addition, the levels of

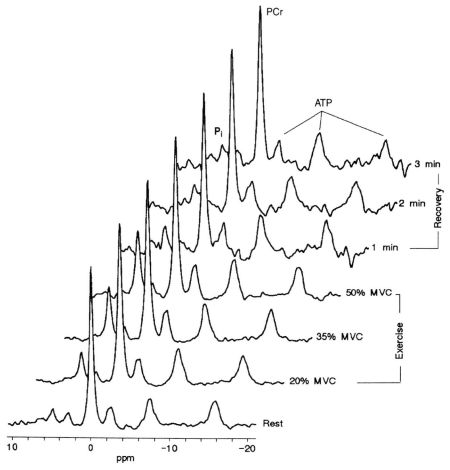

Figure 5.2. Evolution of ^{31}P spectra from human gastrocnemius muscle at rest, during a standardised steady-state exercise and during post-exercise recovery. Twenty free induction decays (FIDs) were accumulated at rest and during recovery, 80 FIDs were recorded at each level of exercise. Spectra were processed at 15 Hz exponential line broadening after removal of the wide component. P_i, inorganic phosphate; PCr, phosphocreatine; MVC, maximal voluntary contraction of the calf muscle; ppm, parts per million.

phosphate metabolites are commonly expressed as relative concentrations.

Most information on metabolic control using ^{31}P-NMR spectroscopy is obtained by studying the transitions from the resting state to different levels of metabolic activation, i.e. during exercise at different levels of work. As shown in Figure 5.2, effort is marked by a progressive decrease in the PCr signal intensity associated with a stoichiometric increase in the P_i peak while the β-ATP peak (only constituted of ATP) remains constant. The pH_i can also

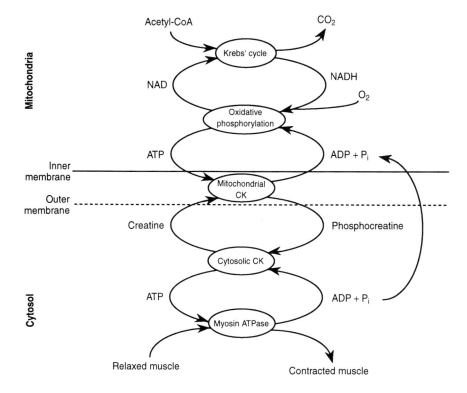

Figure 5.3. Schematic representation of the main biochemical reactions involved in muscle bioenergetics. CK, creatine kinase.

decrease during exercise. These changes are correlated with the intensity of the work performed at every level of exercise. All these changes are inverted during the post-exercise recovering period.

Biochemical information from a ^{31}P-NMR study

During the contraction–relaxation cycle of skeletal muscle, ATP hydrolysis is the only mechanism providing the energy required for the interaction of the myofilaments, and for calcium uptake by the sarcoplasmic reticulum. These two major ATP-utilising systems consume about 70 and 30%, respectively, of the available chemical energy. As the ATP level is low in skeletal muscle (5.5 mmol/kg wet wt) it must be continuously produced at the rate required by the level of energy demand. The term ATP flux is suitable because the rate of energy utilisation by ATPases will be matched by the rate of ATP synthesis.

The ATP-producing systems include both mitochondrial oxidative phosphorylation with the associated Krebs cycle and glycolysis. Phosphocreatine is regarded as an 'energy shuttle' between the sites of mitochondrial ATP supply and myofibrillar utilisation, not as an energy storage in skeletal muscle (Bessman & Geiger, 1981; Figure 5.3). This assumption is based on the localisation of different isoforms of the enzyme creatine kinase (CK) and on the enzymatic activity of CK which is 5 to tenfold higher than that of myosin ATPase.

Three majors biochemical reactions are, therefore, involved in skeletal muscle bioenergetics and the energy transfer from the site of production to the site of utilisation (Figure 5.3):

Oxidative phosphorylation:
$$3 \text{ ADP} + 3 \text{ P}_i + \text{NADH} + \text{H}^+ + \tfrac{1}{2}\text{O}_2 \rightleftharpoons 3 \text{ ATP} + \text{NAD}^+ + \text{H}_2\text{O} \tag{2}$$

Transfer of a phosphoryl group to ADP or creatine (CK reaction):
$$\text{PCr} + \text{ADP} + \text{H}^+ \rightleftharpoons \text{ATP} + \text{Cr} \tag{3}$$

ATP hydrolysis (myosin ATPase):
$$\text{ATP} + \text{H}_2\text{O} \rightleftharpoons \text{ADP} + \text{P}_i + \text{H}^+ \tag{4}$$

Under aerobic conditions mitochondrial respiration is the principal site of ATP supply. In resting muscle the rate of mitochondrial respiration is reduced to a very low level (state 4), producing the small amount of ATP needed to maintain the steady state of the resting cell. Under these conditions the ADP level is also very low. When ATP is hydrolysed during the contraction, ADP and P_i are produced in equal amounts and transported into the mitochondria where respiration is stimulated to produce ATP (state 3).

As seen in Eqn 2, ADP, P_i, NADH and O_2 are substrates for oxidative phosphorylation defining three regulating factors: the phosphorylation state, the redox state and the O_2 concentration. The phosphorylation state is believed to be the principal rate controlling factor in most circumstances (Connett *et al.*, 1990). The concentration of cytosolic free ADP, being in the micromolar range is below the sensitivity of NMR *in vivo*. Chance *et al.* (1985) have shown that the ADP concentration can be calculated from the CK reaction (Eqn 3) assuming that this is at equilibrium and that the value of pH_i, cytosolic free P_i and PCr concentrations are known, giving the equation:

$$[\text{ADP}] = [\text{Cr}]\,[\text{ATP}] \,/\, \kappa[\text{PCr}]\,[\text{H}^+] \tag{5}$$

where κ is the CK equilibrium constant. The proton concentration can be calculated from the shift of P_i from PCr. At constant pH_i and constant ATP, if the change in creatine concentration is equal to the change in P_i concentration, the cytosolic free ADP level becomes equivalent to the P_i/PCr ratio: [ADP] $\approx P_i$/PCr. Therefore, the P_i/PCr ratio will increase in proportion to the intensity of work (or ATPase activity), providing an index of oxidative muscle capacity. In isolated rat heart mitochondria, the rate of ATP production, equal to the rate of ATP breakdown by added ATPase, has been shown to be related to the P_i/PCr ratio (Gyulai *et al.*, 1985). When the rate of cellular energy utilisation exceeds the rate of aerobic ATP production, as occurs during strenuous exercise or when the O_2 supply is limited, the anaerobic pathway of glycolysis yields supplementary ATP production but also generates H^+ and lactate. This is then reflected by intracellular acidosis.

The ADP control of oxidative phosphorylation does not yield to a linear equation but to a Michaelis–Menten relation:

$$V/V_{max} = 1/\{1 + K_m/[ADP]\} \tag{6}$$

where V is the rate of ATP utilisation, V_{max} the maximum velocity of the ATP production via the oxidative phosphorylation, K_m the affinity constant and [ADP] the concentration of the regulatory substrate estimated by the P_i/PCr ratio. The K_m value of ADP is 20 μM which corresponds to a P_i/PCr value of about 0.6. This means that the pool of ATP can be regulated within narrow limits as 50% of the maximum velocity of the ATP synthesis is obtained with only 20 μM change of ADP corresponding to 0.25% change of the ATP pool. The plot of work rate versus P_i/PCr ratio then yields a rectangular hyperbola or a linear curve at low-level exercise (Chance *et al.*, 1985). However, this convenient analysis requires work performed at a constant level to overcome the relatively slow time resolution of ^{31}P-NMR compared with that of bioenergetic changes (Chance *et al.*, 1981).

Much information on energy metabolism can also be obtained from the study of post-exercise recovery. After exercise, the accumulated regulatory ADP continues to stimulate mitochondrial respiration at a high rate to synthesise ATP. Consequently, the cytoplasmic phosphocreatine pool is replenished through the CK equilibrium (Eqn 3). The PCr resynthesis rate depends entirely on mitochondrial respiration because the absence of metabolic recovery has been shown when the muscle is made ischaemic after exercise by the rapid inflation of a sphygmomanometer cuff (Taylor *et al.*, 1983). The rate of PCr resynthesis is, therefore, regarded as an index of mitochondrial function. This can be fitted by a single exponential function enabling the calculation of $t_{1/2}$ for PCr. The rate of PCr resynthesis, however, could be affected by the level of intracellular acidosis and ATP depletion; this, in turn, may depend in part on the motivation of the subject or how strenuous the exercise protocol is (Arnold *et al.*, 1984; Taylor *et al.*, 1986). Some methodological precautions, therefore, have to be taken in order to study the muscular bioenergetics using ^{31}P-NMR spectroscopy.

Exercise design during ^{31}P-NMR spectroscopy

One major problem during ^{31}P-NMR studies of muscle bioenergetics concerns the quantification of the in-magnet exercise. Different solutions have been adopted by research groups to solve this problem, according mainly to the muscle(s) in which they are interested. Transcutaneous nerve stimulation in humans can be only used where a small muscle mass is involved in the effort, e.g. tibialis anterior (Helpern *et al.*, 1989). For a larger exercising muscle mass, a method of monitoring and quantifying the level of exercise needs either an internal metabolic reference, e.g. decrease in pH_i (Bendahan *et al.*, 1990) or PCr (Duboc *et al.*, 1987), or an external mechanical reference requiring an appropriate ergometer.

For example, calf muscle can be exercised by pressing a pedal (active plantar flexion) against a given load (Reutenauer *et al.*, 1991). The pedal is connected to a strain gauge and to a displacement transducer. Force, displacement and pedal frequency are transmitted to a graphic recorder and sampled with an analogue-to-digital convertor to be stored in a computer. This allows calculation of the pedal velocity and power output at each pedal motion. The resistance force can also be obtained by connecting the pedal with a piston linked with a hydraulic system (Gonzáles de Suso *et al.*, 1993).

The exercise procedure has to be accurately designed in accordance with the aim of the bioenergetic study: whether the exercise is to be exhaustive and even ischaemic to determine the anaerobic response, or whether it should reach a non-fatiguing submaximal steady state in order to evaluate the aerobic component. Exhaustive exercise does not take place at steady-state energy equilibrium (Chance *et al.*, 1981), precluding the use of the P_i/PCr ratio as an index of mitochondrial respiration. On the other hand, a steady-state exercise condition maintains the exercising skeletal muscle over a long period of time allowing very good ^{31}P-NMR spectra to be obtained during transitions from the resting state to a number of different activated states. Therefore, a graded steady-state submaximal exercise protocol has to yield a linear relationship between P_i/PCr and work, an absence of marked progressive intracellular acidosis and a steady ATP level in normal subjects (Sapega *et al.*, 1987).

Additional information can be obtained from the determination of blood flow coupled with the metabolic and mechanical measurements. Indeed, the measured metabolic NMR parameters result both from circulatory and cellular activities. The control of one component is the only way to separate them, using either total ischaemia or direct blood flow measurement, e.g. by using venous occlusion plethysmography coupled with ^{31}P-NMR (Minotti *et al.*, 1989).

Clinical application of ^{31}P-NMR spectroscopy

It is beyond the scope of the present chapter to present fully the clinical aspects involved in ^{31}P-NMR spectroscopy (see Gutierrez & Andry, 1989; Barbiroli, 1992). Most studies have focused on the description of direct muscle alterations: muscular enzyme deficiencies, mitochondrial myopathy and muscular dystrophy as well as the consequences of peripheral vascular disease, muscle denervations and chronic heart failure.

Two clinical applications of ^{31}P-NMR spectroscopy are worthy of specific mention as they go beyond a restrictive description of muscle impairment. First, the ^{31}P-NMR spectroscopy could be used as a diagnostic tool for the detection of MH susceptibility because elevated resting P_i/PCr and phosphodiesters (PDE)/PCr ratios as well as slow post-exercise recovery rate of PCr have been reported in MH-susceptible patients (Olgin *et al.*, 1991; Payen *et al.*, 1991, 1993*a*). Second, the potential use of ^{31}P-NMR spectroscopy as a method for the determination of tissue oxygenation and the local effects of therapeutic measures in critically ill patients (Gutierrez & Andry, 1989). For instance, the effects of oxygen inhalation on muscle bioenergetics have been studied in patients with chronic hypoxaemia as well as in normal subjects (Payen *et al.*, 1993*b*).

Exertional heat stroke and ^{31}P-NMR spectroscopy

Methods

Investigation of post-exertional heat stroke patients by ^{31}P-NMR has been reported (Payen *et al.*, 1992). Thirteen men were investigated six months after well-documented episodes of exertional heat stroke (Table 5.1) during a graded non-exhausting standardised exercise protocol involving calf muscles in a 2.35 Tesla 35 cm horizontal bore magnet coupled to a spectrometer (Bruker Spectrospin, Wissembourg, France). This group with exertional heat stroke was compared with a group of 16 age-matched healthy male volunteers. To stress the calf muscles, the subject was asked to perform 360 flexions of the foot (active plantar flexion) with a regular frequency against three consecutive graded loads corresponding to 20, 35 and 50% of the maximal voluntary contraction (MVC) of the calf muscle. The pedal revolved around an axis at the level of the calcaneum and its displacement was limited between stops allowing a 30° plantar flexion. With a motion frequency of $\approx 0.5\,Hz$, each level of exercise (i.e. 120 active plantar flexions) lasted about four minutes. The pedal was linked to a strain gauge and to a displacement transducer to

Table 5.1. *Situational factors and characteristics of 13 heat stroke victims*

Subject	Type of exercise	Distance completed (km)	Tre max (°C)	Mental status and duration (h)	CK (units/L)
A	CF	8	42	coma (0.5)	1600
B	CF	40	40	coma (>1.0)	2800
C	MT	8	42	coma(>1.0)	(-)
D	MT	8	41	coma (0.5)	600
E	CF	8	40	coma (<0.1)	1000
F	CF	9	40	coma(<0.1)	200
G	CF	9	42	coma (1.0)	800
H	MT	8	41	coma (>1.0)	10000
I	MT	8	42	coma(>1.0)	146000
J	CF	11	40	coma (<0.1)	400
K	MT	6	41	disoriented	8100
L	MT	8	40.4	coma (<0.1)	800
M	MT	11	41.4	coma(1.0)	14000

Tre, rectal temperature; CK, serum creatine phosphokinase level (normal range 30–150 units/L); MT, military training with battledress and load of 12 kg; CF, competitive foot race with shorts and t-shirt.

measure velocity and effective power output for each pedal motion. Differences in muscle mass were taken into account by relating power outputs to the cross-sectional calf muscle area (W/cm^2). Each leg was studied, one at a time, after being placed on a platform which contained a 6 cm diameter inductively coupled coil below the gastrocnemius muscle.

The ^{31}P spectra (40.6 MHz) were obtained at rest, during exercise and after recovery. Spectral analysis was based on the integrated measurement of phosphomonoesters (PME), P_i, PCr and βATP peaks. In addition, leg tissue blood flow was determined by venous occlusion plethysmography during the NMR procedure. The entire apparatus used in our laboratory is shown in Figure 5.4. Both groups were comparable as regards body mass, height, VO$_{2max}$, MVC and cross-sectional area of the calf muscle. The most 'impaired' leg as regards muscle metabolism was systematically chosen in the exertional heat stroke group for comparison with the control group.

Results

The evolution of P_i/PCr and intracellular pH (pH$_i$) from rest to the end of the exercise is shown in Figures 5.5 and 5.6. Effective power output was comparable at each level of exercise between the two groups: at 50% MVC, the mean power output was 0.40 ± 0.03 (mean $\pm$ SE) versus 0.39 ± 0.03 W/cm^2 in

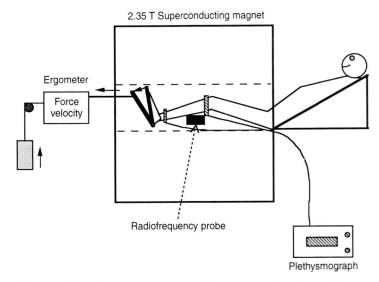

Figure 5.4. Magnet, exercise and venous occlusion plethysmography flow apparatus.

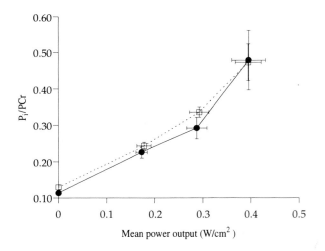

Figure 5.5. Relationship between the effective mean power output (W/cm^2) and the inorganic phosphate to phosphocreatine (P$_i$/PCr) ratio at rest and during the course of exercise at 20, 30 and 50% of maximal voluntary contraction of the calf muscle in 13 exertional heat stroke (filled circles) and 16 control (open squares) subjects. Values are mean ± SE. Adapted with permission from Payen *et al.* (1992).

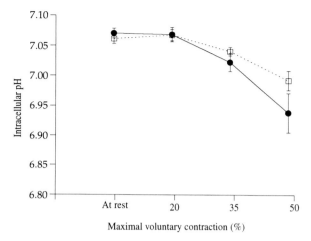

Figure 5.6. Intracellular pH at rest and during the course of exercise at 20, 35 and 50% of maximal voluntary contraction of the calf muscle in 13 exertional heat stroke (filled circles) and 16 control (open squares) subjects. Values are mean ± SE. Adapted with permission from Payen *et al.* (1992).

exertional heat stroke and control groups, respectively. For a comparable level of exercise, no significant differences were found between the two groups in P_i/PCr (Figure 5.5), pH_i (Figure 5.6) and relative ATP at rest as well as during the whole exercise. At 50% MVC, pH_i was 6.94 ± 0.03 versus 6.99 ± 0.02, P_i/PCr was 0.48 ± 0.08 versus 0.47 ± 0.05, respectively. In addition, the changes in leg blood flow from the rest period to the end of the exercise were not significantly different between exertional heat stroke and control subjects: 2.79 ± 0.49 versus 3.45 ± 0.51, respectively. Finally, the rate of PCr resynthesis during recovery was not significantly different between the two groups: $t_{1/2}$ PCr $= 0.58 \pm 0.07$ versus 0.50 ± 0.05 minutes, respectively.

The linear relationship between P_i/PCr and work, the absence of marked progressive intracellular acidosis and the steady ATP level observed in the control group illustrate satisfactory prerequisites to study muscle oxidation metabolism (Sapega *et al.*, 1987). Under these conditions, the similar metabolic results between exertional heat stroke and control groups reflect a comparable capacity of ATP resynthesis from oxidative phosphorylation as the power outputs were similar at the three levels of exercise. The contribution of anaerobic metabolism as reflected by changes in pH_i at the end of exercise was moderate and similar in both groups. Thereby, no evidence of an impairment of muscle energy metabolism was shown in the post-exertional heat stroke group during this kind of steady-state submaximal exercise performed in a room maintained at 20 °C.

Opposite results obtained in forearm muscle during an exhaustive exercise under ischaemia had been previously reported in abstract form (Kozak-Reiss *et al.*, 1988). Thirteen post-exertional heat stroke patients exhibited a lower pH_i at the end of exercise (6.13 ± 0.04) than that of ten controls (6.67 ± 0.04). The effort was not mechanically quantified, however, and the decrease in PCr which served here as an internal standard was also greater in the exertional heat stroke group than in the control group. This could suggest either a difference in the intensity of exercise between both groups or a true muscle energy metabolism impairment in the exertional heat stroke group.

Discussion

This apparent discrepancy between ^{31}P-NMR results from muscle energy metabolism in post-exertional heat stroke patients requires comment. First, it is difficult to state that skeletal muscle abnormalities detected after such a severe muscle injury marked by functional and structural damage (Armstrong, 1984; McCully & Faulkner, 1985) existed prior to exertional heat stroke. Muscle investigations of victims of exertional heat stroke could not easily distinguish between the predisposing factor or residual injury. Studies of post-exertional patients should be performed after a long time delay from exertional heat stroke, usually up to four to six months. Such a delay should allow resolution of any clinical symptoms or physical detraining imposed by physicians (Armstrong *et al.*, 1990).

Second, our study did not demonstrate an impairment in muscle energy metabolism as a predisposing factor that could be related to the occurrence of exertional heat stroke in young men. The exercise protocol and NMR measurement methodology had been successfully used previously in our laboratory in the investigation of other pathologies (Payen *et al.*, 1993*a,b*; Wuyam *et al.*, 1992). This kind of exercise, however, is submaximal and muscle abnormalities may be only detected at a higher level of exercise; therefore, another patient with exertional heat stroke has recently been studied during intensive exercise, reaching 65 and 80% MVC. No energy metabolic differences between his results and those of control subjects have been found (unpublished data). The investigation of both legs in the exertional heat stroke group enabled us to detect no marked leg metabolic asymmetry in all but one exertional heat stroke patient: for a similar power output at 50% MVC, the P_i/PCr ratio reached 1.34 and pH_i dropped to 6.68 in the right leg while normal metabolic values were obtained in the left ($P_i/PCr = 0.38$, $pH_i = 7.05$). This leg metabolic asymmetry was still present six months later without any clinical complaint. Neither neurological nor vascular limb pathologies have been found using electromyography, lumbar NMR imaging and pulsed Doppler. No evidence of myopathy was found on histological and biochemical examination of a muscle biopsy performed on the right leg (L. Bourdon, personal communication).

None of our exertional heat stroke patients exhibited ^{31}P-NMR abnormalities which had been previously reported in MH-susceptible patients (Olgin *et al.*, 1991; Payen *et al.*, 1991, 1993*a*). In addition, two exertional heat stroke patients were tested for MH using the contracture test and the results were negative according to the European MH group protocol. Similar observations were reported by others (Krivosic-Horber *et al.*, 1991). Only on the basis of these results, it remains highly speculative to state definite conclusions about the relationship between exertional heat stroke and MH. Additional investigations in exertional heat stroke victims, i.e. studies of calcium channels and molecular genetics, would be most useful to elucidate this point.

Finally, no differences were shown in exercise-induced changes in leg blood flow between exertional heat stroke and control subjects. One mechanism that could affect muscle blood flow and thermoregulatory/exercise performance is potassium depletion (Knochel & Schlein, 1972; Hubbard *et al.*, 1987). At the time of examination, none of our exertional heat stroke patients exhibited signs of potassium depletion as assessed by blood samples and electrocardiogram.

In conclusion, energy metabolism of gastrocnemius muscle is replenished six months after a severe muscle injury. This adds to the small database about the long-term recovery of post-exertional heat stroke patients. In a recent study, nine out of ten subjects exhibited normal heat acclimatisation responses, thermoregulation and physical performance within six months following exertional heat stroke (Armstrong *et al.*, 1990). Further ^{31}P-NMR studies are needed to confirm our results, especially those investigating the effects of higher levels of exercise. They could also specify the exact relationship between exertional heat stroke and MH.

Acknowledgements

We thank Michel Decorps, Christoph Segebarth and MacDonald Beckley for their critical review of the manuscript.

References

Armstrong, R. B. (1984). Mechanisms of exercise-induced delayed onset muscular soreness: a brief review. *Medicine and Science in Sports and Exercise*, **16**, 529–38.

Armstrong, L. E., De Luca, J. P. & Hubbard, R. W. (1990). Time course of recovery and heat acclimation ability of prior exertional heat stroke patients. *Medicine and Science in Sports and Exercise*, **22**, 36–48.

Arnold, D. L., Matthews, P. M. & Radda, G. K. (1984). Metabolic recovery after exercise and the assessment of mitochondrial function *in vivo* in human skeletal muscle by means of ^{31}P-NMR. *Magnetic Resonance in Medicine*, **1**, 307–15.

Barbiroli, B. (1992). ^{31}P MRS of human skeletal muscle. In *Magnetic Resonance Spectroscopy in Biology and Medicine*, 1st edn, ed. J. D. de Certaines, W. M. M. J. Bovée & F. Podo, pp. 369–86. Oxford, Pergamon Press.

Bendahan, D., Confort-Gouny, S., Kozak-Reiss, G. & Cozzone, P. J. (1990). Heterogeneity of metabolic response to muscular exercise in humans. New criteria of invariance defined by *in vivo* phosphorous-31 NMR spectroscopy. *FEBS Letters*, **272**, 155–8.

Bessman, S. P. & Geiger, P. J. (1981). Transport of energy in muscle: the phosphorylcreatine shuttle. *Science*, **211**, 448–52.

Bourdon, L. & Canini, F. (1995). On the nature of the link between malignant hyperthermia and exertional heatstroke. *Medical Hypotheses*, **45**, 268–70.

Chance, B., Eleff, S., Leigh, J. S., Sokolow, D. & Sapega, A. (1981). Mitochondrial regulation of phosphocreatine/inorganic phosphate ratios in exercising human muscle: a gated ^{31}P NMR study. *Proceedings of the National Academy of Sciences of the USA*, **78**, 6714–8.

Chance, B., Leigh, J. S., Clark, B. J., Maris, J., Kent, J., Nioka, S. & Smith, D. (1985). Control of oxidative metabolism and oxygen delivery in human skeletal muscle: a steady-state analysis of the work/energy cost transfer function. *Proceedings of the National Academy of Sciences of the USA.*, **82**, 8384–8.

Connett, R. J., Honig, C. R., Gayeski, T. E. J. & Brooks, G. A. (1990). Defining hypoxia: a systems view of VO_2, glycolysis, energetics and intracellular PO_2. *Journal of Applied Physiology*, **68**, 833–42.

Denborough, M. A., (1982). Heat stroke and malignant hyperpyrexia. *Medical Journal of Australia*, **1**, 204–5.

Duboc, D., Jehenson, P., Tran Dinh, S., Marsac, C., Syrota, A. & Fardeau, M. (1987). Phosphorus NMR spectroscopy study of muscular enzyme deficiencies involving glycogenolysis and glycolysis. *Neurology*, **37**, 633–71.

Edwards, R. H. T., Harris, R. C., Hultman, E., Kaijser, L., Koh, D. & Nordesjö, L. O. (1972). Effect of temperature on muscle energy metabolism and endurance during successive isometric contractions, sustained to fatigue, of the quadriceps muscle in man. *Journal of Physiology*, **220**, 335–52.

Epstein, Y. (1990). Heat intolerance: predisposing factor or residual injury? *Medicine and Science in Sports and Exercise*, **22**, 29–35.

Gadian, D. G. (1982). *Nuclear Magnetic Resonance and its Application to Living Systems*. Oxford, Clarendon Press.

Gonzáles de Suso, J. M., Bernús, G., Alonso, J., Alay, A., Capdevila, A., Gili, J., Prat J. A. & Arús, C. (1993). Development and characterisation of an ergometer to study the bioenergetics of the human quadriceps muscle by ^{31}P NMR spectroscopy inside a standard MR scanner. *Magnetic Resonance in Medicine*, **29**, 575–81.

Gutierrez, G. & Andry, J. M. (1989). Nuclear magnetic resonance measurements. Clinical applications. *Critical Care Medicine*, **17**, 73–82.

Gyulai, L., Roth, Z., Leigh, J. S. & Chance, B. (1985). Bioenergetics studies of mitochondrial oxidative phosphorylation using ^{31}phosphorus NMR. *Journal of Biological Chemistry*, **260**, 3947–54.

Hackl, W., Winkler, M., Mauritz, W., Sporn, P. & Steinbereithner, K. (1991). Muscle biopsy for diagnosis of malignant hyperthermia susceptibility in two patients with severe exercise-induced myolysis. *British Journal of Anaesthesia*, **66**, 138–40.

Helpern, J. A., Kao, W., Gross, B., Kensora, T. G. & Welch, K. M. A. (1989). Interleaved ^{31}P NMR with transcutaneous nerve stimulation: a method of monitoring compliance-independent skeletal muscle metabolic response to exercise. *Magnetic Resonance in Medicine*, **10**, 50–6.

Hopkins, P. M., Ellis, F. R. & Halsall, P.J. (1991). Evidence for related myopathies in exertional heat stroke and malignant hyperthermia. *Lancet*, **338**, 1491–2.

Hubbard, R. W. (1990). Heatstroke pathophysiology: the energy depletion model. *Medicine and Science in Sports and Exercise*, **22**, 19–28.

Hubbard, R. W., Matthew, C. B., Durkot, M. J. & Francesconi, R. P. (1987). Novel approaches to the pathophysiology of heatstroke: the energy depletion model. *Annals of Emergency Medicine*, **16**, 1066–75.

Jessen, C. (1987). Thermoregulatory mechanisms in severe heat stress and exercise. In *Heat Stress: Physical Exertion and Environment*, ed. J. R. S. Hales & D. A. B. Richards, pp. 1–18. Amsterdam, Elsevier Science Publishers.

Kielblock, A. J. (1987). Strategies for the prevention of heat disorders with particular reference to the efficacy of body cooling procedures. In *Heat Stress: Physical Exertion and Environment*, ed. J. R. S. Hales & D. A. B. Richards, pp. 489–97. Amsterdam, Elsevier Science Publishers.

Knochel, J. P. & Schlein, E. M. (1972). On the mechanism of rhabdomyolysis in potassium depletion. *Journal of Clinical Investigation*, **51**, 1750–8.

Kozak-Reiss, G., Gascard, J.-P., Hervé, P., Jehenson, P., Syrota, A. (1988). Malignant and exercise hyperthermia: investigation of 73 subjects by contracture tests and P31 NMR spectroscopy. *Anesthesiology*, **69**, 415 (abstract).

Kozlowski, S., Brzezinska, Z., Kruk, B., Kaciuba-Uscilko, H., Greenleaf, J. E. & Nazar, K. (1985). Exercise hyperthermia as a factor limiting physical performance: temperature effect on muscle metabolism. *Journal of Applied Physiology*, **59**, 766–73.

Krivosic-Horber, R., Adnet, P. & Reyford, H. (1991). Relationship between exercise-induced myolysis and malignant hyperthermia. *British Journal of Anaesthesia*, **67**, 221 (letter).

McCully, K. K. & Faulkner, J. A. (1985). Injury to skeletal muscle fibres of mice following lengthening contractions. *Journal of Applied Physiology*, **59**, 119–26.

Minotti, J. R., Johnson, E. C., Hudson, T. L., Sibbitt, R. R., Wise, L. E., Fukushima, E. & Icenogle, M. V. (1989). Forearm metabolic asymmetry detected by ^{31}P-NMR during submaximal exercise. *Journal of Applied Physiology*, **67**, 324–9.

Moon, R. B. & Richards, J. H. (1973). Determination of intracellular pH by ^{31}P magnetic resonance. *Journal of Biological Chemistry*, **248**, 7276–8.

Olgin, J., Rosenberg, H., Allen, G., Seestedt, R. & Chance, B. (1991). A blinded comparison of noninvasive, *in vivo* phosphorus nuclear magnetic resonance spectroscopy and the *in vitro* halothane/caffeine test in the evaluation of malignant hyperthermia susceptibility. *Anesthesia and Analgesia*, **72**, 36–47.

Payen, J.-F., Bosson, J.-L., Bourdon, L., Jacquot, C., Le Bas, J.-F., Stieglitz, P. & Benabid, A. L. (1993*a*). Improved noninvasive diagnostic testing for malignant hyperthermia susceptibility from combination of metabolites determined *in vivo* with ^{31}P-magnetic resonance spectroscopy. *Anesthesiology*, **78**, 848–55.

Payen, J.-F., Bourdon, L., Mezin, P., Jacquot, C., Le Bas, J.-F., Stieglitz, P. & Benabid, A. L. (1991). Susceptibility to malignant hyperthermia detected noninvasively. *Lancet*, **337**, 1550–1.

Payen, J.-F., Bourdon, L., Reutenauer, H., Melin, B., Le Bas, J.-F., Stieglitz, P. & Cure, M. (1992). Exertional heat stroke and muscle metabolism: an *in vivo* [31] P-MRS study. *Medicine and Science in Sports and Exercise*, **24**, 420–5.

Payen, J.-F., Wuyam, B., Levy, P., Reutenauer, H., Stieglitz, P., Paramelle, B. & Le Bas, J.-F. (1993*b*). Muscular metabolism during oxygen supplementation in patients with chronic hypoxemia. *American Review of Respiratory Disease*, **147**, 592–8.

Reutenauer, H., Payen, J.-F., Laurent, D., Le Bas, J.-F., Rossi, A. & Benabid, A. L. (1991). A simple ergometer for human calf muscular metabolism study using ^{31}P NMR spectroscopy. *Revue Européenne de Technologie Biomédicale*, **13**, 127–30.

Richards, D. A. B. & Richards, C. R. B. (1987). Physiological factors predisposing to physical exhaustion. In *Heat Stress: Physical Exertion and Environment*, ed. J. R. S. Hales & D. A. B. Richards, pp. 419–26. Amsterdam, Elsevier Science Publishers.

Rome, L. C. & Kushmerick, M. J. (1983). Energetics of isometric contractions as a function of muscle temperature. *American Journal of Physiology*, **244**, C100–9.

Sapega, A. A., Sokolow, D. P., Graham, T. J. & Chance, B. (1987). Phosphorus nuclear magnetic resonance: a non-invasive technique for the study of muscle bioenergetics during exercise. *Medicine and Science in Sports and Exercise*, **19**, 410–20.

Segal, S. S., Faulkner, J. A. & White, T. P. (1986). Skeletal muscle fatigue *in vitro* is temperature dependent. *Journal of Applied Physiology*, **61**, 660–5.

Taylor, D. J., Bore, P. J., Styles, P., Gadian, D. G. & Radda, G. K. (1983). Bioenergetics of intact human muscle: a ^{31}P nuclear magnetic resonance study. *Molecular Biology in Medicine*, **1**, 77–94.

Taylor, D. J., Styles, P., Matthews, P. M., Arnold, D. A., Gadian, D. G., Bore, P. & Radda, G. K. (1986). Energetics of human muscle: exercise-induced ATP depletion. *Magnetic Resonance in Medicine*, **3**, 44–54.

Wuyam, B., Payen, J.-F., Levy P., Bensaîdane, H., Reutenauer, H., Le Bas, J.-F., Benabid, A. L. (1992). Metabolism and aerobic capacity of skeletal muscle in chronic respiratory failure related to chronic respiratory disease. *European Respiratory Journal*, **5**, 157–62.

6

Investigation of exertional heat stroke
3: *In vitro* skeletal muscle contracture testing

P. M. HOPKINS, P. J. HALSALL and F. R. ELLIS

In vitro contracture testing and malignant hyperthermia

Following the demonstration that freshly exercised, cut muscle bundles from patients who had survived malignant hyperthermia (MH) reactions demonstrated an increased sensitivity to the contracture-inducing effects of caffeine *in vitro* (Kalow *et al.*, 1970) and the similar study that described the abnormal *in vitro* contracture response to halothane of muscle bundles from relatives of patients who had fatal MH reactions (Ellis *et al.*, 1971), *in vitro* contracture tests (IVCT) using halothane and caffeine on muscle samples taken at open biopsy have become generally accepted as the 'gold standard' for the diagnosis of susceptibility to MH. These tests are described in more detail in Chapter 11.

Relationship between exertional heat stroke and malignant hyperthermia

Exertional heat stroke is a life-threatening syndrome of raised body core temperature with marked rhabdomyolysis, hyperkalaemia and metabolic acidosis leading to acute renal, cardiac and haemostatic failure (Knochel, 1989; Chapter 3).

MH is a pharmacogenetic disorder of skeletal muscle that is triggered when a susceptible individual receives suxamethonium or one of the volatile anaesthetic agents (halothane, enflurane, isoflurane; Chapter 8). These drugs cause a rise in skeletal muscle myoplasmic calcium ion concentration (Iaizzo *et al.*, 1988) which leads to muscle rigidity, hypermetabolism (pyrexia, hypoxia and metabolic acidosis) and sarcolemmal disruption (hyperkalaemia, myoglobinaemia).

MH shows some resemblance to the porcine stress syndrome (Chapter 14), for example in the response to anaesthetic agents, but the pig condition is notable for awake episodes when the animal is physically stressed. It has often been postulated (but never proven) that MH is in fact a human stress syndrome and that heat stroke may be one manifestation of this (Wingard & Gatz, 1978).

It is with this background that several groups have undertaken the investigation of individuals who have suffered episodes of heat stroke for their susceptibility to MH. The first such investigations to be reported were those carried out by Denborough on one individual (Denborough, 1982). Unfortunately, this is only a brief report in letter form and the details of the methods employed for the IVCT (at a time when there were no published standards), as well as the details of the results obtained are omitted. The clinical history, however, was typical of heat stroke (Chapter 2) and the IVCT 'showed the increased sensitivity to caffeine and halothane which is diagnostic of the myopathies which predispose to malignant hyperpyrexia'. Since 1982, the date of this report, it has been demonstrated that increased sensitivity to the contracture-inducing effects of caffeine and halothane is not specific to MH, with small contractures developing in muscle samples from some patients with myopathies that are not associated with MH (Heiman-Patterson *et al.*, 1988; Lehmann-Horn & Iaizzo, 1990; Heytens *et al.*, 1992; Hopkins *et al.*, 1993). An informed opinion on Denborough's case cannot, therefore, be made without the detailed results of the IVCT. One other explanation for the abnormal IVCT results obtained in this case which may not have been apparent at the time is the relatively short time interval of less than two months between the episode of severe heat stroke with rhabdomyolysis and the subsequent IVCT. Although biochemical indices of muscle function had returned to within normal limits, these only reflect recovery of the integrity of plasma membrane function and residual damage of other functional elements of the muscle cells may still be present. This is important as muscle damaged, even as a secondary effect, may respond abnormally to IVCT (Hopkins *et al.*, 1993).

Gronert *et al.* (1980) had previously reported an unusual case of a 42-year-old man who, although he had not suffered an episode of heat stroke per se, had avoided physical exertion for 20 years because it resulted in 'aching joints, malaise, fever and soaking sweats'. He was also troubled by intermittent fever. Electromyography and serum creatine kinase were normal and the man was referred for muscle biopsy and IVCT. Tests at this time were non-standardised and can therefore only be reported in relation to the experience of those using them. Thus the response to halothane was normal, while that to caffeine and to a combination of caffeine and halothane were considered abnormal. There can, in fact, be little dispute that the caffeine response was abnormal as 90% of peak tension (that tension produced by 32 mmol caffeine) developed in re-

sponse to only 0.5 mmol caffeine. The combined halothane/caffeine test, however, is now known to produce a high incidence of false positive results (Ellis *et
al.*, 1992).

On the basis of these IVCT results the diagnosis of MH susceptibility was
made, the symptoms, according to Gronert and colleagues, being 'manifestations of an awake MH reaction'. Subsequently, the symptoms responded to a
small oral dose of dantrolene (1.1 mg/kg), with any increase in dosage interestingly causing exaggerated muscle weakness. The authors considered these
responses to dantrolene as further supportive evidence for the diagnosis of
MH.

Investigation of the patient's family followed, with his son and daughter
having normal IVCT responses and normal resting serum creatine kinase
(CK) levels. The patient's father, however, had a persistently raised serum CK
of 10–20 times normal: unfortunately he refused to undergo muscle biopsy.

The Austrian MH unit were referred three patients for investigation following exercise-induced reactions, two of which have been reported (Hackl *et al.*,
1991). The first patient presented to hospital 24 hours after exercise (a military
entrance test) with muscle pain and dark urine: during the exercise the thigh
muscles felt painful and swollen, and he was also subjectively hot. Investigations in hospital revealed a mild pyrexia of 37.8 °C and serum CK of 64 800
IU/L. The patient subsequently made a full recovery and was later referred for
IVCT. The tests, carried out according to the European Malignant Hyperthermia Group (EMHG) protocol (EMHG, 1984), produced abnormal contracture responses to both halothane and caffeine.

The second Austrian case was one of fulminant exertional heat stroke with
loss of consciousness, tachycardia, hypotension, pyrexia of 41.7 °C, hypoxaemia, metabolic acidosis, rhabdomyolysis and coagulopathy with platelet
consumption. Subsequent IVCT, however, produced normal responses both
to halothane and to caffeine.

In 1991 we reported the results of our investigations of two servicemen who
have suffered episodes of heat stroke for their susceptibility to MH (Hopkins
et al., 1991*a*). The first case was that of a 19-year-old recruit who collapsed
after 7.5 miles of alternate forced march and running while carrying 15 kg of
equipment, as well as a rifle, and wearing boots, lightweight trousers, combat
jacket and a steel helmet. His rectal temperature was 41 °C and he was treated
with sponging and intravenous fluids. Initial biochemistry results were not
obtained, but 90 minutes following the collapse the serum potassium, blood
gases and pH were normal. CK was raised at 2329 IU/L (ref. 28–205 IU/L),
rising to 35 000 IU/L by the next day; a specimen of urine sent at this stage was
negative for myoglobin. The ambient temperature at the time of the incident

was 22.5 °C with a relative humidity of 73%. The victim had no recognised predisposing factors (Chapter 2).

Eleven months following this incident the subject attended for diagnostic muscle biopsy and IVCT. In addition to testing with halothane and caffeine according to the protocol of the EMHG (1984), a ryanodine contracture test was performed (Hopkins *et al.*, 1991*b*). The response to caffeine was within normal limits (0.2 g contracture at 4 mM caffeine) but there was an abnormal response to halothane (0.2 g contracture at 2% halothane) which, according to the EMHG protocol is classified as MH equivocal (MHEh), but is invariably interpreted as indicating clinical susceptibility to MH. The additional ryanodine contracture test did not, however, support the diagnosis of MH.

Subsequently, both parents of the subject attended for identical diagnostic procedures. His mother had a normal response to all tests, but his father showed a similar abnormal response to halothane (MHEh) with normal caffeine and ryanodine results.

The second case was that of a 23-year-old soldier who had two documented episodes of heat intolerance. The first occurred on a hot day after he had run six miles wearing vest, trousers, boots and carrying a rifle. He collapsed but remained conscious and responded to intravenous fluid therapy. The second incident occurred five years later following eight miles of running in full battle dress carrying 15 kg of equipment. On this occasion consciousness was lost for approximately 45 minutes and the axillary temperature recorded at 39 °C. Of note in his family history was that his maternal grandfather had died in his sixties with a late-onset myopathy. No other member of the family was thought to have been similarly affected.

This man attended for muscle biopsy and IVCT with halothane, caffeine and ryanodine eight months after the second episode of heat stroke. The response to caffeine was within normal limits (0.2 g at 3 mmol caffeine) but again the response to halothane was abnormal (0.3 g at 2% halothane). In this case the response to ryanodine was abnormal, but not typical for MH muscle. He was classified as MHEh.

IVCT were performed on the parents and brother of this second soldier. The results for his mother were all normal, while his father and brother both had a normal response to caffeine and halothane but with a similar abnormal response to ryanodine.

In both victims there was a normal response to caffeine but an abnormal contracture on exposure of the muscle to halothane. This type of *in vitro* response is seen with muscle of MH-susceptible individuals, but has also been demonstrated in the muscle of patients with other muscle diseases (Heiman-Patterson *et al.*, 1988; Lehmann-Horn & Iaizzo, 1990; Heytens *et al.*, 1992;

Hopkins *et al.*, 1993). The heat stroke victims' muscle, however, differed from MH-susceptible muscle in its response to ryanodine (Hopkins *et al.*, 1991*b*). These studies suggest that both heat stroke victims have an underlying skeletal muscle abnormality that is probably distinct from MH but which involves a similar deregulation of control of myoplasmic calcium ion concentration, which leads to both the *in vitro* contracture in response to drugs and the clinical heat stroke syndrome in response to extreme exertion.

The family investigations support the concept of an inherited component to this demonstrated muscle abnormality. This is most clearly evident in the first case where the father of the victim had identical abnormal pharmacological responses. The evidence in the second case is not so clear, but this could also result from a dominantly inherited abnormality that is expressed to a greater degree in the heat stroke victim than in his father and brother. This would be analogous to the situation in MH where susceptible members of the same family display considerable heterogeneity with respect to the *in vitro* responses.

Most recently Kozak-Ribbens *et al.* (1994) have presented the results of IVCT performed on 55 patients with a history of exertional heat stroke. Although the details of the heat stroke reactions and IVCT results are not available to us, the patients were classified according to the EMHG protocol as shown in Table 6.1 (see also Chapter 11).

Histological and histochemical analysis, however, revealed that several of the patients with abnormal IVCT results had clear evidence of other myopathies: the anomalies included type 2 atrophy and carnitine palmitoyl transferase deficiency. Two of the patients classified as MHS were children of parents with mitochondrial myopathies.

Does an abnormal IVCT response always indicate MH susceptibility?

In answering this question it is first necessary to define MH. Over the past 30 years many definitions have been proposed with little consensus between workers in the field. It may seem obvious but any such definition can only be as precise and complete as allowed by knowledge at the time. Confusion has also arisen because some have attempted a definition of MH purely as a clinical syndrome without any regard to the underlying pathological nature of the condition. MH is a complex condition and this is reflected in our definition which we justify below. In reaching a definition of such a complex condition it is necessary to include both negative and positive findings. We will then go on to define MH susceptibility.

Table 6.1. In vitro *contracture test results in 55
patients with a history of exertional heat stroke*

MHS	16
MHEh	2
MHEc	11
MHN	36
Total	55

MH, malignant hyperthermia; S, susceptible, Ec,
(equivocal (caffeine positive); Eh, equivocal
equivocal (halothane positive); N, normal.
Source: Kozak-Ribbens, *et al.* (1994).

Steps in reaching a definition of malignant hyperthermia

1. The clinical reaction of MH is a hypermetabolic response manifesting during anaesthesia, with features including hypercapnoea, tachycardia, acidosis, hypoxia, progressive pyrexia and muscle rigidity.
2. The above finding can, however, occur as a result of other conditions, for example sepsis, thryotoxicosis, phaeochromocytoma and cerebral ischaemia. The definition should then be refined to exclude such pathologies and this can be achieved by stipulating that the anaesthetic reaction is the result of an underlying inherited disorder of skeletal muscle.
3 We can go further in describing the nature of this disorder of skeletal muscle as, under carefully controlled conditions (such as those described in the EMHG protocol), muscle fascicles from survivors of MH reactions have consistently abnormal IVCT responses to halothane and also, early studies suggest, to ryanodine. The responses to caffeine are also often abnormal. Inclusion of IVCT criteria in the definition of MH allows us to distinguish MH from other myopathies in which an anaesthetic reaction similar to that of MH occurs (there are, after all, only a limited number of ways diseased muscle can react). Although abnormal IVCT responses do occur in muscle from some patients with these diseases there is no consistent relationship between the clinical reaction and the abnormal laboratory result, i.e. muscle from those who have had a reaction invariably does not react abnormally to IVCT.
4. We must therefore positively exclude those with other recognised myopathies in our definition of MH.

Our definition of MH therefore reads: an inherited disorder of skeletal muscle that can be pharmacologically triggered to produce a potentially fatal combination of hypermetabolism, muscle rigidity and muscle breakdown that is diagnosed by abnormal IVCT responses and the exclusion of other myopathies.

There are families, however, who are generally accepted to have MH who would not be encompassed by this definition. These are families with central core disease and abnormal IVCT typical of MH. This is probably a unique situation likely to result from the close association of the gene for central core disease and one of the genetic loci for MH (Chapter 13).

Malignant hyperthermia susceptibility

This is the term applied to those thought to have the muscle abnormality underlying MH. Although in the future this diagnosis is likely to be made with precision by identifying one of the (as yet undetermined) genetic abnormalities we must have clinically applicable criteria that can be used until genetic diagnosis can be validated. These criteria are that the patient, or relative, has had an anaesthetic reaction compatible with MH and that the patient has abnormal IVCT responses.

Are exertional heat stroke and MH different expressions of the same disease?

To a certain extent we are, as yet, not in a position to give a complete answer to this vital question. Evidence for this assertion can be summarised as follows:

1. Studies of the porcine stress syndrome (Chapter 14) have shown that a single abnormality can cause both exertion-induced and anaesthetic-induced reactions.
2. The clinical manifestations are remarkably similar.
3. Excised muscle bundles from survivors of both syndromes have abnormal IVCT responses, indicating a skeletal muscle abnormality.
4. Investigation by IVCT of family members of survivors of both syndromes indicate an inherited underlying muscle abnormality. In the case of MH, the evidence for an inherited susceptibility is, of course, much stronger (Chapter 13).

Evidence against exertional heat stroke and MH being manifestations of the same abnormality may be summarised as follows:

1. There are no reports of individuals who have had both fulminant exertional heat stroke and MH reactions. Moreover, there are many MH susceptible individuals who have undertaken severe exercise without developing heat stroke. Although heat stroke victims have had uneventful general anaesthesia, the numbers are small and it is known that MH susceptible individuals do not detectably react during every anaesthetic they receive (Ellis *et al.*, 1986).

2. Although IVCT responses are abnormal in survivors of exertional heat stroke and MH, there may be important differences in the nature of these abnormalities. The cardinal feature of MH muscle with the IVCT is that it develops a contracture (as defined in the EMHG protocol) in response to halothane. Supportive evidence is found in approximately 85% of cases with contracture development in response to low concentrations of caffeine. More recently, early contracture development in response to ryanodine has been found to be a very consistent finding in MH-susceptible individuals (Hopkins *et al.*, 1991*b*, 1993: Lenzen *et al.*, 1993). The first feature of the IVCT responses of the heat stroke victims that is worthy of note is the force of contracture developed. While the response to halothane (and in some cases caffeine) is above the threshold value, in those cases where we have the details, the maximum force was at the lower end of the range of abnormality: similar results have been obtained with IVCT carried out on muscle samples taken from patients with a variety of myopathies. The second feature has become apparent in our studies incorporating the ryanodine responses, where there is a lack of consistency between the responses to halothane and ryanodine in the muscle of the heat stroke victims – a feature that is also present in their relatives.

Conclusions

There is a high incidence of abnormal IVCT responses in muscles from individuals with a history of exertional heat stroke, suggesting that one or more skeletal muscle abnormalities are responsible for a significant proportion of exertional heat stroke cases. There is evidence that at least some of these abnormalities may be inherited. Present evidence suggests that exertional heat stroke and MH myopathies are distinct. The risks of anaesthesia with suxamethonium and/or the volatile anaesthetics for those with exertional heat stroke myopathy are unknown, although it seems unlikely that MH susceptibility renders an individual prone to heat stroke.

References

Denborough, M. A. (1982). Heat stroke and malignant hyperpyrexia. *Medical Journal of Australia*, **1**, 204–5.

Ellis, F. R., Halsall, P. J. & Harriman, D. G. F. (1986). The work of the Leeds Malignant Hyperpyrexia Unit 1971–1984. *Anaesthesia*, **41**, 809–15.

Ellis, F. R., Halsall, P. J. & Hopkins, P. M. (1992). Is the K-type halothane/caffeine responder susceptible to malignant hyperthermia? *British Journal of Anaesthesia*, **69**, 468–70.

Ellis, F. R., Harriman, D. G. F., Keaney, N. P., Kyei-Mensah, K. & Tyrrell, J. J.

(1971). Halothane induced muscle contracture as a cause of hyperpyrexia. *British Journal of Anaesthesia*, **43**, 721–2.

European Malignant Hyperpyrexia Group. (1984). A protocol for the investigation of malignant hyperpyrexia susceptibility. *British Journal of Anaesthesia*, **56**, 1267–9.

Gronert, G. A., Thompson, R. L. & Onofrio, B. M. (1980). Human malignant hyperthermia: awake episodes and correction by dantrolene. *Anesthesia and Analgesia*, **59**, 377–8.

Hackl, W., Winkler, M., Mauritz, W., Sporn, P. & Steinbreithner, K. (1991). Muscle biopsy for diagnosis of malignant hyperthermia susceptibility in two patients with severe exercise-induced myolysis. *British Journal of Anaesthesia*, **66**, 138–40.

Heiman-Patterson, T., Rosenberg, H., Fletcher, J. E. & Tahmoush, A. J. (1988). Halothane-caffeine contracture testing in neuromuscular diseases. *Muscle and Nerve*, **11**, 453–7.

Heytens, L., Martin, J. J., Van de Kelft, E. & Bossaert, L. L. (1992). *In vitro* contracture tests in patients with various neuromuscular diseases. *British Journal of Anaesthesia*, **68**, 72–5.

Hopkins, P. M., Ellis, F. R. & Halsall, P. J. (1991a). Evidence for related myopathies in exertional heat stroke and malignant hyperthermia. *Lancet*, **338**, 1491–2.

Hopkins, P. M., Ellis, F. R & Halsall, P. J. (1991b). Ryanodine contracture: a potentially specific *in vitro* diagnostic test for malignant hyperthermia. *British Journal of Anaesthesia*, **66**, 611–13.

Hopkins, P. M., Ellis, F. R. & Halsall, P. J. (1993). Comparison of *in vitro* contracture testing with halothane, caffeine and ryanodine in patients with malignant hyperthermia and other neuromuscular disorders. *British Journal of Anaesthesia*, **70**, 397–401.

Iaizzo, P. A., Klein, W. & Lehmann-Horn, F. (1988). Fura-2 detected myoplasmic calcium and its correlation with contracture force in skeletal muscle from normal and malignant hyperthermia susceptible pigs. *Pflügers Archiv*, **411**, 648–53.

Kalow, W., Britt, B. A., Terreau, M. E. & Haist, C. (1970). Metabolic error of muscle metabolism after recovery from malignant hyperthermia. *Lancet*, **2**, 895–98.

Knochel, J. P. (1989). Heat stroke and related heat stress disorders. *Disease of the Month*, **35**, 301–77.

Kozak-Ribbens, G., Rodet, L., Petrognani, R., Figarella-Branger, D., Desnuelle, C., Pellisier, J. F., Cozzone, P. J. & Aubuert, M. (1994). Hyperthermie d'effort: resultats des explorations de 55 patients. *Minerva Anestesiologica*, **60**(Suppl. 3), 177–81.

Lehmann-Horn, F. & Iaizzo, P. A. (1990). Are myotonias and periodic paralyses associated with susceptibility to malignant hyperthermia? *British Journal of Anaesthesia*, **65**, 692–7.

Lenzen, C., Roewer, N., Wappler, F., Scholz, J., Kahl, J., Blank, M., Rumberger, E., Schulte, A. M. & Esch, J. (1993). Accelerated contractures after administration of ryanodine to skeletal muscle of malignant hyperthermia susceptible patients. *British Journal of Anaesthesia*, **71**, 242–6.

Wingard, D. W. & Gatz, E. E. (1978). Some observations on stress susceptible patients. In *The Second International Symposium on Malignant Hyperthermia*. J. A. Aldrete & B. A. Britt ed. pp. 363–72. New York, Grune and Stratton.

7

Future research in exertional heat stroke

P. M. HOPKINS

Introduction

The preceding chapters have defined exertional heat stroke, described its epidemiology and clinical and pathophysiological features. Chapters 4, 5 and 6 have described some of the approaches used to investigate exertional heat stroke. Much progress has been made in identifying environmental and other extrinsic factors that predispose individuals to the development of exertional heat stroke. It is clear, however, that some individuals appear to be intrinsically at greater risk than others in the same environmental conditions and in the absence of known external factors.

Heat stroke results from an inability to lose excessive heat. In classical heat stroke the excessive heat is gained from the environment and illness develops when the capacity to lose heat is exceeded: the degree of hydration appears to be a key factor in determining when this occurs. Exertional heat stroke differs in that heat is also generated by the muscular activity and it is differences in metabolic activity of the skeletal muscle that seem to predispose some individuals to be at greater risk of developing exertional heat stroke. In extreme conditions anybody subjecting themselves to significant physical exertion is potentially susceptible, hence the protocol of the British Army described in Chapter 1. Some individuals may subject themselves to predisposing factors (again detailed in Chapter 1), making the development of exertional heat stroke more likely in less extreme conditions. It is the remaining heat stroke victims, i.e. those with few or no predisposing factors, who develop the condition in relatively temperate conditions who perhaps warrant the majority of research effort. This is because, unlike those who appear to be less susceptible, exertional heat stroke can not always be avoided by limiting predisposing factors and avoiding exercise in extreme conditions.

I would like to use this brief chapter to propose a scheme of multidisciplinary research designed to identify and investigate these more susceptible individuals. The proposals are not intended to be exhaustive in their detailed description of potential experiments but indicate areas that are likely to steer later research in the most fruitful directions.

The human physiology laboratory

Epidemiological data (Chapter 1) give an indication of the incidence of heat stroke episodes. Inevitably these occur in different environmental conditions and it is impossible to determine what role, if any, was played by an individual's inherent susceptibility. In the laboratory situation standardised patterns of exercise can be performed in controlled conditions enabling direct comparisons to be made between individuals. It would thus be possible to define population characteristics of a range of variables measured in response to the exercise. Although many subjects are likely to be required it would be of great interest to determine whether the distribution of any such characteristic in the population was bimodal.

^{31}P nuclear magnetic resonance spectroscopy

This is potentially a hugely important tool in any area of research involving muscle. Payen and Stieglitz (Chapter 5) provide an excellent account of the theory behind the method and describe their early findings in heat stroke victims. They could not demonstrate any statistically significant differences from normal patients but it must be remembered that the number of patients investigated so far is small and that heat stroke victims are likely to represent a heterogeneous group. It would be interesting to observe whether subjecting the limb to stress (ishaemic, heat, pharmacological) would produce greater abnormalities in heat stroke victims.

In vitro *muscle physiology and biochemistry*

As described in Chapter 6 several groups have reported abnormal responses of skeletal muscle from heat stroke victims when tested with the *in vitro* contracture test protocols as used in the investigation of malignant hyperthermia susceptibility. The drugs used in these tests have proved useful in delineating abnormal responses in heat stroke patients despite being chosen for their efficacy in a condition triggered by anaesthetic drugs rather than by a combination of environmental heat and exercise. In our studies the addition of a ryanodine contracture test increased the information obtained from these studies. This raises the possibility that there are further, or alternative, drugs that may be more specific contracture-inducing agents in muscle from heat stroke victims; such drugs might include adrenergic stimulants and/or phosphodiesterase inhibitors. These additional studies may, in turn, provide evidence for potential defects underlying increased susceptibility to exertional heat stroke that can be investigated using appropriate electrophysiological or subcellular biochemical techniques. Whatever the range of experiments used, there is much to be learnt about the aetiological role of skeletal muscle pathologies in exertional heat stroke from investigating more victims by muscle biopsy and subsequent physiological testing.

Molecular genetic studies

It now seems likely that an increased predisposition to the development of exertional heat stroke may be genetically inherited (Chapter 6). This possibility opens up a further line of investigation of abnormalities underlying this predisposition. The type of study that could be used would follow those used in the investigation of the molecular genetics of malignant hyperthermia (Chapter 13). A necessary prerequisite in the initial linkage studies would, however, require many members of a family to be characterised for muscle abnormalities. At present there are no such families who have been sufficiently investigated.

Section 2

Malignant hyperthermia

8

Clinical presentation of malignant hyperthermia

P. J. HALSALL

Introduction

Nowadays the term malignant hyperthermia (MH) is something of a misnomer. The rise in temperature associated with MH is a late and sometimes absent sign. Better monitoring facilities indicate other abnormalities, in particular a rising end-tidal CO_2 and an unexplained persistent tachycardia, occur well before the core temperature begins to rise. In 1960, however, when MH was first described pyrexia was the most impressive clinical feature and the name certainly reflects the dramatic and potentially fatal outcome of an MH reaction.

Fortuitously the first case reported by Denborough & Lovell (Denborough *et al.*, 1960, 1962) enabled both the clinical signs and the mode of inheritance as an autosomal dominant gene or genes, to be described. Undoubtedly MH has accounted for a significant proportion of unexpected, un- explained anaesthetic deaths prior to its recognition.

The first case reported in 1960 involved a young man who was terrified of having general anaesthesia for a fractured tibia and fibula because 11 relatives (out of 24 having had general anaesthesia), including cousins, uncles and aunts, had died during general anaesthesia, all except one undergoing minor surgical procedures. These deaths were thought to be related to ether anaesthesia, so he was anaesthetised with thiopentone, nitrous oxide, oxygen and halothane. Within 10 minutes he developed a tachycardia, low blood pressure, cyanosis and became very hot and sweaty. Anaesthesia was terminated and active cooling instituted and he recovered after about two hours. Extensive investigations, e.g. chest radiograph, thyroid function tests, urinary catecholamine studies and porphyrins were entirely normal. A subsequent spinal anaesthetic caused no problems. Examination of the records of the deceased relatives showed temperatures of 42–43°C with no postmortem abnormalities.

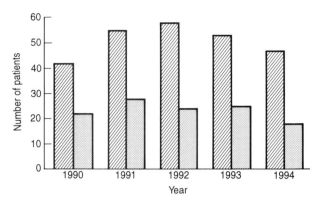

Figure 8.1. The yearly referral rate of probands (1990–1994) indicating the proportion proved MH susceptible (MHS). (▨), Total cases; (▨), MHS.

In the ensuing years further cases were reported and with the development of *in vitro* contracture test (IVCT) screening, specialised centres were set up enabling clinical cases to be collated. It became apparent that MH could present in a variety of ways ranging from the classical fulminant description to relatively mild forms and also some unexpected presentations.

Even within the short history of MH the pattern of presentation has changed as anaesthetists have become more knowledgeable and aware of the problem. It is now rare for fulminant reactions to develop as the suspected diagnosis is made early in the development of the reaction enabling treatment to be instituted at an early stage. Thus, many of the signs associated with MH may be attenuated or absent. This awareness, together with the availability of intravenous dantrolene, has contributed to the fall in mortality rate. Originally, the mortality rate was 70–80% but is now about 2–3% in the UK, reflecting one death per year over recent years, although the incidence of new referrals remains roughly the same (Figure 8.1) as previously reported (Ellis *et al.*, 1986; Halsall & Ellis, 1993). This improvement in the mortality rate is seen worldwide.

The incidence of MH is difficult to estimate but is generally accepted to be in the order of 1 in 10 000 to 20 000. In the UK this represents between 20 and 30 new cases (i.e. probands) identified every year. All races are affected. In socio-economic terms MH is the major cause of unexpected anaesthetic morbidity and mortality in young fit patients. An intriguing aspect is that male probands occur about twice as frequently as females (Figure 8.2) and the commonest age group is 10–30 years, the incidence dropping dramatically in older age groups (Figure 8.3).

MH reactions are more common in certain types of operative procedure,

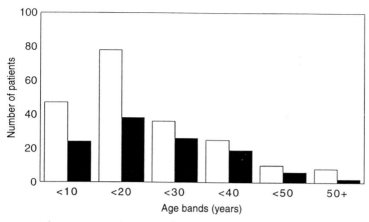

Figure 8.2. The male/female ratio of malignant hyperthermia-susceptible probands. (□), Males 66%, (■), females 34%.

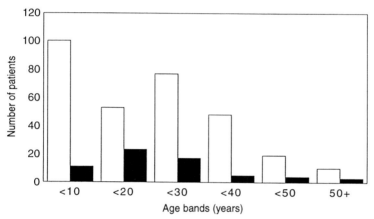

Figure 8.3. Age distribution of malignant hyperthermia-susceptible probands. (□), Total; (■), deaths.

such as trauma, orthopaedic, dental, ear, nose and throat, and eye surgery. This finding led to the suggestion that there was an increased incidence of musculoskeletal abnormalities (e.g. squints) in MH susceptible patients and that 'stress' associated with trauma was a predisposing factor. Great care, however, should be taken when interpreting the above epidemiological findings. A simple explanation may be that this group of patients is exposed to the 'triggering' anaesthetic agents more frequently because of the favoured anaesthetic technique. The male preponderance may reflect the differing lifestyles of the sexes, males presenting more frequently with minor trauma and for orthopaedic procedures. Nevertheless, even accounting for this there remains an underlying unexplained higher incidence of male probands. Family studies of relatives with a 50% chance of MH support an autosomal dominant pattern of inheritance (Ellis *et al.*, 1986).

Preoperative presentation

Patients susceptible to MH are usually impossible to identify before operation, except in a few circumstances. It should be emphasised that previous uneventful exposure to general anaesthesia, even with the known triggering agents, does not exclude the possibility of MH. Many probands, including those who have died from fulminant MH, have had previous anaesthesia (Halsall *et al.*, 1979). The reason for this inconsistency of response remains a mystery. Despite this, clearly the preoperative assessment of a patient should include questions relating to previous exposure to anaesthesia and the family anaesthetic history. A family history of an unexplained, unexpected anaesthetic death/cardiac arrest is often significant (see later).

It has been suggested that MH is associated with a multiplicity of abnormalities, particularly musculoskeletal in origin. Indeed, Britt (1988) lists 25 conditions predisposing to MH, including such features as poor dental enamel, dyslexia, as well as squints, hernias, scoliosis and arthrogryphosis multiplex. In the latter condition, it has been shown that such patients may develop a hypermetabolic response to anaesthesia, which is unrelated to MH (Hopkins *et al.*, 1991). A review of our own patients ($n = 2500$) does not indicate the presence of any abnormal features; indeed, the MH-susceptible group appear remarkably 'normal' (Ellis, presented at the Munich International MH Workshop, 1991).

The King–Denborough syndrome is also said to be associated, although as this diagnosis is not precise, the association with MH is uncertain. The King–Denborough syndrome is said to be a recessive trait, and includes such features as down-slanting palpebral fissures, ptosis, low set ears, malar and mandibular hyperplasia, short stature, scoliosis, cryptorchidism, mildly progressive myopathy and contractures (King & Denborough, 1973).

Muscle diseases, e.g. muscular dystrophy, cause anaesthetic problems in their own right, and the inconsistent minor IVCT contractures reported in these patients probably reflect the diseased muscle rather than true MH (Lehmann-Horn & Knorr-Held, 1990; Lehmann-Horn & Iaizzo, 1990). The only clearly associated muscle disorder is central core disease (CCD) (Brownell, 1989), although interestingly this is not an invariable association. CCD presents as weakness which may be mild and unrecognised by the patients to more severe weakness, wasting and scoliosis.

Other conditions said to be associated with MH are sudden infant death syndrome (SIDS), neuroleptic malignant syndrome (NMS) and heat stroke. A postulated increased incidence of MH in parents of SIDS (Denborough *et al.*, 1982) has not been substantiated by a three-part study involving the incidence of MH in SIDS, the incidence of SIDS in MH susceptible parents and IVCT studies in SIDS parents (Ellis *et al.*, 1988).

NMS produces a similar clinical picture to an MH reaction, occurring in response to neuroleptic drugs, e.g. halo-peridol and phenothiazines, and dantrolene is an effective treatment. The MH centre in Lille has made a particular study of patients with the NMS and found all to be MH normal (Krisovic-Harker & Adnet, 1989; Chapter 15).

Heat stroke victims present with similar features to an MH crisis. An association has been proposed, but so far not confirmed and further studies in these patients are needed (Hopkins *et al.*, 1991; Section 1).

The role of stress in the aetiology of MH is difficult to assess. A similar, but probably recessive condition, occurs in pigs which can develop marked reactions leading to death without anaesthesia, known as the porcine stress syndrome (PSS; Chapter 14). In a series of porcine studies it was suggested that α agonist activity precipitated MH in pigs, whereas β adrenergic stimulation (Hall *et al.*, 1977; Lister *et al.*, 1976) exerted some protection. The suggestion that unexplained sudden death unrelated to anaesthesia is more common in MH families (Wingard, 1974) has never been substantiated. Stress was thought a potential factor in triggering an MH reaction because of the possible association of trauma and MH reactions. It is well known that MH patients do not react to the triggering drugs on each occasion, leading to the theory that for a reaction to occur three factors need to be present: the inherited predisposition, exposure to the triggering drugs and a third missing factor. It was easy to select 'stress' as this missing factor.

In summary, MH can only be suspected before the operation if there is a history of CCD, a personal or family history of MH or an unexplained, unexpected anaesthetic death/cardiac arrest.

Presentation of a malignant hyperthermia crisis

Unfortunately there is no symptom or sign that is unique to MH. The diagnosis depends on the combination of characteristic signs with particular reference to the timing of events. A crisis can develop in a variety of ways ranging from a fulminant life-threatening or fatal event with major metabolic derangements such that a crisis is often described as a 'metabolic storm' to one with mild signs and symptoms (see later). The clinical diagnosis can therefore often be difficult and because of the potentially fatal nature of a reaction, anaesthetists will intervene early in order to abort the response. Thus characteristic signs may well be absent.

Characteristic signs seen in malignant hyperthermia

1. Masseter muscle spasm
2. Generalised muscle rigidity
3. Unexplained increasing persistent tachycardia that may lead to arrhythmias
4. Unexplained tachypnoea or increasing hypercarbia
5. Difficulty in maintaining oxygen saturation
6. Increasing core temperature usually greater than 2 °C per hour and maybe up to 5 °C per hour.

Apart from masseter muscle spasm following the administration of suxamethonium, a combination of increasing tachycardia and hypercarbia are the earliest signs of the development of MH.

Laboratory abnormalities include:

1. Metabolic acidosis
2. Hyperkalaemia
3. Marked increase in creatine kinase (CK); initial and 24 hours later. CK is slow to appear in the serum, hence the later estimation is essential
4. Myoglobinuria (first specimen of urine) which may lead to renal failure if gross. Indeed postoperative renal failure can be the presenting sign
5. Rarely evidence of disseminated intravascular coagulopathy.

A clear contemporaneous record is essential when assessing the likelihood of MH as the cause of the abnormal reaction. The onset of abnormalities may occur dramatically almost immediately after induction or may have an insidious onset depending on the anaesthetic technique used. For example it may take up to two hours of anaesthesia using a small concentration of enflurane, as part of a balanced anaesthetic technique, before any abnormalities develop.

The important implications of an MH diagnosis to both the patient and their family mean that a suspicious reaction can not be ignored and should be referred for expert opinion. Nevertheless, there are mimics of MH that should be considered as they can usually be eliminated from the differential diagnosis by straightforward investigations.

'Light anaesthesia' may account for tachycardia and tachypnoea, pyrexia may result from an infective process either caused by the condition requiring surgery or by a concurrent infection and can easily be excluded by differential white blood cell count and other appropriate investigations, e.g. chest radiograph. A presentation comprising predominantly of the metabolic signs of MH may be due to thyrotoxicosis or phaeochromocytoma which can be excluded by thyroid function tests and urinary ca echolamine studies respectively. A predominantly muscle-sign presentation may be due to a muscle disease, particularly the myotonias that can be very mild and asymptomatic. These can be excluded by resting CK estimations, electromyographic (EMG) studies and neurological assessment. As already discussed, a variety of muscle diseases cause problems with anaesthesia in their own right and although some of the symptoms may suggest the clinical diagnosis of MH the only accepted association is with CCD (Lehmann-Horn & Knorr-Held, 1990).

Occasionally, MH presents after an operation with evidence of rhabdomyolysis, i.e. discoloured urine and sometimes renal failure, without any apparent intraoperative problem. Histological examination of the muscle as well as IVCT studies is important in these patients to exclude underlying muscle pathology.

Classification of the clinical presentation

There is no currently universally accepted method for the classification of the various presentations of clinical MH reactions. Britt originally grouped patients as 'rigid' or 'non-rigid' (Britt & Kalow, 1970) but this method has not been followed despite a general agreement that the clinical signs fall into two distinct categories, metabolic and muscle in origin. More recently Halsall and colleagues (Ellis *et al.*, 1990) have published the clinical presentation of 402 probands on the basis of a classification system first proposed by Ørding & Ranklev (personal communication). At present an attempt to devise a more objective MH scoring system based on the Delphi consensus method is underway. Clinical information is often sparse, records are not available and relevant investigations incomplete, so that it is virtually impossible to define strict objective criteria when classifying individual patient reactions. Nevertheless, it is usually possible to gain an overall impression of the MH crisis such that a proband can be allocated to one of eight mutually exclusive categories.

A Fulminant/classical
  This is a life-threatening event which includes a multiplicity of marked metabolic and muscle anomalies requiring very active treatment.
B Moderate
  This group includes both metabolic and muscle signs but the situation does not appear life-threatening and the treatment required included the withdrawal of trigger agents and only a single dose of dantrolene.
C Mild signs only of mild metabolic derangements without muscle signs.

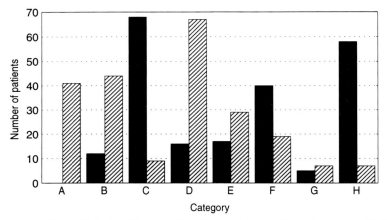

Figure 8.4. Incidence of malignant hyperthermia susceptibility in the eight categories of clinical presentation as defined in Table 8.1. (■), MH negative; (▨), MH-susceptible.

D Masseter muscle spasm with evidence of muscle involvement, i.e. high CK and myoglobinuria.
E Masseter muscle spasm with accompanying metabolic disturbance, e.g. arrhythmia and increasing core temperature.
F Masseter muscle spasm alone.
G Unexplained anaesthetic death or cardiac arrest.
H Other, e.g. postoperative pyrexias, rhabdomyolysis, renal failure, suspect family history.

These classifications correlate well with the IVCT results (Figure 8.4) and an incidence of MH susceptibility can be given for each group (Table 8.1). Interestingly, one patient in the fulminant group was apparently MHN (negative). This patient, a 16-year-old male, died. Both parents were MHN although the father suspected he was not the natural father. Many years later the deceased boy's child was screened, proving to be clearly MH-susceptible (MHS).

Groups A–C

Patients with these presentations are straightforward and require no further comment.

Masseter muscle spasm (Groups D, E and F)

This is a controversial topic not least because masseter muscle spasm (MMS) is a subjective sign. This difficulty is compounded by the demonstration of

Table 8.1. *Shows the probability of malignant hyperthermia in each category of clinical presentation*

Clinical category	Incidence of MHS (%)
A. Fulminant	96
B. Moderate	88
C. Mild	14
D. MMS and muscle signs	76
E. MMS and metabolic signs	56
F. MMS alone	28
G. Unexplained anaesthetic death/cardiac arrest	66
H. Others, e.g. postoperative pyrexias, renal failure	7

MHS, malignant hyperthermia susceptibility.

reduced mouth opening and a short period (less than one minute) of increased jaw tone following the administration of suxamethonium in both children (Van Der Spek *et al.*, 1987) and adults (Leary & Ellis, 1990). Clearly MMS is difficult to define and relies on the interpretation of the attendant anaesthetist. It may be that MMS represents an extreme of a normal distribution.

It has been described as the most common manifestation of MH and is certainly one of the earliest signs, making tracheal intubation difficult or impossible, although chest-inflation is usually not impaired. The incidence of MMS in MH-susceptible probands has been variously reported; 80% by Britt & Kalow (1970), 64% by Ellis & Halsall (1984), 50% by Rosenberg & Fletcher (1986). Two studies (Schwartz *et al.*, 1984; Carroll, 1987) reported a very high incidence of MMS in children. In the latter study no patient had muscle confirmation of their suspected clinical MH reaction and in the former study all patients tested were claimed to be MH susceptible, however, MH testing in this case was by the now discredited calcium uptake technique (Nararajan *et al.*, 1987). Another review of children presenting with MMS showed 50% to be susceptible to MH (Christian *et al.*, 1989). As already stated the incidence of MH susceptibility in probands who develop MMS correlates well with further corroborative evidence of muscle involvement, e.g. very high CK values and myoglobinuria. In addition, MH-susceptible patients frequently describe very severe muscle stiffness and immobility persisting for several days.

When MMS appears to be the only presenting sign (group F), the incidence of MH susceptibility is low (28%). This group, however, would include patients in whom other abnormalities may have been present, but not recorded. We strongly recommend that MMS should still be regarded as an indicator of MH susceptibility.

Group G

In view of the high incidence of MH susceptible probands in this group, a family history of an unexplained unexpected anaesthetic cardiac arrest/death (group G), should alert the anaesthetist to the possibility of MH, and attempts should be made to elicit further information.

Group H

The very low incidence of MH susceptibility in group H (others), in which by far the largest numerical group was the postoperative pyrexias, prompted further study of this particular group. From 30 patients, some of whom described dramatic events 'packed in ice', fanned, admitted to an intensive care unit, recurrent episodes, family history, all were quite clearly MH normal. Thus a postoperative pyrexia alone, without intraoperative problems, assuming a reasonable standard of intraoperative monitoring, does not warrant screening for MH susceptibility (Halsall & Ellis, 1992). The other presentations in this group, an unexpected postoperative renal failure and myoglobinuria, are highly indicative of MH or possibly other muscle pathology.

The character of MH has changed since its first recognition. The mortality has significantly decreased and the clinical signs are usually less florid. These changes have been brought about by the vigilance and knowledge of anaesthetists and the availability of monitoring facilities. Further inroads into the significance of the variety of presentations will only be made when the relevant clinical investigations are complete in all patients.

Fortunately MH is rare, but the occurrence of new cases remarkably remains the same. Until such time as there is a routine preoperative blood test for MH susceptibility, the mortality and morbidity for an MH crisis will continue to depend solely on the skills of the anaesthetist.

References

Britt, B. A. (1988). Hereditary and epidemiological aspects of malignant hyperthermia. In *Malignant Hyperthermia: Current Concepts.*, ed. F. Nalda, S. Gottman., H. J. Khambatta, pp. 19–39. Normed Verlag, Bad Homberg.

Britt, B. A. & Kalow, W. (1970). Malignant hyperthermia: a statistical review. *Canadian Anaesthetists Society Journal*, **59**, 273–31.

Brownell, A. K. W. (1989). Malignant hyperthermia: relationship to other diseases. *British Journal of Anaesthesia*, **60**, 303–8.

Carroll, J. B. (1987). Increased incidence of masseter spasm in children with strabismus anesthetized with halothane and succinylcholine. *Anesthesiology*, **66**, 680–5.

Christian, A. S., Ellis, F. R. & Halsall, P. J. (1989). Is there a relationship between masseteric muscle spasm and malignant hyperpyrexia? *British Journal of Anaesthesia*, **62**, 540–4.

Denborough, M. A., Forster, J. F. A. & Lovell, R. R. A. (1960). Anaesthetic deaths in a family. *Lancet*, **ii**, 45.

Denborough, M. A., Forster, J. F. A., Lovell, R. R. A. Maplestone, P. A. & Villiers, J. D. (1962). Anaesthetic deaths in a family. *British Journal of Anaesthesia*, **34**, 395–6.

Denborough, M. A., Galloway, G. J. & Hopkinson, K. C. (1982). Malignant hyperthermia and sudden infant death. *Lancet*, **2**, 1068.

Ellis, F. R. & Halsall, P. J. (1984). Suxamethonium spasm; a differential diagnostic conundrum. *British Journal of Anaesthesia*, **56**, 381–4.

Ellis, F. R., Halsall, P. J. & Christian, A. S. (1990). Clinical presentation of suspected malignant hyperthermia due to anaesthesia in 402 probands. *Anaesthesia*, **45**, 838–41.

Ellis, F. R., Halsall, P. J. & Harriman, D. G. F. (1986). The work of the Leeds Malignant Hyperthermia Unit, 1971–84. *Anaesthesia*, **41**, 809–15.

Ellis, F. R., Halsall, P. J. & Harriman, D. G. F. (1988). Malignant hyperthermia and sudden infant death syndrome. *British Journal of Anaesthesia*, **60**, 28–30.

Hall, G. M., Lucke, J. N. & Lister, D. (1977). Porcine MH. V: fatal hyperthermia in Pietran pig associated with infusion of adrenergic agonists. *British Journal of Anaesthesia*, **49**, 855–962.

Halsall, P. J., Cain, P. A. & Ellis, F. R. (1979). Retrospective analysis of anaesthesia received by patients before malignant hyperpyrexia was recognised. *British Journal of Anaesthesia*, **51**, 949–54.

Halsall, P. J. & Ellis, F. R. (1992). Does post-operative pyrexia indicate malignant hyperthermia susceptibility? *British Journal of Anaesthesia*, **68**, 209–230.

Halsall, P. J. & Ellis, F. R. (1993). Malignant hyperthermia. In *Bailliere's Clinical Anaesthesiology*, vol.7, No.2. *The Anaesthetic Crisis*, ed. McD. Fisher, pp. 343–56. Bailliere Tindall. London.

Hopkins, P. M., Ellis, F. R. & Halsall, P. J. (1991*a*). Hypermetabolism in arthrogyphosis multiplex congenita. *Anaesthesia*, **46**, 374–5.

Hopkins, P. M., Ellis, F. R. & Halsall, P.J. (1991*b*). Evidence for related myopathies in exertional heat stroke and malignant hyperthermia. *Lancet*, **338**, 1491–2.

King, J. O. & Denborough, M. A. (1973). Anaesthetic induced malignant hyperpyrexia in children. *Journal of Pediatrics*, **83**, 37–40.

Krisovic-Horber, R. & Adnet, P. J. (1989). Malignant hyperthermia and neurolept malignant syndrome. *Beitrage zur Anaesthesiologie und Intensivmedizin*, **27**, 108–13.

Leary, N. P. & Ellis, F. R. (1990). Masseteric muscle spasm as a normal response to suxamethonium. *British Journal of Anaesthesia*, **64**, 488–92.

Lehmann-Horn, F. & Iaizzo, P. A. (1990). Are myotonias and periodic paralysis associated with susceptibility to malignant hyperthermia? *British Journal of Anaesthesia*, **65**, 692–7.

Lehmann-Horn, F. & Knorr-Held, S. (1990). Muscle diseases relevant to the anaesthetist. *Acta Anaestheologica Belgica*, **41**, 113–18.

Lister, D., Hall, G. M. & Lucke, J. N. (1976). Porcine MH. *III*: adrenergic blockade. *British Journal of Anaesthesia*, **48**, 831–7.

Nararajan, K. Fishbein, W. N., Muldoon, S. M. & Pezeshkar, G. (1987). Calcium uptake in frozen muscle biopsy sections compared with other predictors of malignant hyperthermia susceptibility. *Anesthesiology*, **66**, 680–5.

Rosenberg, H. & Fletcher, J. E. (1986). Masseter muscle rigidity and MH susceptibility. *Anesthesia and Analgesia*, **65**, 163–4.

Schwartz, L., Rockoff, M. A. & Kola, B.V. (1984). Masseter spasm with anesthesia: incidence and complications. *Anesthesiology*, **61**, 722–5.

Van der Spek, A. F. L., Fang, W. B., Ashton-Miller, L. T. A., Stohler, S., Coulson, D. S. & Schork, M. A. (1987). The effects of suxamethonium on mouth opening. *Anesthesiology*, **67**, 459–65.

Wingard, W. W. (1974). Malignant hyperthermia: a human stress syndrome? *Lancet*, **iv**, 1450–1.

9

Clinical management of malignant hyperthermia

G. A. GRONERT and J. F. ANTOGNINI

Introduction

Malignant hyperthermia (MH) can have an exceedingly rapid course with physiological changes and hypermetabolism, manifested as increased carbon dioxide and lactic acid production. Cell permeability increases with the release of creatine phosphokinase (CK) and myoglobin, with the ominous sequela of renal failure. Other sequelae include cerebral oedema, disseminated intravascular coagulation (DIC) and electrolyte abnormalities. Successful treatment of MH requires discriminate, quick action and specific attention to each of these problems. The introduction of dantrolene in 1979 dramatically increased the survival of patients who develop episodes of MH. This chapter discusses the clinical management of MH and the management of patients who are MH susceptible.

Treatment of a malignant hyperthermia crisis

The response to and treatment of a suspected MH episode or an actual MH episode will depend on the clinical presentation. MH presentations can be arbitrarily separated into (1) fulminant, (2) abortive, (3) masseter spasm and (4) atypical (Ørding, 1985; Ranklev-Twetman, 1990).

Fulminant

In the past, MH episodes were often fulminant, primarily because of the late recognition of the syndrome. Most anaesthesiologists today are trained to recognise an MH episode and utilize a capnograph and so it is unusual to have a fulminant occurrence of MH. Treatment of fulminant cases of MH requires a quick response and teamwork. The metabolic derangements of MH, i.e.

Table 9.1. *Drug use in malignant hyperthermia*

Contraindicated	Safe
Halothane	Opiates
Enflurane	Barbiturates
Isoflurane	Propofol
Desflurane	Etomidate
Sevoflurane	Ketamine
Succinylcholine	Amide/ester local anaesthetics
Curare (weak depolariser)	Calcium
	Noradrenaline
	Adrenaline
	Digoxin/digitoxin

Table 9.2. *Treatment of a malignant hyperthermia crisis*

1. Stop all triggering anaesthetic agents, hyperventilate with 100% O_2 (more than 10 L/min) to obtain a normal $PaCO_2$
2. Administer dantrolene 2–3 mg/kg intravenously, and repeat every five minutes as needed for a response, up to a total of 10 mg/kg
3. Give $NaHCO_3$ 2–4 mEq/kg. Administer additional $NaHCO_3$ as needed for ongoing acidosis
4. Cool patient via: (1) intravenous iced saline, (2) surface cooling, and (3) lavage body cavities with sterile iced saline. Stop at 38–39 °C to avoid cooling below 37 °C
5. Place urinary catheter to monitor urine volume and colour. If cola-coloured, centrifuge; if the plasma is clear, then the coloration is due to intact red blood cells; if the plasma remains cola-coloured after centrifugation, then either rhabdomyolysis or haemolysis has occurred, and forced alkaline diuresis is mandated
6. Monitor blood gases, electrolytes, serum and urine myoglobins, and coagulation studies. Hyperkalaemia may occur; treat with $NaHCO_3$, insulin, glucose and calcium

severe acidosis, hyperkalaemia and profound hyperthermia, wreak havoc within the cells of the body and can eventually lead to end-organ damage and death. Dantrolene is the key to the treatment in these cases. Dantrolene halts the hypermetabolic process in the muscle, which reverses the secondary manifestations of MH, such as hyperkalaemia, acidosis, increased CK, DIC etc. Dantrolene must be administered quickly because the falling cardiac output will decrease perfusion to the tissues, including muscle.

Dantrolene acts by inhibiting the release of calcium from the sarcoplasmic reticulum. Dantrolene was originally developed as a urinary antibiotic, but its muscle relaxant properties were discovered through further investigation of its actions. It was also found to have little or no effect on cardiac or smooth muscles. In 1975 Harrison reported the use of dantrolene in malignant hyperthermic swine (Harrison, 1975). This important study established that dantrolene could act specifically in muscle to reverse the metabolic process that occurred with porcine MH, and that dantrolene might be an important agent in the management of human MH. In a non-randomised multicentre study, Kolb *et al.* (1982) demonstrated the efficacy of dantrolene in human MH; because of ethical and practical considerations, this study could not be performed in a blinded and placebo controlled fashion. The marked response, however, of patients who received dantrolene during treatment for MH indicated that dantrolene could dramatically reverse the metabolic derangements of human MH. Subsequent clinical experience further indicated that dantrolene is probably the single most important treatment modality in human MH. When administered acutely, dantrolene has limited side-effects, although it can cause some muscle weakness. There is enough muscle tone to maintain adequate coughing, deep breathing and airway control. Dantrolene 20 mg is mixed with 88 mg sodium hydroxide and 2 g mannitol, and it must be dissolved in sterile water. Heating the bottle in warm water will help in solubilising the dantrolene. Dantrolene is administered in an initial dose of 2 mg/kg, and this may be repeated every five to ten minutes to a total of approximately 10 mg/kg.

Other treatments for MH include the following:

1. Stop all anaesthetic triggering drugs and ventilate with 100% oxygen. Ventilation should be adjusted and increased to obtain a normal arterial CO_2. High flows of oxygen will eliminate inhalational agents from the anaesthesia machine, so that valuable time should not be wasted changing the machine.
2. Anaesthesia can be maintained with nitrous oxide and non-triggering agents, such as propofol, barbiturates, midazolam, opiates, non-depolarising muscle relaxants etc.
3. Sodium bicarbonate should be given in doses of approximately 2–4 mEq/kg. Additional bicarbonate can be guided by blood gas analysis.
4. The patient should be cooled using a variety of techniques, including surface cooling and cooling of body cavities with cold, sterile fluids. It is rare to be able quickly to place a patient on cardiopulmonary bypass and cool by that technique. Cooling measures should be discontinued when the temperature has reached 38–39 °C, as the temperature will continue to drift downward.
5. Laboratory investigations include examination of urine for myoglobinuria and blood tests for liver enzymes, DIC, electrolytes and arterial blood gases.

Because the release of myoglobin can adversely affect kidney function and can indeed result in acute renal failure, the administration of a diuretic, such as mannitol or furosemide (frusemide) is warranted.

Many of the adverse consequences of MH, including hyperkalaemia, DIC and cardiac arrhythmias, will abate once treatment has been initiated with dantrolene. Although specific therapy for each of these and other secondary problems of MH is indicated, the primary goal of treating MH is administration of dantrolene. Those agents which have no specific role in MH, and in fact may be contraindicated, include the calcium antagonists, such as verapamil, nifedipine and diltiazem. These drugs can interact with high dose dantrolene and result in severe hyperkalaemia. (Saltzman *et al*, 1984; Rubin & Zablocki, 1987; Yoganathan *et al.*, 1988). The cooling measures outlined above are important not only in terms of preventing the sequelae of MH, but because hyperthermia itself appears to be a triggering factor for MH in susceptible pigs (Ørding *et al.*, 1985) and may, therefore, be important in man.

Once stabilised, the patient should be observed in an intensive care unit for at least 24 hours, with continued close monitoring of vital signs and adequacy of urine output. Serial CKs should be obtained, and dantrolene 2 mg/kg should be administered every 8–12 hours according to clinical and metabolic signs. This dosing regimen will maintain adequate plasma levels of dantrolene because the half-life of dantrolene is approximately ten hours. Once the patient is stabilised and there has been no end-organ malfunction or the damage has resolved, the patient may be discharged home with instructions to undergo muscle biopsy.

Abortive

All the signs of MH are non-specific, and it is sometimes difficult to establish a correct diagnosis. Arrhythmias, tachycardia, temperature elevation, rigidity, rhabdomyolysis, hypoxaemia, hypercarbia and acidosis can all result from numerous other entities. In fact, the presence of only one of these signs makes MH an unlikely diagnosis. Ellis *et al.* (1990) described the presentation of MH in 402 probands; these patients underwent contracture testing to determine MH susceptibility. Those who were classified as having had fulminant classical MH, i.e. marked hypermetabolism and abnormal muscle activity with metabolic acidosis, temperature greater than 38.8 °C, muscle rigidity and CK greater than 1500 IU/L, had a 96% chance of being MH susceptible. Those patients who had a moderate presentation had an 88% chance of being MH susceptible. Those patients with a mild presentation (i.e. pH greater than 7.30

and temperature less than 38.5 °C), however, had only a 14% chance of being MH susceptible. The presence of masseter spasm, in conjunction with other signs, also made MH susceptibility more likely, as did an unexplained anaesthetic death as a result of cardiac arrest. Interestingly, the least likely factors were postoperative pyrexia and postoperative rhabdomyolysis. These results are discussed in more detail in Chapter 8. In a similar study, Larach *et al* described the presentation in 48 patients who had suspected MH and who underwent muscle biopsy (Larach *et al*, 1987). This smaller study corroborates that by Ellis *et al* (1990) in that more than one sign was necessary to reasonably predict MH susceptibility. For example, in seven patients in whom masseter rigidity, acidosis or temperature elevation were the sole adverse anaesthetic events, the muscle biopsy was negative (Larach, *et al.*, 1987).

MH susceptible patients have varied responses to triggering agents, for unexplained reasons. This may be related to the use of adjunctive agents such as barbiturates, non-depolarising muscle relaxants, tranquilisers and depressants, all of which delay the onset of MH (Gronert & Milde, 1981a). Halsall *et al.* (1979) reviewed prior anaesthetics in 73 patients with MH. Many of these patients had received triggering agents prior to the diagnosis of MH, and these exposures were uneventful. The lack of response could not be attributed, in many cases, to other agents, as halothane and succinylcholine were often the only agents used. Thus, an MH susceptible patient may have an absolutely normal response to triggering agents, or may have a fulminant episode, or something in between. Treatment must necessarily be dictated by the clinical situation because of these considerations.

In those cases in which there may be only subtle changes in physiological variables, such as tachycardia and increased expired CO_2, as mentioned above, the likelihood that these represent MH is low and supports the decision that no specific therapy need be taken. More common causes of these signs, such as inadequate levels of the components of anaesthesia (hypnosis, analgesia and muscle relaxation) should be actively excluded. Other conditions which may mimic subtle MH include patients who have had a preoperative fever, patients with intracranial pathology, i.e. with free blood in the CSF, those with bacteraemia, thyrotoxicosis or phaeochromocytoma, and patients in whom heat loss is diminished, as could occur in a small paediatric patient whose body is covered with drapes. If no other cause for the signs can be found the possibility of MH should not be ignored and the patient should subsequently be referred to an MH testing centre. In these mild cases observation and close monitoring is probably the most important thing to do and dantrolene is not indicated. If, however, there is a continued deterioration in the patient's status with increasing CO_2, acidosis, hyperkalaemia, etc., then all triggering agents should be stopped and dantrolene administered, because its acute risk is minimal.

Masseter muscle spasm

A current area of intense interest and research is masseter muscle spasm (MMS) following administration of succinylcholine. MMS manifests as marked jaw muscle tension in conjunction with muscle flaccidity elsewhere. This entity was originally thought to be highly associated with MH (Gronert, 1980), but more recent data indicate that normal jaw muscle can have fairly marked increases in tension following succinylcholine (Smith *et al.*, 1990; Van der Spek *et al.*, 1990). This is related to the presence of slow tonic fibres that undergo a contracture in response to a depolarising drug, such as succinylcholine. The likelihood of MH increases with the severity of MMS spasm and, when rigidity is present elsewhere in the body, then MH is very likely. In these cases the anaesthetic should be discontinued immediately and dantrolene administered. If possible, the surgery should also be stopped, but if this is not possible, then anaesthesia should be continued with non-triggering agents.

In those patients who have only isolated masseter spasm, the correct course of treatment is not well defined. In one study, 57 patients continued to receive a triggering agent after the diagnosis of MMS, but no patient developed fulminant MH (Littleford *et al.*, 1991). Eventual contracture testing, however, revealed that some of these patients were MH susceptible. In addition, several of these patients had marked rises in CK. Of interest, normal children can respond to succinylcholine with a significant elevation in serum myoglobin (Brustowicz *et al.*, 1987). These findings suggest that patients who have MMS be closely monitored, including end-tidal CO_2, visual inspection of urine for myoglobin, venous or arterial blood gases and electrolytes. If changes suggestive of MH occur, then treatment for MH should begin without delay. Again, the response depends on the clinical manifestation. In a patient in whom the jaw is impossible to open, the procedure should probably be stopped, although the use of dantrolene at this point is probably optional. The patient can usually be ventilated easily by mask; if necessary dantrolene will relax the jaw muscles, but non-depolarising muscle relaxants will not. MMS will usually subside after 10–15 minutes. If the jaw is tight but not impossible to open, then some would continue the anaesthetic using non-triggering agents; others would decide to stop the procedure. All of these patients, if possible, should be evaluated for MH susceptibility with a muscle biopsy. This will definitively answer the question as regards each individual patient, and it would also expand our knowledge base regarding the association of MMS and MH. It is of great interest that some patients with MMS have been given succinylcholine on subsequent anaesthesia, with no development of MMS (Ørding *et al.*, 1991).

Atypical

Recent reports indicate that sudden cardiac arrest can occur in apparently otherwise healthy paediatric patients (Rosenberg & Gronert, 1992). In such a case, a young boy may undergo an anaesthetic induction with halothane and succinylcholine. Within minutes a serious arrhythmia occurs, such as brady-cardia, which then deteriorates to ventricular fibrillation or asystole. In these cases marked hyperkalaemia has been observed and is probably related to the massive breakdown of muscle with the resultant release of potassium, myo-globin and CK. Further evaluation in these patients has revealed the presence of an inapparent myopathy, such as Duchenne's. These cases probably do not represent true MH, but represent a final common pathway of muscle break-down, hyperkalaemia, hypermetabolism, etc. If this occurs, immediate efforts should be undertaken to treat the hyperkalaemia, including administration of calcium, bicarbonate, insulin and glucose. Dantrolene treatment seems appro-priate, particularly as its side-effects are minimal. Surviving patients should undergo muscle biopsy to determine the relationship between this entity and MH, and to examine the muscle for histological/histochemical abnormalities.

Anaesthesia for susceptible patients

Anaesthesia for MH susceptible patients is fairly straightforward and will be discussed in detail below. What is not clear, however, is which patients need to be considered MH susceptible.

It is not uncommon for a patient to report a family history of problems with anaesthesia. Quite often the details of this problem are not available; occa-sionally the patient reports that 'there was a fever after the operation'. How should this information be handled? As previously noted, by itself post-operative fever is unlikely to indicate MH. Halsall & Ellis reported that, in 30 patients who had only postoperative fever, MH contracture testing indicated that none of the patients was MH susceptible (Halsall & Ellis, 1992). Other data from the North American MH Registry show a low evidence of MH susceptibility. Thus, a history of postoperative fever by itself probably does not warrant alteration of anaesthetic management.

Cases which more strongly suggest MH warrant further investigation. This should include examination of the pertinent records. It is common for the patient to misunderstand or misinterpret the events of prior surgery and anaesthesia and subsequently report these details inaccurately. Thus, what may have been reported by the patient to be a significant problem with a postoperative fever and other intraoperative problems may in fact have been a normal course. If, however, the records indicate that MH may be a real possibility, then it is appropriate to obtain resting CKs on the patient and any siblings and the mother and father. While an elevated CK is suggestive of MH in this situation, a normal value does not exclude MH. In many of these cases it may be appropriate to have the patient evaluated by a centre that performs muscle biopsy. If the patient refuses biopsy or undergoes a biopsy and is shown to be MH susceptible, then a trigger-free anaesthetic is utilised.

In the past, prophylactic dantrolene was routinely administered to MH susceptible patients undergoing anaesthesia. Quite often this consisted of oral dantrolene, but subsequent work demonstrated the uncertainty of predictive blood levels, unless high doses were used, and unpleasant side-effects; therefore intravenous administration was recommended. Prophylactic dantrolene should be given to an obstetrical patient after the cord is clamped. This prevents passage to the foetus, which is particularly susceptible to the weakening effects of dantrolene (Shime *et al.*, 1988). Clinical experience over the past several years has indicated, however, that virtually all MH patients can undergo a trigger-free anaesthetic without the use of prophylactic dantrolene. A rare hypermetabolic response during a non-triggering anaesthetic responded to dantrolene (Pollock *et al.*, 1992).

General anaesthesia for the MH susceptible patient can include any of the non-triggering agents such as nitrous oxide, barbiturates such as thiopentone and methohexitone, opioids such as fentanyl and morphine, and non-depolarising muscle relaxants. Benzodiazepines, such as midazolam and diazepam, and propofol and etomidate are also excellent choices. None of these agents is thought to cause MH. Nitrous oxide has infrequently been incriminated as a trigger of MH, but its routine use in MH susceptible patients and the lack of effect in MH susceptible swine (Gronert & Milde, 1981*b*) suggest that it is safe in these situations. All of the volatile agents, such as halothane, isoflurance and enflurane, have been associated with MH and must be avoided. The newer inhalation agents such as desflurane and sevoflurane must not be used as they have been reported to cause MH. Depolarising muscle relaxants such as succinylcholine must likewise be avoided. Curare should also be avoided because of a weak depolarising effect noted in denervated muscle.

While awake triggering of MH can occur in pigs, human awake MH is not well documented. There are only a few reports of human awake MH, but a common factor is anxiety and stress (Gronert *et al.*, 1980). It seems prudent, therefore, to allay anxiety and administer sedative agents prior to anaesthetic induction.

Regional anaesthesia can be safely used in MH patients, and any of the local anaesthetics may be used. In the past, amide local anaesthetics were considered contraindicated in MH because of their ability to cause *in vitro* muscle contractures, but this phenomenon occurs also in normal muscle and was solely the result of high concentrations of the drugs in the bath. The routine use of amide local anaesthetics for the evaluation of MH susceptibility vindicates the use of these anaesthetics in MH (Berkowitz & Rosenberg, 1985).

Reversal of non-depolarising muscle relaxants does not appear to be a triggering factor of MH. Ørding *et al.* (1991) reported the use of neostigmine plus glycopyrrolate in patients who are MH susceptible. None of these patients developed MH. Thus, these important drugs in anaesthetic practice may be administered in MH susceptible patients.

The anaesthesia machine must be prepared for a patient who is MH susceptible and is to undergo anaesthesia. In the past this frequently involved a machine solely dedicated to such patients, or a machine flushed with high flows of oxygen for 12–24 hours. This made it difficult to treat MH patients who required emergency surgery and in whom the 12–24 hour waiting period was ill-advised. In point of fact, virtually all anaesthetic machines can be prepared in a simple fashion and in a minimal amount of time (Beebe & Sessler, 1988). Anaesthetic vaporisers are removed, taped off or drained. All of the rubber components such as the fresh gas hose, circuit and reservoir bag, and anaesthetic ventilator bellows are replaced. Fresh soda lime should also be used, although contaminated soda lime actually produces little residual anaesthetic. The machine can then be flushed with oxygen at 10 L/min for five to ten minutes. These steps will ensure that a minuscule amount of volatile anaesthetic is delivered to the patient.

Yentis *et al.* (1992) retrospectively reviewed the charts of 303 children who were labelled MH susceptible and had undergone surgery with trigger-free anaesthetics. Of these, 25 children had biopsy proven MH but no intra- or postoperative problems. Of the remaining 275 patients none had had MH episodes. These data suggest that MH susceptibility by itself does not warrant admission to hospital after an operation, i.e. outpatient procedures are feasible.

Routine monitoring when anaesthetising MH susceptible patients includes capnography and temperature. A slight 2–3 °C temperature decrease is not unreasonable because hypothermia appears to partially prevent MH. (Nelson, 1990).

Numerous syndromes and diseases have been associated with MH. Some of these are well documented, others are not. The King–Denborough syndrome is a genetic disorder with short stature, low set ears and musculo-skeletal anomalies, such as malar hypoplasia, kyphoscoliosis and pectus carinatum. Myopathy is usually also present. This disorder has been associated with MH, and therefore any patient with this diagnosis must be considered MH susceptible (Steenson & Torkelson, 1987).

Central core disease is a myopathy that may present as weakness in infancy but may diminish as the patient grows older. Characteristic biopsy findings include central cores extending through multiple sections of mitochondria, indicating the absence of certain oxidative enzymes. The genetic component is carried on chromosome 19 near the MH locus and is invariably associated with MH (Haan *et al.*, 1990; but see Chapter 8).

Duchenne dystrophy is X-linked, while MH is autosomal dominant. Nonetheless, it has been associated with MH, although contracture testing has been normal in these patients (Gronert *et al.*, 1992). It is probable that some of the MH episodes were in fact a manifestation of cell membrane disruption and cell breakdown with subsequent rhabdomyolysis, hyperkalaemia and acidosis. Although these may not be true MH episodes, they behave in a similar fashion and treatment with dantrolene is indicated.

Patients with myotonias may respond to succinylcholine with contractures, but actual MH episodes in myotonic patients are unlikely and disputed (Lehmann-Horn & Iaizzo, 1990). These contractures, which may be confused with MH, do not have any of the serious metabolic abnormalities that accompany MH.

Sudden infant death syndrome (SIDS) has been reported to occur in association with MH; however, Ellis *et al.* in 1988 described a series of patients, some of whom were MH susceptible, some who had a family history of SIDS, and some parents of children with SIDS, who underwent muscle biopsy. There proved to be no association between MH and SIDS, and therefore it is not indicated to change anaesthetic management in a patient who has a family history of SIDS.

Neuroleptic malignant syndrome (NMS) has also been associated with MH. This is on the basis, for the most part, of some common clinical presenting signs. In NMS, adverse reactions can occur to commonly used psychotropic drugs. There may be hyperthermia, muscle rigidity, extrapyramidal manifestations and altered consciousness. These occur via a central mechanism and are not related to a direct muscle effect. The syndrome is slow to progress, unlike MH, which occurs rapidly (Hermesh *et al.*, 1988). There were 32 procedures performed in which triggering agents were used, with no occurrence of MH. Another study examined contracture responses in NMS and determined that

NMS contractures were normal (Adnet *et al.*, 1989). These data indicate that it is unlikely that NMS is related to MH and that anaesthetic plans need not be altered. Interestingly, dantrolene may be helpful in treating NMS. NMS may also be treated with electroshock therapy (Addonizio *et al.*, 1987).

A rare patient may have unexplained and otherwise asymptomatic CK elevations that defy diagnosis. Lingaraju & Rosenberg described a series of seven patients who were referred for MH evaluation as part of their workup for asymptomatic CK elevations (Lingaraju & Rosenberg, 1991). Three of these seven patients had positive muscle biopsies. The CK in these patients ranged from 350 to over 2000 IU/L. None of the patients had had an MH episode, however. Thus, it is unclear what the true incidence of MH susceptibility is in these patients.

Summary

The course of treatment in MH is dictated by the clinical situation. In mild cases, where MH suspicion is low, no specific therapy is indicated. In fulminant cases dantrolene must be administered and specific therapy undertaken to minimise organ damage and to maximise outcome. Anaesthesia for susceptible individuals is easily accomplished because of the many drugs that can be safely administered to these patients. Further research will be required to delineate the relationship between certain disorders and MH.

References

Addonizio, G. & Susman, V. L. (1987). ECT as a treatment alternative for patients with symptoms of neuroleptic malignant syndrome. *Journal of Clinical Psychology*, **48**, 102–5.

Adnet, P. J., Krivosic-Horber, R. M., Adamantidis, M. M., Haudecoeur, G., Adnet-Bonte, C. A., Saulnier, F. & Dupuis, B. A. (1989). The association between the neuroleptic malignant syndrome and malignant hyperthermia. *Acta Anaesthesiologica Scandinavica*, **33**, 676–80.

Beebe, J. J. & Sessler, D. I. (1988). Preparation of anesthesia machines for patients susceptible to malignant hyperthermia. *Anesthesiology*, **69**, 395–400.

Berkowitz, A. & Rosenberg, H. (1985). Femoral block with mepivacaine for muscle biopsy in malignant hyperthermia patients. *Anesthesiology*, **62**, 651–2.

Brustowicz, R. M., Moncorge, C. & Koka, B. V. (1987). Metabolic responses to tourniquet release in children. *Anesthesiology*, **67**, 792–4.

Ellis, F. R., Halsall, P. J. & Christian, A. S. (1990). Clinical presentation of suspected malignant hyperthermia during anaesthesia in 402 probands. *Anaesthesia*, **45**, 838–41.

Ellis, F. R., Halsall, P.J., Harriman, D. G. F. (1988). Malignant hyperpyrexia and sudden infant death syndrome. *British Journal of Anaesthesia*, **60**, 28–30.

Gronert, G. A. (1980). Malignant hyperthermia. *Anesthesiology*, **53**, 395–423.

Gronert, G. A., Fowler, W., Cardinet, G. H. III, Grix, A. Jr., Ellis, W. G. & Schwartz, M. Z. (1992). Absence of malignant hyperthermia contractures in Becker–Duchenne dystrophy at age 2. *Muscle and Nerve*, **15**, 52–6.

Gronert, G. A. & Milde, J. H. (1981a). Variations in onset of porcine malignant hyperthermia. *Anesthesia and Analgesia*, **60**, 499–503.

Gronert, G. A. & Milde, J. H. (1981b). Hyperbaric nitrous oxide and malignant hyperpyrexia. *British Journal of Anaesthesia*, **53**, 1238, (letter).

Gronert, G. A., Thompson, R. L. & Onofrio, B. M. (1980). Human malignant hyperthermia: awake episodes and correction by dantrolene. *Anaesthesia and Analgesia*, **59**, 377–8.

Haan, E. A., Freemantle, C. J., McCure, J. A., Friend, K. L. & Mulley, J. C. (1990). Assignment of the gene for central core disease to chromosome 19. *Human Genetics*, **86**, 187–90.

Halsall, P. J., Cain, P. A. & Ellis, F. R. (1979). Retrospective analysis of anaesthetics received by patients before susceptibility to malignant hyperpyrexia was recognised. *British Journal of Anaesthesia*, **51**, 949–54.

Halsall, P. J. & Ellis, F. R. (1992). Does postoperative pyrexia indicate malignant hyperthermia susceptibility? *British Journal of Anaesthesia*, **68**, 209–10.

Harrison, G. G. (1975). Control of the malignant hyperpyrexic syndrome in MHS swine by dantrolene sodium. *British Journal of Anaesthesia*, **47**, 62–5.

Hermesh, H., Aizenberg, D., Lapidot, M. & Munitz, H. (1988). Risk of malignant hyperthermia among patients with neuroleptic malignant syndrome and their families. *American Journal of Psychiatry*, **145**, 1431–4.

Kolb, M. E., Horne, M. L. & Martz, R. (1982). Dantrolene in human malignant hyperthermia: a multicenter study. *Anesthesiology*, **56**, 254–62.

Larach, M. G., Rosenberg, H., Larach, D. R. & Broennle, A. M. (1987). Prediction of malignant hyperthermia susceptibility by clinical signs. *Anesthesiology*, **66**, 547–50.

Lehmann-Horn, F. & Iaizzo, P. A. (1990). Are myotonias and periodic paralyses associated with susceptibility to malignant hyperthermia? *British Journal of Anaesthesia*, **65**, 692–7.

Lingaraju, N. & Rosenberg, H. (1991). Unexplained increases in serum creatine kinase levels: its relation to malignant hyperthermia susceptibility. *Anesthesia and Analgesia*, **72**, 702–5.

Littleford, J. A., Patel, L. R., Bose, D., Cameron, C. B. & McKillop, C. (1991). Masseter muscle spasm in children: implications of continuing the triggering anaesthetic. *Anesthesia and Analgesia*, **72**, 151–160.

Nelson, T. E. (1990). Porcine malignant hyperthermia: critical temperatures for *in vivo* and *in vitro* responses. *Anesthesiology*, **73**, 449–54.

Ørding, H. (1985). Incidence of malignant hyperthermia in Denmark. *Anesthesia and Analgesia*, **64**, 700–4.

Ørding, H., Hald, A. & Sjontoft, E. (1985). Malignant hyperthermia triggered by heating in anaesthetised pigs. *Acta Anaesthesilogica Scandinavica*, **29**, 698–701.

Ørding, H., Hedengran, A. M. & Skovgaard, L. T. (1991). Evaluation of 119 anaesthetics received after investigation for susceptibility to malignant hyperthermia. *Acta Anaesthesiologica Scandinavica*, **35**, 711–16.

Ørding, H. & Nielsen, V. G. (1986). Atracurium and its antagonism by neostigmine (plus glycopyrrolate) in patients susceptible to malignant hyperthermia. *British Journal of Anaesthesia*, **58**, 1001–4.

Pollock, N., Hodges, M. & Sendall, J. (1992). Prolonged malignant hyperthermia in the absence of triggering agents. *Anaesthesia and Intensive Care*, **20**, 520–3.

Ranklev-Twetman, E. (1990). Malignant hyperthermia: the clinical syndrome. *Acta Anaesthesiologica Belgica*, **41**, 79–82.

Rosenberg, H. & Gronert, G. A. (1992). Intractable cardiac arrest in children given succinylcholine. *Anesthesiology*, **77**, 1054 (letter).

Rubin, A. S. & Zablocki, A. D. (1987). Hyperkalemia, verapamil and dantrolene. *Anesthesiology*, **66**, 246–49.

Saltzman, L. S., Kates, R. A., Corke, B. C., Norfleet, E. A. & Heath, K. R. (1984). Hyperkalemia and cardiovascular collapse after dantrolene and verapamil administration in swine. *Anesthesia and Analgesia*, **63**, 473–8.

Shime, J., Gare, D., Andrews, J. & Britt, B. (1988). Dantrolene in pregnancy: lack of adverse effects on the fetus and newborn infant. *American Journal of Obstetrics and Gynecology*, **159**, 831–4.

Smith, C. E., Saddler, J. M., Bevan, J. C., Donati, F. & Bevan, D. R. (1990). Pretreatment with non-depolarising neuromuscular blocking agents and suxamethonium-induced increases in resting jaw tension in children. *British Journal of Anaesthesia*, **64**, 577–81.

Steenson, A. J. & Torkelson, R. D. (1987). King's syndrome with malignant hyperthermia: potential outpatient risks. *American Journal of Diseases of Children*, **141**, 271–3.

Van der Spek, A. F. L., Reynolds, P. I., Fang, W. B., Ashton-Miller, J. A., Stohler, C. S. & Schork, M. A. (1990). Changes in resistance to mouth opening induced by depolarising and non-depolarising neuromuscular relaxants. *British Journal of Anaesthesia*, **64**, 21–7.

Yentis, S. M., Levine, M. F. & Hartley, E. J. (1992). Should all children with suspected or confirmed malignant hyperthermia susceptibility be admitted after surgery? A 10-year review. *Anesthesia and Analgesia*, **75**, 345–50.

Yoganathan, T., Casthely, P. A. & Lamprou, M. (1988). Dantrolene-induced hyperkalemia in a patient treated with diltiazem and metoprolol. *Journal of Cardiothoracic Anesthesia*, **2**, 363–4.

10

Pathophysiology of malignant hyperthermia

J. E. FLETCHER and H. ROSENBERG

Background

What is malignant hyperthermia?

We reserve the term malignant hyperthermia (MH) for the anaesthesia-induced MH syndrome in humans. The syndrome usually includes several or all of the following signs: temperature elevation, muscle rigidity, acidosis, muscle breakdown (elevated potassium and creatine kinase (CK) values, myoglobinuria) and arrhythmias. We emphasise that we are defining a syndrome and that a similar syndrome most likely can be a common final pathway for any one of several different protein defects. The analogous syndrome in pigs will be specifically referred to as the porcine stress syndrome (PSS).

Problems with understanding malignant hyperthermia

Human MH has not been an easy problem to solve for several reasons. In most cases humans who are MH susceptible appear perfectly normal in the absence of anaesthetics and have no histological evidence of a muscle disorder. It is difficult, therefore, to phenotype those individuals with only mild signs sugges-tive of MH during anaesthesia, as these could result from a number of perioperative complications unrelated to MH. The only convincing case is a full-blown life-threatening episode of MH, and these are rare owing to the discontinuation of triggering anaesthesia on early signs of MH. We are forced to rely on the outcome of the *in vitro* contracture test (IVCT) for diagnosing MH and, while the test appears to be sufficiently sensitive, it may not be as specific as we would desire. Another reason is the recently identified hetero-geneity of the syndrome that forces us to consider how defects in any one of several different proteins may share the same final pathway (i.e. myoplasmic Ca^{2+} elevation), with either the same or some variation in severity of the syndrome. The variability inherent in MH and PSS probably results from up- and downregulation of one or more modulating processes that appear to be under regulation by the primary defect. Furthermore, the functions of a variety of proteins that are not the primary defect are indirectly altered in MH muscle, perhaps also resulting from the widespread influence of one or more second messenger systems. Even understanding the pathophysiology of PSS has been very elusive, although it may be caused by a single mutation in all cases, most likely due to these modulators and second messengers.

Species susceptible to malignant hyperthermia

The human MH syndrome was first identified in 1960 by Denborough & Lovell (see Gronert, 1980). The proband had a family history of anaesthesia-related deaths that supported the MH syndrome as an inherited disorder. The PSS had been a problem in the pork industry prior to the identification of the MH syndrome, as the meat from susceptible swine was unmarketable. The identification of the similarities between human MH and the PSS in the response to triggering anaesthesia was a major advance in the field of MH. This provided an animal model for studies that could not possibly be conducted in humans or with human tissue. Other animals proposed for studying MH have been horses, which have not proven to be a practical model, and dogs, which might prove to be an interesting model if further developed.

Overview of the pathophysiology of malignant hyperthermia

One very complete review by Gronert (1980) is recommended for details of the early studies and controversies in MH and PSS. Three major areas are the focus of intense study, as judged simply by the number of publications. These are the Ca^{2+} release channel of skeletal muscle, the presence of a general membrane defect and the modulation of Ca^{2+} regulation by fatty acids. However, several other interesting and potentially important areas are being studied, including 1,4,5-inositol trisphosphate (IP_3) metabolism, a defect in the antioxidant defence system, the dihydropyridine receptor and the Na^+ channel.

It is now clear that more than one protein can be responsible for human MH. In contrast, a single nucleotide base exchange in the Ca^{2+} release channel, or ryanodine receptor, of skeletal muscle appears to account for PSS in all strains of swine tested. This mutation (a thymine for cytosine substitution at position 1843 in the porcine genomic DNA) results in a cysteine[615] for arginine[615] substitution in the amino acids comprising the Ca^{2+} release channel.

It is possible that a defect in the Ca^{2+} release channel might also be responsible for some cases of human MH.

It is also necessary to invoke one or more factors that modulate the expression of the MH defect, as humans and swine do not always exhibit the MH, despite exposure to adequate amounts of triggering agent. These factors may be a normal process that is up- or downregulated by the primary mutation in MH. In some cases, the modulating system may be the primary defect (actual genetic mutation) in MH. It might be possible to target the modulator for prophylaxis and therapeutics because the occurrence of the MH syndrome and PSS syndromes is completely dependent on the modulator. A better understanding of what the consequences of the modulators are on proteins with altered function may help to explain many of the mysteries of MH.

Important clinical and biochemical considerations for a hypothesis

Spectrum of responses

There are several features of MH that have caused considerable confusion in the field. First, there is a spectrum of presentations that can occur, ranging from relatively minor intraoperative complications to a rapid temperature rise, muscle rigidity, acidosis, arrhythmias and death. Some cases have a greater latency to onset and are not manifest until several hours after the operation. Second, MH does not always occur in response to triggering agents. This is a well-established observation in human MH and similar observations have been reported in swine. Young PSS-susceptible pigs experience a period of several weeks where they cannot be triggered (Cheah *et al.*, 1986). Also, while most investigators would agree that PSS is a more consistently triggered syndrome than the human MH syndrome, even adult swine occasionally do not respond to a prolonged halothane and suxamethonium (succinylcholine) challenge (Fletcher *et al.*, 1993*a*). The term MH may be a misnomer, as sometimes patients show no signs of temperature elevation. Finally, many cases do not exhibit rigidity, which is sometimes incorrectly considered a hallmark sign of the syndrome.

Association of malignant hyperthermia with muscle disorders

There are a number of muscle disorders that have been associated with MH, such as the myotonias. In most cases the episode does not fit the classical definition of MH. The important question is whether the muscle disorders per se predispose the patients to an MH or MH-like episode, or whether only a subpopulation of patients with these disorders will be susceptible to MH, perhaps because of a unique defect in the protein responsible for the muscle disorder. Not all patients with a particular muscle disorder have problems with anaesthetics. Another possibility is that a modulator of MH must be coinherited with the muscle disorder. It is unclear, therefore, whether the positive diagnostic contracture test, or the abnormal signs during an anaesthetic in patients with muscle disorders reflect true MH.

Agents associated with a hypersensitive response of malignant hyperthermia muscle

The main triggering agents are the halogenated volatile anaesthetics (halothane, enflurance, isoflurane, methoxyflurane, desflurane) and the depolarising neuromuscular blocking agents (primarily suxamethonium (succinylcholine)). Cyclopropane and ether are also regarded as triggering agents. Controversy surrounds a few other agents. The halogenated volatile anaesthetics and the depolarising neuromuscular blocking agents are not only structurally dissimilar, but they do not even share the same primary mechanism of action. Halothane and succinylcholine act synergistically *in vivo* to increase serum CK values and *in vitro* to induce contractures in skeletal muscle. Also, halothane and Bay K 8644, a calcium and sodium channel agonist, also act in synergy *in vitro* (Adnet *et al.*, 1991). Bay K 8644 is of special interest as it appears to exhibit more of a synergy with halothane in MH rather than normal muscle (Adnet *et al.*, 1991). This may prove to be useful both in better discriminating MH muscle diagnostically and in understanding the pathophysiology of MH. An additional agent, caffeine, is used for diagnostic testing. While halothane and caffeine both cause release of Ca^{2+} from the sarcoplasmic reticulum, they do not act by identical mechanisms. Ryanodine has also been reported to be more effective in inducing contractures in MH than in normal muscle, although these studies are in the early stages.

Agents antagonising the malignant hyperthermia syndrome

Dantrolene is the most effective antagonist of the MH syndrome. In isolated muscle preparations, dantrolene antagonises halothane- and caffeine-induced contractures (Okumura *et al.*, 1980). Dantrolene has some drawbacks, including poor aqueous solubility and, at the doses required for MH, mild muscle weakness and gastrointestinal disturbances. Although dantrolene blocks Ca^{2+} release from the sarcoplasmic reticulum, its exact mechanism has not been satisfactorily identified. There is some controversy as to whether dantrolene antagonises Ca^{2+} release in skinned fibre and isolated terminal cisternae-containing preparations that may relate to the specific conditions of the assay. Azumolene, a more soluble dantrolene analogue, is also very effective in antagonising *in vivo* episodes of MH. Curare, a non-depolarising neuromuscular blocking agent, antagonises the onset of MH to suxamethonium (succinylcholine), but not to halothane *in vivo* and antagonises contractures to suxamethonium *in vitro*. A second non-depolarising neuromuscular blocking agent, pancuronium, offers partial protection to an *in vivo* halothane challenge. Also, thiopental at high doses delays the onset of an MH episode in swine.

The contracture test for diagnosis of human malignant hyperthermia

The IVCT is reviewed in Chapter 11. There are some observations, however, that are highly relevant for understanding the pathophysiology of MH. There can be considerable variability in response between fibre bundles from the same biopsy specimen. This finding would suggest that the MH mutation is not manifest homogeneously throughout the skeletal muscle mass. The contracture response to halothane exhibits a curious temperature dependence that is difficult to explain. That is, the contractures to halothane observed in MH muscle at 37 °C are greatly attenuated or abolished at 25 °C (Nelson, 1990; Fletcher, 1994). There appears to be no association between the magnitude of the contracture response in the diagnostic test and the severity of an MH episode, as a positive contracture test can be obtained at a time when PSS susceptible swine will not exhibit a response to triggering anaesthetics (Fletcher *et al.*, 1993*a*). It is possible that *in vivo* drug treatment will influence the outcome of the contracture response, as has been observed in horses and rats, suggesting that the defect in MH can be normalised. For example, in one pig susceptible to PSS, exposure to phenytoin (50 mg/kg orally per day for two days and 25 mg/kg per day for the next five days) the *in vitro* contracture response to caffeine was reduced by 63%, whereas the *in vitro* contracture response to halothane was unaffected (unpublished data).

Genetics : dominant human malignant hyperthermia and recessive porcine stress syndrome

Any one of several different proteins can cause human MH (for a review see MacLennan & Phillips, 1992) and only one of the two chromosomes (one from each parent) is required to be defective for MH susceptibility. In contrast, a single genetic mutation in the Ca^{2+} release channel appears to account for all known PSS (for a review, see MacLennan & Phillips, 1992) and both alleles must be defective for PSS susceptibility (MacLennan & Phillips, 1992; Fletcher *et al.*, 1993*a*). The PSS mutation results in a cysteine for arginine substitution at position 615 in the protein. In contrast to MH susceptible humans carrying only one defective allele, heterozygote swine exhibit a negative contracture test for MH (Fletcher *et al.*, 1993*a*) and exhibit no signs of MH when administered triggering anaesthetics (Fletcher *et al.*, 1993*a*).

MH susceptible humans inherit the disorder in a dominant pattern (the equivalent of a heterozygote pig), and so differences in the physiological 'background' have been evoked as a possible explanation for the radically different responses between heterozygote pigs and MH susceptible humans. The same rationale has been used to explain the differences in response between strains of homozygous PSS swine. While this is possible, it is highly speculative and without experimental support regarding MH or PSS.

Tissues expressing the malignant hyperthermia defect

Tissues other than skeletal muscle

There seems to be a difference between swine and humans in the extent to which the MH or PSS defect is expressed throughout the organism. This is not completely surprising as the primary defects are not identical. In the pig the defect is manifest in red blood cells as an increased osmotic fragility (for references, see Fletcher, 1994) and increased peroxidation (Duthie & Arthur, 1993). Evidence exists for primary expression of the defect in cardiac muscle in PSS susceptibles, but this has been controversial. Hepatic cells are also affected in PSS susceptibles (Duthie & Arthur, 1993). In humans the expression of the defect appears to be restricted to skeletal muscle. For example, the osmotic fragility of red blood cells appears normal (Fletcher,1994). Human MH appears to be confined to skeletal muscle, so we will focus on mechanisms in that tissue.

Skeletal muscle

The MH and PSS defects are expressed in skeletal muscle, as evidenced by the IVCT for MH susceptibility. They appear to be expressed in type I and type II fibres (Adnet *et al.*, 1993). The distributions and amounts of protein in whole skeletal muscle and in isolated sarcoplasmic reticulum appear to be normal by electrophoretic analysis. Minor proteins, however, could be significantly altered and this would not be detected by the methodologies employed. On the basis of the *in vitro* contracture response to halothane, the defect is not uniformly expressed in the skeletal muscle mass (Fletcher, 1994).

Organelles in skeletal muscle expressing the malignant hyperthermia defect

General

General agreement now points to enhanced Ca^{2+} release from MH or PSS sarcoplasmic reticulum in response to triggering agents as a major turning point in the syndrome. The manner in which this occurs is not certain and may not necessarily involve a component of excitation–contraction coupling as an initiating factor. It is clear, regardless of the primary cause of MH, that the defect is manifest directly or indirectly in several organelles, including the sarcoplasmic reticulum, mitochondria and the sarcolemma.

Sarcoplasmic reticulum

Elevated myoplasmic Ca^{2+} appears to play a crucial role in MH. The mechanisms for controlling Ca^{2+} levels reside primarily in the sarcoplasmic reticulum. The major functional units and their associated terminology are reviewed in Figure 10.1. A variety of methods can be employed to study Ca^{2+} regulation in skeletal muscle and these are reviewed in Figure 10.2.

Several investigators have identified altered function of the sarcoplasmic reticulum in PSS, even in the absence of anaesthetics. These would include a low threshold of Ca^{2+}-induced Ca^{2+} release in the presence (Nelson, 1983; Ohnishi *et al.*, 1983; Fletcher *et al.*, 1993 *a*) or absence (Mickelson *et al.*, 1986) of ATP, Mg^{2+} and the influence of the Ca^{2+} pump. In brief, this means that less added Ca^{2+} is required to open the Ca^{2+}- regulated Ca^{2+} release channel in terminal cisternae-containing preparations from PSS susceptibles and this finding is independent of the Ca^{2+} uptake mechanisms or a stimulator (ATP) or inhibitor (Mg^{2+}) of the Ca^{2+} release channel. Also observed for PSS Ca^{2+}-induced Ca^{2+} release are an enhanced rate of release from skinned fibres (Kim *et al.*, 1984) and terminal cisternae (Mickelson *et al.*, 1989). The maximum amount of Ca^{2+} released is similar for PSS and normal vesicles (Nelson, 1983; Kim *et al.*, 1984). The effect of temperature on the threshold of Ca^{2+}-induced Ca^{2+} release in the absence of anaesthetics is slight (Nelson, 1990) relative to the much more dramatic effects of temperature on halothane-induced contractures of MH muscle (Fletcher, 1994; Nelson, 1990). Ca^{2+} uptake is not believed to be

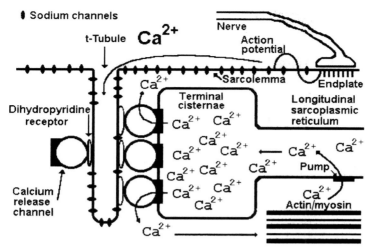

Figure 10.1. The action potential generated at the endplate region of the neuromuscular junction is propagated down the sarcolemma into the t-tubules to the dihydropyridine receptors by the opening of voltage-dependent sodium channels. The dihydropyridine receptors in skeletal muscle function as voltage sensors and are coupled to the Ca^{2+} release channels which are shown as large circles. When the Ca^{2+} release channels are opened, the available terminal cisternae Ca^{2+} stores are released and the levels of myoplasmic Ca^{2+} are elevated. The Ca^{2+} then interacts with the troponin–tropomyosin complex associated with actin and allows interaction of actin with myosin for mechanical movement. The Ca^{2+} signal is terminated by pumping the Ca^{2+} into the longitudinal sarcoplasmic reticulum by an ATP-driven process. A defect in either of two general processes (increased Ca^{2+} release or decreased Ca^{2+} uptake) could therefore account for an increase in myoplasmic Ca^{2+}.

significantly affected in MH or PSS muscle (Louis *et al.*, 1992). In human MH, the Ca^{2+} release process appears to be less affected than that in PSS muscle. For example, the threshold of Ca^{2+}-induced Ca^{2+} release in terminal cisternae-containing fractions is not altered in human MH (Fletcher *et al.*, 1990, 1991, 1993*b*) under the same conditions (pyrophosphate present) in which a decrease has been reported for PSS susceptibles (Fletcher *et al.*, 1991, 1993*b*). A slightly greater amount of Ca^{2+}-induced Ca^{2+} release (13%) in MH muscle has been reported by one group (McSweeney & Heffron, 1990). An additional difference between porcine and human muscle regarding Ca^{2+} regulation in the absence of anaesthetics is the segregation of the threshold of Ca^{2+}-induced Ca^{2+} release into two populations: one unique to the normal swine and the other unique to the MH susceptible swine (Nelson, 1983; Ohnishi *et al.*, 1982; Fletcher *et al.*, 1991). In contrast to porcine muscle both populations of thresholds of Ca^{2+}-

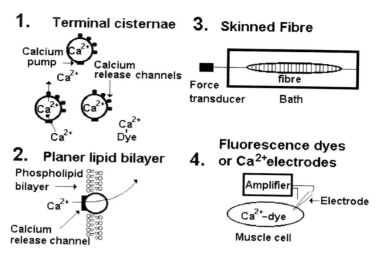

Figure 10.2. Skeletal muscle can be homogenised and resealed portions of the terminal cisternae containing the Ca^{2+} release channel can be recovered by a series of centrifugation steps. These vesicles can take up Ca^{2+} from the bathing medium by means of the ATP-driven Ca^{2+} pump and can subsequently release Ca^{2+} by opening of the Ca^{2+} release channels. Ca^{2+} levels in the extravesicular medium can be monitored spectrophotometrically by a number of dyes (usually metalochrome indicators such as arsenazo III or antipyrylazo III). Alternatively, $^{45}Ca^{2+}$ and filtration of the vesicles can be used. The amount of calcium released is usually determined by the decrease in radioactivity retained on the filters that contain the vesicles. Both the spectrophotometric and radioisotopic approaches allow monitoring of Ca^{2+} uptake and Ca^{2+} release and these processes can be dissociated pharmacologically with the Ca^{2+} release channel blocker, ruthenium red. The terminal cisternae method allows the overall response of a large population of channels to be examined and may best reflect the overall responsiveness of the muscle. It is possible to incorporate the Ca^{2+} release channel into artificial lipid bilayers (i.e. planer lipid bilayer) and monitor the Ca^{2+} current as an electrical charge movement through as few as one channel at a time. While this method can provide very useful detailed information on the opening and closing of individual Ca^{2+} release channels, it does not provide an indication of the overall responsiveness of the muscle in which both Ca^{2+} uptake and Ca^{2+} release are participating. A third approach involves skinned fibre preparations in which the sarcolemma is removed either mechanically, or made permeable chemically, and the function of the sarcoplasmic reticulum and myofibrils (actin and myosin) is monitored by the contractile response of the fibre. This preparation has an interesting advantage in that type I and type II fibres can be distinguished (for references see Adnet *et al*., 1993). This method only examines one muscle fibre at a time. This might be a disadvantage in MH or PSS skeletal muscle, as the defect is not uniformly expressed throughout the tissue. Lastly, the cytoplasmic Ca^{2+} levels can be monitored in intact muscle either with fluorescence dyes or Ca^{2+} electrodes. The former can monitor a muscle mass, while the latter examines individual fibres. Both approaches can be used with cell culture systems.

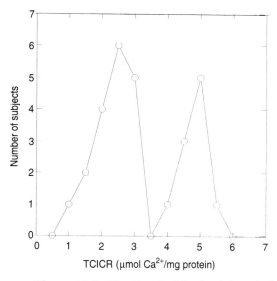

Figure 10.3. The threshold of calcium-induced calcium release (TCICR) in skeletal muscle terminal cisternae-containing preparations from 28 human subjects diagnosed by the halothane and caffeine contracture test as not being susceptible to MH. The values for the population at the low end are similar to those observed in swine with PSS and the values at the high end are similar to those for control swine. Adapted from Fletcher *et al.* (1993*b*).

induced Ca^{2+} release are observed with about equal frequency in normal human muscle (Figure 10.3; Fletcher *et al.*, 1993*b*).

As regards anaesthetic action, the rate of halothane-induced Ca^{2+} release is abnormally high in PSS-susceptibles (Kim *et al.*, 1984; Louis *et al.*, 1992). In contrast, in human MH muscle (McSweeney & Heffron, 1990) the dose–response curves for halothane-induced Ca^{2+} release are normal when the amount of Ca^{2+} release is monitored. The concentration of Ca^{2+} in the assay medium greatly influences the rate and amount of Ca^{2+} release by halothane (Mickelson *et al.*, 1986). It is believed, therefore, that the differences observed in halothane-induced Ca^{2+} release actually result from an acceleration in Ca^{2+}-induced Ca^{2+} release by halothane. The effects of halothane on the amount of Ca^{2+} released appear to be more dramatic on normal than on MH muscle at physiological levels of Ca^{2+} (30–100 mmol; Mickelson *et al.*, 1986). There is no effect of temperature on the rate of halothane-induced Ca^{2+} release (Louis *et al.*, 1992), as is observed with halothane-induced contractures of MH muscle (Nelson, 1990; Fletcher, 1994).

In terminal cisternae-containing preparations examined with pyrophosphate to load Ca^{2+} into the vesicles, halothane at clinically relevant concentrations can not induce a sustained opening of the Ca^{2+} release channel if physiological levels of ATP and Mg^{2+} are included (Fletcher *et al.*, 1991, 1993*b*). Transient openings of the Ca^{2+} release channel at lower than normal concentrations of halothane have been reported for PSS terminal cisternae preparations under similar conditions, but in which oxalate was used in place of pyrophosphate (Ohnishi *et al.*, 1983). The addition of fatty acids to MH or normal vesicles (human, porcine or equine) markedly (about 20 to 30-fold) decreases the concentration of halothane required (into the clinical range) for the sustained opening of the Ca^{2+} release channel in the presence of ATP, Mg^{2+} and pyrophosphate (Fletcher *et al.*, 1991, 1993*b*). Unlike all the previous studies of Ca^{2+} release, there is an absolute temperature-dependence (occurs at 37 °C, not at 25 °C) of the fatty acid enhancement of halothane-induced Ca^{2+} release (Fletcher *et al.*, 1993*b*), which is consistent with the temperature dependence of halothane-induced contractures of MH muscle (Nelson, 1990; Fletcher, 1994).

Mitochondria

Mitochondria oxidise a variety of substrates to generate the form of energy (ATP) most useful for driving cellular reactions and these reactions are reviewed in Figure 10.4. Defects in mitochondrial function do not appear to initiate the MH syndrome. The mitochondria, however, provide an interesting model in which to examine some biochemical consequences of the MH defect and they may participate as the syndrome progresses. The results obtained with mitochondria may seem contradictory; however, this is only because the outcome is very dependent on the experimental conditions. The most consistent findings suggest that a temperature close to the physiological range and the addition of Ca^{2+} are crucial for unmasking differences between normal and MH or PSS-susceptible muscle mitochondria. The ADP-stimulated oxidation of a variety of substrates, including succinate, appears to be normal at either 25 °C or 37–40 °C (Cheah & Cheah, 1981; Cheah *et al.*, 1989). In contrast, a low threshold for uncoupling of Ca^{2+}-stimulated succinate oxidation in the absence of ADP is observed in PSS (Cheah & Cheah, 1981) and human MH (Cheah *et al.*, 1989) muscle at 40 °C that is not observed at 25 °C (Cheah & Cheah, 1981; Cheah *et al.*, 1989). The mitochondria, therefore, may become uncoupled as the syndrome progresses, and then would not generate enough ATP to sustain the ATP-driven Ca^{2+} pump. This temperature dependence of mitochondrial uncoupling is similar to the temperature dependence of halothane-induced contractures of skeletal muscle *in vitro* noted above. Fatty acids have been suggested to be involved in Ca^{2+}-stimulated uncoupling of

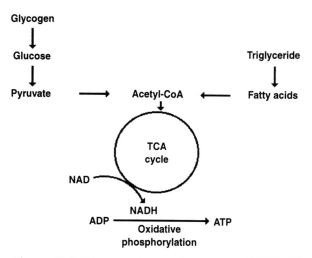

Figure 10.4. There are two main sources of ATP. First pyruvate, which is the final stage of glycolysis, is converted to acetylCoA through the pyruvate dehydrogenase complex. Second, fatty acids, derived from the diet or from adipose or intramuscular stores (triglycerides), are converted to acetylCoA through β-oxidation of fatty acids. Fatty acids are a major energy source in skeletal muscle and their oxidation can account for up to 80% of the oxidative energy consumed by resting muscle. The acetylCoA from both sources is converted to NADH by the tricarboxylic acid (TCA) cycle (Krebs cycle). The NADH is then converted to ATP through oxidative phosphorylation. Within the TCA cycle several intermediates can be oxidised, including succinate, fumarate, malate, citrate and others. Oxygen is consumed in the phosphorylation of ADP to ATP and this is referred to as state 3, or active, respiration. In the absence of ADP respiration is minimal and this is referred to as the state 4, or idling, rate of oxygen consumption. It is possible to uncouple the utilisation of oxygen from the generation of ATP. When mitochondria become uncoupled they consume oxygen even in the absence of ADP, and usually at a higher rate than normal respiration occurring in the presence of ADP. Calcium can also stimulate respiration in the presence of a substrate that can be oxidised, such as succinate.

mitochondria. This suggestion was based on the excess production of free fatty acids in MH mitochondria and the antagonism of Ca^{2+}-induced uncoupling of succinate oxidation by bovine serum albumin, which binds and removes free fatty acids from the mitochondrial membrane (Cheah & Cheah, 1981; Cheah *et al.*, 1986, 1989). Phospholipase A_2 activity was originally suggested as the source of fatty acids, as this is the most significant source of free fatty acids in normal mitochondrial incubates (Cheah & Cheah, 1981; Cheah *et al.*, 1986). It now appears that skeletal muscle triglyceride-associated metabolism is the source of free fatty acids in MH and PSS muscle (Fletcher *et al.*, 1989, 1990).

Sarcolemma

The sarcolemma maintains the membrane potential of the muscle cell and acts as a permeability barrier to Na^+, Cl^- and Ca^{2+}. Skeletal muscle, in most cases, does not require extracellular Ca^{2+} for nerve- or electrically-evoked contractility. In contrast, halothane-induced contractures (Adnet *et al.*,1991) require extracellular Ca^{2+}. A breakdown in this barrier could result in a large influx of Ca^{2+} from the extracellular medium. Also, opening specific Ca^{2+} channels (e.g. dihydropyridine receptors) in the sarcolemma would allow the entry of extracellular Ca^{2+}. The dihydropyridine receptors in skeletal muscle, however, do not normally appear to act as Ca^{2+} channels in the same manner that they do in other tissues. There is a report of altered dihydropyridine receptor binding characteristics. Also, the Na^+ channel function is altered in human MH (Wieland *et al.*, 1989, 1992*b*).

General membrane defect

The MH and PSS defects are manifest in several different membranes in many different ways. Various probes used to detect membrane fluidity or microviscosity have detected differences between PSS and control skeletal muscle (Thomas *et al.*, 1991). The phase transition temperature, which is a reflection to some extent of the lipid environment in membranes, is altered in PSS skeletal muscle mitochondria (Cheah & Cheah, 1981). Minor differences in lipid composition have been reported in skeletal muscle from pigs (Fletcher *et al.*, 1988; Duthie & Arthur, 1993). These differences may depend on extraction techniques (Fletcher *et al.*, 1988), diet, lipid peroxidation (Duthie & Arthur, 1993), altered triglyceride-associated fatty acid metabolism (Fletcher *et al.*, 1989, 1990) or the use of different strains of swine for control and PSS groups. The functions of a large number of proteins are altered, perhaps owing to secondarily altered physical characteristics of the membrane, so the nondescript term 'general membrane defect' has been used to characterise the pervasive influence of the MH defect. It is important to consider that at least some of the changes in membrane composition could occur only on disruption of the tissue (Fletcher *et al.*, 1988).

Specific proteins with altered function in malignant hyperthermia

Calcium release channel

The Ca^{2+} release channel of skeletal muscle is encoded by a different gene (chromosome 19q13.1) from that in cardiac muscle and brain (chromosome 1) and is the primary means of releasing the sarcoplasmic reticulum stores of Ca^{2+} (MacLennan & Phillips, 1992). The Ca^{2+} release channel is an extremely large homotetramer in which the subunits are about 560 000 molecular weight (MW) each. The Ca^{2+} release channel has a binding site for the contracture-inducing plant alkaloid ryanodine and is, therefore, also referred to as the ryanodine receptor.

The function of the Ca^{2+} release channel is definitely altered in PSS muscle. Many of the functional studies are described under 'Sarcoplasmic reticulum'. Also, the K_d, but not the B_{max}, of ryanodine binding to the Ca^{2+} release channel is reduced in PSS muscle (Mickelson *et al.*, 1988; Hawkes *et al.*, 1992). The observed K_d of ryanodine binding actually appears to be an average of ryanodine binding to two or more interconvertible states (differing in affinity) of the channel (Hawkes *et al.*, 1992). The K_d values are usually different for normal (predominantly low affinity) and PSS susceptible (predominantly high affinity) swine. In agreement, MH-like values for the threshold of Ca^{2+}-induced Ca^{2+} release are frequently found in normal humans (Fletcher *et al.*, 1993*b*). These differences in K_d, therefore, may reflect the presence or absence in the muscle of a modulator of the Ca^{2+} release channel function. This modulator is tightly associated with the Ca^{2+} release channel, as the high proportion of high affinity ryanodine binding sites is retained even after the tissue is homogenised and the Ca^{2+} release channel is highly purified (Shomer *et al.*, 1993). High salt conditions abolish differences between PSS and normal ryanodine binding (Shomer *et al.*, 1993), most likely by greatly increasing the percentage of the high affinity ryanodine binding sites in normal muscle. While one group has reported a decreased antagonistic effect of high concentrations of Ca^{2+} on ryanodine binding in PSS (Mickelson *et al.*, 1988; Shomer *et al.*, 1993), this has not been observed by others (Hawkes *et al.*, 1992) and may relate to the use of different strains of swine for the control and PSS groups.

Subtle changes in the function of the Ca^{2+} release channel have been observed in PSS (Shomer *et al.*, 1993) and MH (Fill *et al.*, 1991; Nelson, 1992) muscle using planer lipid bilayer approaches. These differences relate primarily to the probability of the Ca^{2+} release channel being in an open state under highly artificial conditions. While differences between normal and PSS susceptibles have been reported in the absence of halothane or caffeine (Shomer *et al.*, 1993), human MH muscle requires the presence of caffeine (Fill *et al.*, 1991) or halothane (Nelson, 1992) to detect the differences. In human MH muscle there appear to be two populations of ion channels, halothane-insensitive and halothane-sensitive (Nelson, 1992). The halothane-sensitive channels have an increased probability of opening in the presence of clinically relevant concentrations of halothane. They do not occur in all MH muscle and both types (or states) of channels can coexist in the same muscle biopsy (Nelson,

1992), as was the case with the K_d of ryanodine binding (Hawkes *et al.*, 1992). One group of subjects classified as phenotype K (MHE in the article) by the diagnostic test for MH has not been demonstrated to exhibit a convincing case for MH susceptibility (Fletcher, 1994). This group has the same caffeine sensitivity of Ca^{2+} channels in planer lipid bilayers as the MH susceptibles (Fill *et al.*, 1991). As suggested by these latter authors (Fill *et al.*, 1991), other factors may influence the expression of such a defect. Whether these subtle differences in Ca^{2+} release channel function in planer lipid bilayers, or the differences in K_d of ryanodine binding, reflect a different acylation or phosphorylation state of the Ca^{2+} release channel should be investigated.

In agreement with the altered function of the Ca^{2+} release channel, there has been a specific mutation identified (Arg^{615} to Cys^{615}) in the protein that is associated with PSS. The porcine mutation, and selective breeding for lean musculature, may account for the tendency of the states of ryanodine binding and the functional states of the Ca^{2+} release channel to be different in most cases in normal and PSS swine. As mentioned above, however, these states are interconvertible and MH-like states can be observed in normal muscle (Fletcher *et al.*, 1990, 1993*b*). Some families with human MH exhibit linkage to the gene encoding the Ca^{2+} release channel (MacLennan & Phillips, 1992). In the few MH families in which the PSS Ca^{2+} release channel mutation has been identified (about 2%), the evidence is not yet convincing for this as the cause of MH. Overall, while the evidence is strong for the defect in the Ca^{2+} release channel as the primary cause of PSS, the Ca^{2+} release channel has been less convincingly demonstrated as the primary cause of human MH (MacLennan & Phillips, 1992; Fletcher *et al.*, 1995).

The sodium channel

Skeletal and cardiac muscle sodium channels have two subunits (α, 220 000 MW; β, 40 000 MW; reviewed in Catterall, 1992). The 'adult' sodium channel in skeletal muscle is encoded by a different gene (chromosome 17 for the α-subunit) than the sodium channel in cardiac muscle (chromosome 3). Sodium channels in skeletal muscle are of two types and these can be differentiated by their sensitivity to tetrodotoxin (TTX), which blocks the channel pore. The first is an 'embryonic', or TTX-insensitive type, which is identical to the cardiac sodium channel, and the second is the adult, or TTX-sensitive type. There are immunologically distinct differences between t-tubule Na^+ channels and those on the surface membrane. Substituting as few as two amino acids in the sodium channel converts its selectivity from Na^+ to Ca^{2+}. It is of interest in this regard that extracellular Ca^{2+} appears to be necessary for halothane-

induced contractures *in vitro* (Adnet *et al.*, 1991). Defects in the sodium channel have been implicated as the cause of other disorders of skeletal muscle, including hyperkalaemic periodic paralysis and paramyotonia congenita.

The function of the sodium channel is abnormal in primary cultures of human MH skeletal muscle (Wieland *et al.*, 1989, 1992*b*). Fatty acids do modulate the function of the skeletal muscle sodium channels from normal patients (Wieland *et al.*, 1992 *a*). Intracellular injection of fatty acids into primary cell cultures of normal human skeletal muscle activates otherwise inactive Na^+ channels of the adult (TTX-sensitive) type (Wieland *et al.*, 1992*a*). In contrast, the adult (TTX-sensitive) Na^+ channels in primary cultures of skeletal muscle from MH susceptible humans are almost all active even without injected fatty acid and the intracellular injection of fatty acids has no further effect (Wieland *et al.*, 1992*b*).

There is also evidence for linkage of MH to chromosome 17 at or near the locus encoding the Na^+ channel α-subunit (Olckers *et al.*, 1992) and the β-subunit is encoded on chromosome 19 (Makita *et al.*, 1994). Additionally, a specific mutation in the Na^+ channel has been associated with a positive MH contracture test (Vita *et al.*, 1995). As with the Ca^{2+} release channel, it is not clear whether the altered function reflects a primary defect in the Na^+ channel protein, or that the function is altered indirectly by processes such as phosphorylation or acylation (Catterall, 1992).

Other proteins

In PSS there are reports of altered acetylcholinesterase activity and dihydropyridine receptor binding. These studies have not been followed-up. One complication in many of these studies is the use of different strains of swine for the PSS and control groups. Therefore, it is difficult to distinguish strain differences from PSS or MH. Enzymes involved in lipid metabolism are discussed below.

Lipid involvement in malignant hyperthermia

General

Lipids are an important component of a cell, both for structure and function. The lipid composition of membranes can have a marked influence on the function of membrane-associated proteins. Several lipid metabolites serve second messenger functions. Finally, fatty acids are the major source of energy in the resting state of skeletal muscle and can also contribute up to 65% of the energy during exercise.

The lipid fraction is comprised primarily of phospholipids, triglycerides, cholesterol (and cholesterol esters), diacylglycerides, monoacylglycerides and free fatty acids. The phospholipids are responsible for the formation of the lipid bilayer and are involved in many aspects of signal transduction. Triglycerides are a storage form of fatty acids that can be used as a source of energy, or for the synthesis of other lipids. Cholesterol can exist in either a free form or as cholesterol ester, which contains a fatty acid. Cholesterol is a component of membranes. Diacylglycerol has been recognised as an important second messenger that activates an important signal transduction enzyme, protein kinase C (Nishizuka, 1992).

Fatty acids

In addition to existing in a free form, fatty acids are esterified to phospholipids, triglycerides, diacylglycerides, monoacylglycerides and cholesterol esters. Free fatty acids are maintained at very low levels in a cell (because they are very toxic) and most of the free fatty acids are bound to fatty acid binding proteins. The metabolism of free fatty acids is reviewed in Figure 10.5.

Fatty acid production is elevated in mitochondrial fractions (Cheah *et al.*, 1986, 1989) from PSS and MH susceptibles. There is an age-related increase in fatty acid production in skeletal muscle that parallels an age-related increase in susceptibility to the PSS (Cheah *et al.*, 1986). The particular assay (spectrophotometric analysis of fatty acid soaps), however, employed for all of the assays demonstrating elevated fatty acid production very likely includes all forms (free, acylCoA, acylcarnitine) of fatty acid. When only free fatty acids are examined, they are at normal levels in human MH (Fletcher *et al.*, 1989) and PSS (Fletcher *et al.*, 1988) muscle. The flux of fatty acids through β oxidation could still be greatly increased, however, without increasing the levels of free fatty acids and this flux from triglycerides probably accounts for the low levels of triglycerides in biopsies of MH or PSS skeletal muscle (Fletcher *et al.*, 1989, 1990). It will be important in the future, therefore, to examine levels of fatty acid metabolites (see AcylCoA and acylcarnitine discussion below) to better understand the aspect of metabolism that is altered in MH and PSS muscle.

The effects of fatty acids on Ca^{2+} release from skeletal muscle sarcoplasmic reticulum are significant but not dramatic in the absence of anaesthetics (Fletcher *et al.*, 1990) and they are not mediated through the Ca^{2+} release channel (unpublished data). The fatty acids, however, act in synergy with

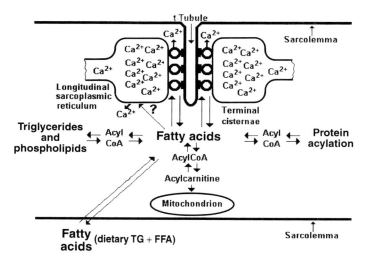

Figure 10.5. Free fatty acids are derived primarily from the blood and are readily incorporated into triglycerides or oxidized (β-oxidation) by the mitochondria for ATP production. Free fatty acids can bind covalently to proteins by two processes of acylation (myristoylation, palmitoylation). Myristoylation is a one-time contranslational (during protein synthesis) event in which myristic acid (14:0) is permanently attached enzymatically to an N-terminal glycine. Palmitoylation is a post-translational (after the protein is synthesised) event that involves a more dynamic transfer of palmitic (16:0), stearic (18:0), oleic (18:1) and linoleic (18:2) acids by acyltransferase enzymes that target these fatty acids primarily to cysteine residues and to a lesser extent to serines and threonines on specific proteins. Free fatty acids are activated to acylCoAs before being metabolised by the mitochondria, used in the synthesis of phospholipids or proteins, or acylated to proteins. Furthermore, acylCoAs are converted to acylcarnitine for transport into the mitochondria prior to β-oxidation. Fatty acids alter the function of a variety of ion channels, including the Ca^{2+} release channel (Fletcher *et al.*, 1990, 1991, 1993b) and Na^+ channel (Wieland *et al.*, 1992a) of skeletal muscle in addition to interacting with the major signalling enzyme, protein kinase C (Nishizuka, 1992), and other proteins.

halothane and decrease the amount of halothane required for sustained Ca^{2+} release by 20 to 30-fold (Fletcher *et al.*, 1991, 1993b). This fatty acid enhancement of halothane-induced Ca^{2+} release, unlike all other studies of Ca^{2+} release, exhibits the same temperature dependence (i.e. only occurs at 37 °C, but not at 25 °C) as halothane-induced contractures of skeletal muscle (Fletcher *et al.*, 1993b) and is mediated through the Ca^{2+} release channel (Fletcher *et al.*, 1993b). While the concentration of fatty acid required for this effect exceeds that of the normal unbound form, halothane can displace fatty acids from fatty acid binding proteins (Dubois & Evers, 1992). It is highly

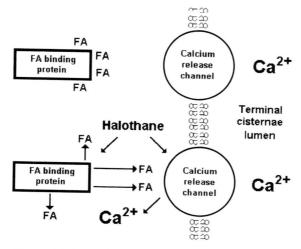

Figure 10.6. The interaction between fatty acids and halothane and the effects on Ca^{2+} release. Normally, even if fatty acids are produced in excess, they would be bound by intracellular fatty acid binding proteins (top) and their free concentrations would be kept at low levels. Under normal conditions, therefore, fatty acids probably do not exert a significant effect on Ca^{2+} release. Halothane can displace fatty acids from fatty acid binding proteins (Dubois & Evers, 1992), however, and would thereby increase the fatty acid concentration at the site of halothane action (bottom). It is very likely, therefore, that high levels of free fatty acids would be reached at the calcium release channels acted on by halothane and that a synergistic action on Ca^{2+} release would ensue (Fletcher *et al.*, 1991, 1993*b*).

likely, therefore, that concentrations greatly exceeding $20\,\mu M$ could be achieved at the site of halothane actions (Figure 10.6). If these levels of free fatty acids are sustained by accelerated triglyceride breakdown, then this would lead to greatly elevated myoplasmic Ca^{2+} levels.

Phosphatidylinositol metabolism

Phosphatidylinositol phospholipids have become of interest since one specific metabolite of phospholipase C action, IP_3, has been demonstrated to be elevated in human MH (Scholz *et al.*, 1991*b*) and PSS muscle (Foster *et al.*, 1989; Scholz *et al.*, 1991*b*). This product of the hydrolysis of phosphatidylinositol 4,5-bisphosphate causes Ca^{2+} release from intracellular stores. While some evidence exists for decreased inositol 1,4,5,-trisphosphate phosphatase activity (Foster *et al.*, 1989), the elevation of all products of phosphatidylinositol hydrolysis (Scholz *et al.*, 1991*a*) would suggest that phospholipase C activity may be elevated in MH. Activation of phospholipase C in skeletal muscle also indirectly elevates free fatty acids by deacylation of the diacylglycerol, which, like IP_3, is a direct product of phospholipase C activity.

Antioxidant defence abnormality

The antioxidant defence abnormality in PSS (for a review, see Duthie & Arthur, 1993) is especially interesting as it could be either the cause or effect of accelerated fatty acid production. In either case, it provides a novel target site for prophylactic and therapeutic intervention. Observations supporting an antioxidant defence abnormality in PSS include the production in plasma of excess thiobarbituric acid reactive substances and conjugated dienes, non-specific markers of peroxidation of unsaturated fatty acids. Although the same is not observed in PSS skeletal muscle a threefold elevation in pentane production does occur and this is another marker of lipid peroxidation. Despite an antioxidant defence abnormality, the levels of skeletal muscle antioxidants and antioxidant enzymes are normal. Excessive peroxidation could contribute to the loss of Ca^{2+} regulation in MH muscle (Duthie & Arthur, 1993).

Working hypothesis for malignant hyperthermia invoking modulators

The evidence for the existence of one or more modulators of the MH syndrome or PSS, including second messengers, has been presented in detail above. This evidence could be summarised as follows: (1) the variability between strains of swine in expression of PSS, (2) the absence of a syndrome in MH or PSS susceptibles in the presence of an adequate triggering agent, (3) the normal dose-response curves for halothane-induced Ca^{2+} release in terminal cisternae-containing preparations in human MH muscle, and (4) widespread protein defects.

The first concept that must be grasped is that there is a difference between carrying the MH mutation and having the full potential for expressing an MH episode. An MH episode is not observed on every challenge even within the same MH humans and even in heterozygous humans (Fletcher *et al.*, 1995) or homozygous PSS-susceptible swine (Fletcher *et al.*, 1993*a*) having the Arg[615] to Cys[615] ryanodine receptor mutation. The primary MH defect may be essential, but it is not sufficient, for the MH syndrome. While variability in expression of gene defects has been attributed to 'environmental factors' by geneticists, in the case of MH these factors may eventually be identified. The identification of these factors is very important, for it provides a novel point of intervention for prophylaxis and treatment of MH, regardless of the specific

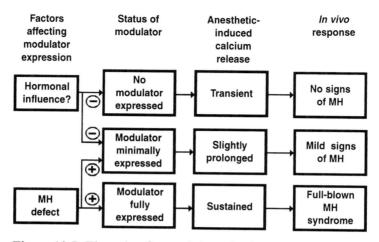

Factors affecting modulator expression	Status of modulator	Anesthetic-induced calcium release	*In vivo* response
Hormonal influence? ⊖	No modulator expressed	Transient	No signs of MH
⊖ ⊕	Modulator minimally expressed	Slightly prolonged	Mild signs of MH
MH defect ⊕	Modulator fully expressed	Sustained	Full-blown MH syndrome

Figure 10.7. The role of a modulator in the MH or PSS syndrome. In this model we have assumed that specific yet-to-be-identified hormones (e.g. steroid or thyroid hormones) downregulate (denoted by the minus sign) the modulator protein. The effects of the modulator can be present or absent without altering the function of skeletal muscle significantly. The modulator protein could be an enzyme that produces, for example, fatty acids or IP_3. The MH defect, in contrast to the hormones, upregulates (denoted by the plus sign) the modulator protein. In the upper row the MH defect has no influence on the modulator (any effects are completely overridden by the hormones) and there is only a slight response to triggering anaesthetics. The MH defect does not lead to the syndrome without the modulator contributing to the response. In the bottom row the hormones (because they are sometimes not present in significant amounts) are having no influence on the modulator and the MH defect has fully upregulated the modulator. In this state the muscle will respond maximally to the triggering agents. In the middle row both the MH defect and the hormones are exerting significant and opposing effects on the modulator, resulting in an intermediate response to the triggering agents.

mutation initiating the syndrome. In the model presented the MH defect is required to 'activate' the modulator. A mutation in the modulator itself, however, could possibly cause MH.

At least two possibilities exist with regard to the inheritance and expression of the modulator. The first possibility is that an individual may have to inherit two mutations to actually exhibit the MH syndrome. One of these mutations would be extremely frequent in the normal population and would serve the modulator function. The second mutation would be the actual MH defect and would result in a positive diagnostic IVCT for MH. The MH syndrome would only result if both defects were coinherited and coexpressed. The second, and more likely, possibility is that the modulator is a normal protein that varies in the degree to which it is transcribed and/or translated (hence its abundance is altered), or the manner in which its activity or function is regulated by cofactors in skeletal muscle. The manner in which the modulator could affect the expression of the MH mutation is shown in Figure 10.7. Two possible modulator systems are triglyceride-associated fatty acid metabolism and IP_3 metabolism.

Conclusions

While some of the pieces of the puzzle regarding the PSS are falling into place, we have much to learn about human MH. The Ca^{2+} release channel mutation resulting in a conversion of Arg^{615} to Cys^{615} appears to account for susceptibility to most or all of the PSS. The expression of this mutation as a syndrome, however, appears to be dependent on a modulator. While some human MH families may also have a defect in the Ca^{2+} release channel, there is convincing evidence that a defect in any one of several proteins may account for the syndrome. A modulator also appears to play a crucial role in the expression of the human MH syndrome and fatty acids and/or IP_3 have been suggested to be involved in this role. The functions of many proteins are altered indirectly in MH and PSS and sorting out cause–effect relationships is difficult, especially with an overriding modulator and activation of second messenger systems which further confuse the puzzle.

References

Adnet, P. J., Bromberg, N. L., Haudecoeur, G., Krivosic, I., Adamantidis, M. M., Reyford, H., Bello, N. & Krivosic Horber, R. M. (1993). Fibre-type caffeine sensitivities in skinned muscle fibers from humans susceptible to malignant hyperthermia. *Anesthesiology*, **78**, 168–77.

Adnet, P. J., Krivosic-Horber, R. M., Adamantidis, M. M., Reyford, H., Cordonnier, C. & Haudecoeur, G. (1991). Effects of calcium-free solution, calcium antagonists, and the calcium agonist BAY K 8644 on mechanical responses of skeletal muscle from patients susceptible to malignant hyperthermia. *Anesthesiology*, 75, 413–19.

Catterall, W. A. (1992). Cellular and molecular biology of voltage-gated sodium channels. *Physiological Reviews*, **72**, S15–48.

Cheah, K. S. & Cheah, A. M. (1981). Mitochondrial calcium transport and calcium-activated phospholipase in porcine malignant hyperthermia. *Biochimica et Biophysica Acta*, **634**, 70–84.

Cheah, K. S., Cheah, A. M., Fletcher, J. E. & Rosenberg, H. (1989). Skeletal muscle mitochondrial respiration of malignant hyperthermia-susceptible patients. Ca^{2+}-induced uncoupling and free fatty acids. *International Journal of Biochemistry*, **21**, 913–20.

Cheah, K. S., Cheah, A. M. & Waring, J. C. (1986). Phospholipase A_2 activity, calmodulin, Ca^{2+} and meat quality in young and adult halothane-sensitive and halothane-insensitive British Landrace pigs. *Meat Science*, **17**, 37–53.

Dubois, B. W. & Evers, A. S. (1992). 19F-NMR spin-spin relaxation (T2) method for characterising volatile anaesthetic binding to proteins. Analysis of isoflurane binding to serum albumin. *Biochemistry*, **31**, 7069–76.

Duthie, G. G. & Arthur, J. R. (1993). Free radicals and calcium homeostasis: relevance to malignant hyperthermia. *Free Radical Biology and Medicine*, **14**, 435–42.

Fill, M., Stefani, E. & Nelson, T. E. (1991). Abnormal human sarcoplasmic reticulum Ca^{2+} release channels in malignant hyperthermic skeletal muscle, *Biophysical Journal*, **59**, 1085–90.

Fletcher, J. E. (1994). Current laboratory methods for the diagnosis of malignant hyperthermia susceptibility. *Anesthesiology Clinics of North America*, **12**, 553–7.

Fletcher, J. E., Calvo, P. A. & Rosenberg, H. (1993a). Phenotypes associated with malignant hyperthermia susceptibility in swine genotyped as homozygous or heterozygous for the Arg^{615} to Cys^{615} ryanodine receptor mutation. *British Journal of Anaesthesia*, **71**, 410–7.

Fletcher, J. E., Mayerberger, S., Tripolitis, L., Yudkowsky, M & Rosenberg, H. (1991). Fatty acids markedly lower the threshold for halothane-induced calcium release from the terminal cisternae in human and porcine normal and malignant hyperthermia susceptible skeletal muscle. *Life Sciences*, **49**, 1651–7.

Fletcher, J. E., Rosenberg H., Michaux, K., Cheah, K. S. & Cheah, A. M. (1988). Lipid analysis of skeletal muscle from pigs susceptible to malignant hyperthermia. *Biochemistry and Cell Biology*, **66**, 917–21.

Fletcher, J. E., Rosenberg, H., Michaux K., Tripolitis, L. & Lizzo, F. H. (1989). Triglycerides, not phospholipids, are the source of elevated free fatty acids in muscle from patients susceptible to malignant hyperthermia. *European Journal of Anaesthesia*, **6**, 355–62.

Fletcher, J. E., Tripolitis, L., Erwin, K., Hanson, S., Rosenberg, H., Conti, P. A. & Beech, J. (1990). Fatty acids modulate calcium-induced calcium release from skeletal muscle heavy sarcoplasmic reticulum fractions: implications for malignant hyperthermia. *Biochemistry and Cell Biology*, **68**, 1195–201.

Fletcher, J. E., Tripolitis, L., Hubert, M., Vita, G. M., Levitt, R. C. & Rosenberg, H. (1995). Genotype and phenotype relationships for mutations in the ryanodine receptor in patients referred for diagnosis of malignant hyperthermia. *British Journal of Anaesthesia*, **75**, 307–10.

Fletcher, J. E., Tripolitis, L., Rosenberg, H & Beech, J. (1993b). Malignant hyperthermia: halothane- and calcium-induced calcium release in skeletal muscle. *Biochemistry and Molecular International*, **29**, 763–72.

Foster, P. S., Gesini, E., Claudianos, C., Hopkinson, K. C. & Denborough, M. A. (1989). Inositol 1,4,5,-trisphosphate phosphatase deficiency and malignant hyperpyrexia in swine. *Lancet*, **1**, 124–6.

Gronert, G. A. (1980). Malignant hyperthermia. *Anesthesiology*, **53**, 395–423.

Hawkes, M. J., Nelson, T. E. & Hamilton, S. L. (1992). [^{3}H]Ryanodine as a probe of changes in the functional state of the Ca^{2+}-release channel in malignant hyperthermia. *Journal of Biological Chemistry*, **267**, 6702–9.

Kim, D. H., Streter, F. A., Ohnishi, S. T., Ryan, J. F., Roberts, J., Allen, P. D., Meszaros, L. G., Antoniu, B. & Ikemoto, N. (1984). Kinetic studies of Ca^{2+} release from sarcoplasmic reticulum of normal and malignant hyperthermia susceptible pig muscles. *Biochimica et Biophysica Acta*, **775**, 320–7.

Louis, C. F., Zualkernan, K., Roghair, T. & Mickelson, J. R. (1992). The effects of volatile anesthetics on calcium regulation by malignant hyperthermia-susceptible sarcoplasmic reticulum. *Anesthesiology*, **77**, 114–25.

MacLennan, D. H. & Phillips, M. S. (1992). Malignant hyperthermia. *Science*, **256**, 789–94.

McSweeney, D. M. & Heffron, J. J. A. (1990). Uptake and release of calcium ions by heavy sarcoplasmic reticulum fraction of normal and malignant hyperthermia-susceptible human skeletal muscle. *International Journal of Biochemistry*, **22**, 329–33.

Mickelson, J. R., Gallant, E. M., Litterer, L. A., Johnson, K. M., Rempel, W. E. & Louis, C. F. (1988). Abnormal sarcoplasmic reticulum ryanodine receptor in malignant hyperthermia. *Journal of Biological Chemistry*, **263**, 9310–5.

Mickelson, J. R., Gallant, E. M., Rempel, W. E., Johnson, K. M., Litterer, L. A., Jacobson, B. A. & Louise, C. F. (1989). Effects of the halothane-sensitivity gene on sarcoplasmic reticulum function. *American Journal of Physiology*, **257**, C781–94.

Mickelson, J. R., Ross, J. A., Reed, B. K. & Louis, C.F. (1986). Enhanced Ca^{2+}-induced calcium release by isolated sarcoplasmic reticulum vesicles from malignant hyperthermia susceptible pig muscle. *Biochimica et Biophysica Acta*, **862**, 318–28.

Makita, N., Bennett Jr., P. B. & George Jr., A. L. (1994). Voltage-gated Na^+ channel β_1 subunit mRNA expressed in adult human skeletal muscle, heart and brain is encoded by a single gene. *Journal of Biological Chemistry*, **269**, 7571–8.

Nelson, T. E. (1983). Abnormality in calcium release from skeletal sarcoplasmic reticulum of pigs susceptible to malignant hyperthermia. *Journal of Clinical Investigation*, **72**, 862–70.

Nelson, T. E. (1990). Porcine malignant hyperthermia: critical temperatures for *in vivo* and *in vitro* responses. *Anesthesiology*, **73**, 449–54.

Nelson, T. E. (1992). Halothane effects on human malignant hyperthermia skeletal muscle single calcium-release channels in planer lipid bilayers. *Anesthesiology*, **76**, 588–95.

Nishizuka, Y. (1992). Intracellular signalling by hydrolysis of phospholipids and activation of protein kinase C. *Science*, **258**, 607–14.

Ohnishi, S. T., Taylor, S. & Gronert, G. A. (1983). Calcium-induced Ca^{2+} release from sarcoplasmic reticulum of pigs susceptible to malignant hyperthermia: the effects of halothane and dantrolene. *FEBS Letters*, **161**, 103–7.

Okumura, F., Crocker, B. D. & Denborough, M. A. (1980). Site of the muscle cell abnormality in swine susceptible to malignant hyperpyrexia. *British Journal of Anaesthesia*, **52**, 377–83.

Olckers, A., Meyers, D. A., Meyers, S., Taylor, E. W., Fletcher, J. E., Rosenberg, H., Isaacs, H. & Levitt, R. C. (1992). Adult muscle sodium channel alpha-subunit is a gene candidate for malignant hyperthermia susceptibility. *Genomics*, **14**,829–31.

Scholz, J., Roewer, N., Rum, U., Schmitz, W., Scholz, H. & Schulte am Esch, J. (1991 *a*). Possible involvement of inositol-lipid metabolism in malignant hyperthermia. *British Journal of Anaesthesia*, **66**, 692–6.

Scholz, J., Troll, U., Schulte am Esch, J., Hartung, E., Patten, M., Sandig, P. & Schmitz, W. (1991*b*). Inositol-1,4,5-trisphosphate and malignant hyperthermia. *Lancet*, **337**, 1361.

Shomer, N. H., Louis, C. F., Fill, M., Litterer, L. A. & Mickelson, J. R. (1993).

Reconstitution of abnormalities in the malignant hyperthermia-susceptible pig ryanodine receptor. *American Journal of Physiology*, **264**, C125–35.

Thomas, M. A., Rock, E. & Viret, J. (1991). Membrane properties of the sarcolemma and sarcoplasmic reticulum of pigs susceptible to malignant hyperthermia. Action of halothane. *Clinica Chimica Acta*, **200**, 201–10.

Vita, G. M., Olckers, A., Jedlicka, A. E., George, A. L., Heiman-Patterson, T., Rosenberg, H., Fletcher, J. E. & Levitt, R. C. (1995). Masseter muscle rigidity associated with glycine[1306]-to-alanine mutation in the adult muscle sodium channel α-subunit gene. *Anesthesiology*, **82**, 1087–103.

Wieland, S. J., Fletcher, J. E. & Gong, Q.-H. (1992a). Differential modulation of a sodium conductance in skeletal muscle by intracellular and extracellular fatty acids. *American Journal of Physiology*, **263**, C308–12.

Wieland, S. J., Fletcher, J. E., Rosenberg, H. & Gong, Q. H. (1989). Malignant hyperthermia: slow sodium current in cultured human muscle cells. *American Journal of Physiology*, **257**, C759–65.

Wieland, S. J., Gong, Q.-H., Fletcher, J. E. & Rosenberg, H. (1992b). Fatty acid activation of silent sodium channels in cultured human skeletal muscle. *Anesthesiology*, **77**, 761 (abstract).

11

Screening for malignant hyperthermia susceptibility

P. J. HALSALL

Introduction

The role of a diagnostic test is to distinguish without overlap, two groups of patients, those affected by the disease/disorder and those unaffected. Many of the tests proposed for malignant hyperthermia (MH) show a population difference between MH susceptible (MHS) patients and MH normal (MHN) patients. Although valuable in furthering the understanding of MH, such tests cannot always be applied as a screening test on individuals. Studies that may have the potential for development as a diagnostic test but are still a research tool are described here, together with the current standard screening test. A full list of all the described but now obsolete tests for MH will not be given, however, as they can be obtained elsewhere (Ørding, 1988).

A biological test will always have a degree of overlap between the two groups and inevitably compromises will need to be made when selecting threshold or cutoff values between normal and affected patients. In the case of MH these threshold values need to avoid a false negative diagnosis as this would lead to the administration of triggering drugs to an individual who is really susceptible to MH with potentially fatal consequences. A false positive MH diagnosis while clearly not desirable is inherently less dangerous. It was with these concepts in mind that the European MH Group (EMHG) developed its *in vitro* contracture test (IVCT) protocol, identifying the potential borderline group as MH equivocal (MHE) (European Malignant Hyperthermia Group, 1984, 1985).

Any screening procedure needs to be validated against the clinical presentation (Ellis *et al.*, 1990) and to follow the expected mode of inheritance in family studies. Denborough's original family clearly shows an autosomal dominant pattern of inheritance (Denborough & Lovell, 1960) and families with more than one proband support this view.

157

In vitro contracture tests

Although MH was described in 1960 by Denborough & Lovell (1960) it was not until 1970 that a potential screening test for MH was described by Kalow *et al.*, (1970). This test involved the exposure of living muscle samples to caffeine and the following year Ellis and coworkers (Ellis *et al.*, 1971) described a similar IVCT using halothane. These two tests now form the basis of routine family screening for MH throughout Europe, North America, Australia, New Zealand and South Africa.

Selection of patients for screening

Patients are referred usually, but not always, because of a suspected MH reaction to anaesthesia. As there is no sign unique to MH, assessment of the clinical presentation can often be very difficult especially when there is lack of recorded data (Ellis *et al.*, 1990). Once the decision has been taken to investigate the suspect reaction then ideally the proband should be tested to confirm or refute the clinical diagnosis. If the proband has died or is too young then the most appropriate close relation, usually the parents, will need to be screened. Most but not all centres do not screen children under 10–12 years. Although the total amount of muscle taken is only 1–2 g, the length of specimen is particularly important, and can be difficult to obtain in small children. This may account for the unsatisfactory results obtained from children in the past, which together with the maturation of muscle tissue has led to the reluctance to screen young children.

The aim of screening is to identify those family members not at risk from MH. In a theoretical family only 11–12% need be screened to identify the 5% at risk. Family screening is organised on the basis of an autosomal dominant pattern of inheritance. Thus relatives with a 50% chance of being affected are screened first (Ellis *et al.*, 1986).

European MH Group protocol for the *in vitro* contracture test (1984, 1985)

Muscle specimens are taken from the vastus medialis muscle around the motor point just above and medial to the knee. This localises the site of muscle samples consistently between patients. The operation is usually performed under a 3-in-1 femoral nerve block or non-triggering general anaesthesia. The samples are dissected *in situ* as fascicles ($30 \times 5 \times 3$ mm approximately) excised and stored at room temperature in carbonated Krebs' solution. The amount of

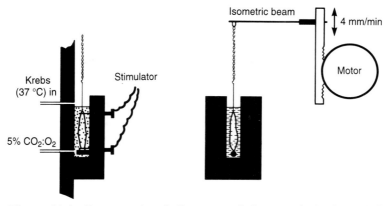

Figure 11.1. Cross-sectional diagrams of the muscle bath used for *in vitro* contracture tests.

muscle taken is of the order of 1g. For contracture testing, fascicles are attached in the tissue bath with one end suspended from a strain gauge transducer by a silk tie. The tissue bath (5 ml) is continuously perfused with carbonated Krebs solution to maintain the pH. Vapourised agents can be introduced via the gas line and agents in solution via the Krebs line (Figure 11.1). During testing the samples are stimulated to indicate the viability. The tests include the exposure of two separate muscle samples to halothane in incremental doses; 0.5, 1, 2% vapouriser settings, equivalent to 0.11, 0.22 and 0.44 mmol in the tissue bath calibrated by gas liquid chromatography. At least one test is static (Figure 11.2) and the other either static or dynamic. Some units are unable to perform the dynamic test and believe it is of no added value. The dynamic test, however, does illustrate several abnormalities thus adding confidence to an abnormal test (Figure 11.3).

Two further specimens are exposed to caffeine also in incremental doses 0.5, 1, 1.5, 2, 3, 4, and 32 mmol (Figure 11.4). Thus the two types of test are duplicated.

The results are regarded as positive if a sustained contracture of 0.2 g or greater is developed with 2% halothane or less and with 2 mmol caffeine or less. If both the halothane and caffeine tests are abnormal the patient is classified as MHS (susceptible), if both are normal the classification is MHN (normal) and MHE (equivocal) if only one type of test is abnormal. To clarify which type of test is abnormal in the MH equivocal group it is further subdivided into MHE(h), reacting to halothane only and MHE(c), reacting to caffeine only. A variation in laboratory standards may account for only one type of MH equivocal result being recorded in any one centre.

As already indicated the MH equivocal group was designated to identify a

(a)

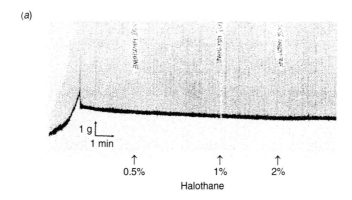

(b)

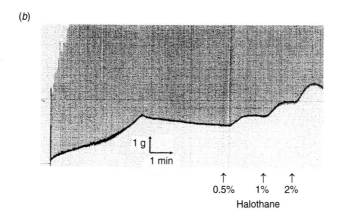

Figure 11.2. The *in vitro* response to increasing concentrations of halothane of muscle from: (*a*) a normal patient, and (*b*) a malignant hyperthermia susceptible patient. Note the increase in baseline tension in (*b*).

possible false positive/borderline result. For clinical purposes MH equivocal patients are treated as MH susceptible, while for research purposes they should be excluded in the first instance, as there is the potential of a doubtful diagnosis. Subsequent experience with the EMHG protocol has shown that the MH equivocal group has remained consistently high, in the order of 17%. It is apparent that some MHE(h) patients are developing marked contractures to halothane whereas others develop only small contractures (e.g. less than 0.5 g). Further family studies suggest that even some MHE(h) patients with poor contractures (less than 0.5 g) are likely to be truly MH susceptible, indicating that it would be unwise to alter the threshold values. It is estimated

(a)

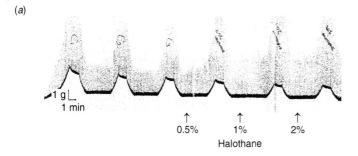

(b)

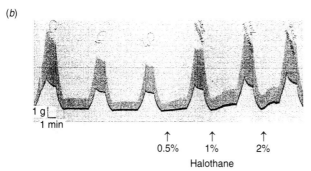

Figure 11.3. Dynamic halothane test. First to third curves: three control curves. Fourth to sixth curves: exposure to 0.5, 1 and 2% halothane, respectively. The curve is composed of four points. Upward deflection: muscle stretched by set amount. Top plateau: muscle rested for one minute at stretched length. Downward deflection: muscle relaxed by set amount. Bottom plateau: muscle rested in relaxed state for three minutes. Halothane perfusion commenced at the start of the three minute period. Each curve is produced by exactly the same amount of mechanical stretch and relaxation. Contracture is measured from the end of the one minute (top plateau) resting period.

that the true false positive rate is of the order of 5% (EMHG unpublished data). To aid interpretation of IVCT results the threshold values should be supplemented by the contracture strength when publishing the MH diagnosis. Indeed, this method of reporting has already been stipulated for genetic linkage studies performed by centres in the EMHG.

Since the formulation of the original protocol various quality control factors have been addressed by the EMHG to obtain greater uniformity between the various laboratories. These include the measurement of the concentration of halothane and caffeine in the tissue bath, characterisation of the tissue bath dynamics, types of muscle samples used from both patients and controls, type of anaesthesia administered to control patients, viability of samples and time to complete IVCT.

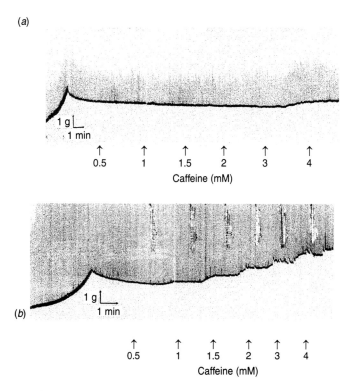

Figure 11.4. The *in vitro* response to increasing concentrations of caffeine of muscle from: (*a*) normal patient and (*b*) a malignant hyperthermia susceptible patient.

Validation of the European Malignant Hyperthermia Group protocol

This has been undertaken in two ways, first by comparing the IVCT results with the clinical presentation of the proband and second by reviewing the data from control cases. No fulminant case of MH from the EMHG has tested MH normal. A small percentage of control patients (1% for halothane and 4% for caffeine) have tested MH equivocal according to the protocol but the contractures were small at 0.2–0.3 g (EMHG unpublished data).

The clinical presentation of MH has been divided into several categories depending on the severity and type of clinical reaction and correlates well with the incidence of positive IVCT results (Ellis *et al.*, 1990). A review of patients with a 50% chance of inheriting MH, i.e. parents, siblings and children of a known case, does demonstrate a 50:50 distribution of positive:negative IVCT results (Ellis *et al.*, 1986). Furthermore, although entirely anecdotal, there have been no reports of MH normal patients reacting adversely to normal general anaesthesia.

North American Malignant Hyperthermia Group protocol

Following the establishment of the European protocol, the North American centres adopted a similar but differing protocol (Larach, 1989; Melton *et al.*, 1989; Rosenberg, 1989). The tests used include:

1. Single dose exposure to 3% halothane.
2. Incremental dose exposure to 0.5, 1, 2, 4, 8 and 32 mmol caffeine.
3. Exposure to the combined 1% halothane and caffeine test. This test is optional. In this test caffeine is added incrementally in the doses 0.25, 0.5, 1, 2, 4 and 32 mM to muscle exposed to 1% halothane.

The interpretation of the results in general is as follows:

1. Halothane test. A positive result is taken to be a contracture of 0.2–0.7 g. The threshold is to be determined by each laboratory as tissue bath concentrations of halothane are not measured.
2. Caffeine test. A positive result for this test is determined in three ways:
   (a) A contracture of 0.2 g or greater with 2 mmol caffeine.
   (b) Measurement of the 'caffeine-specific' concentration (CSC), i.e. the concentration of caffeine needed to produce a net increase in tension of 1 g should be less than 4 mmol.
   (c) Greater than 7% of the maximum contracture achieved with 32 mM should occur at 2 mmol or less.
3. Combined halothane/caffeine test. A contracture of 1 g or more should occur at a concentration of 1 mmol caffeine or less in the presence of 1% halothane.

Only one test needs be abnormal for the patient to be labelled as MH susceptible. A borderline/equivocal group as in the European protocol has been recently introduced, so the NAMHG interpretation of the IVCT results now achieves the subtlety of the EMHG protocol. Larach in a review of control data from the centres using the NAMHG protocol makes particular mention of the lack of quality controls in using the protocol and consequently a lack of uniformity in the standards set for the IVCT. It was estimated that a half to a quarter of control patients had a positive IVCT result equivalent to a false positive diagnosis, depending on which combination of the 5 tests were used (Larach *et al.*, 1992).

Various European centres have assessed the alternative interpretations of the caffeine test and the 3% halothane test. It was found that the false positive rate was increased to 6% for halothane and 5% for the CSC interpretation of the caffeine test. In addition there was also a false negative rate of 7% for the CSC caffeine interpretation in fulminant cases of MH. Consequently, the EMHG continues to use 2% halothane and 2 mmol caffeine threshold values (pooled EMHG data presented at the Munich Workshop, 1991).

Specificity of the *in vitro* contracture test

A variety of neuromuscular disorders such as myotonia, muscular dystrophies, familial periodic paralysis, have produced mildly abnormal but inconsistent responses to the IVCT (Heiman-Patterson *et al.*, 1988, Lehmann-Horn & Iaizzo, 1990). Furthermore, some patients with muscle disorders react abnormally to anaesthesia with an 'MH-like' reaction. It is generally accepted that these positive IVCT results reflect the lack of specificity of the IVCT on abnormal muscle and does not indicate that such patients are also susceptible to MH. The only exception is central core disease which is associated, although not invariably, with MH (Heytens *et al.*, 1992).

Other *in vitro* contracture tests

Although several tests have been described in the past (Ørding, 1988) they are no longer in common usage and will not be described here. There are two tests of current interest.

Combined halothane/caffeine test

Much controversy surrounds this test which is said to identify a separate group of MH susceptible patients known as the K-type (Nelson *et al.*, 1983). Such patients react normally to all other *in vitro* tests. Positive results, however, are seen in a significant number of control patients (Rosenberg, 1981; Nelson *et al.*, 1983) and it correlates poorly with the halothane and caffeine tests used separately (Ellis *et al.*, 1992). It contributes little to the diagnosis of MH and is no longer used by the EMHG although its use remains optional in the NAMHG protocol where its use is advocated strongly by some centres.

Ryanodine test

Ryanodine is a plant alkaloid with a high binding affinity for the foot process structure linking the gap between the sarcoplasmic reticulum and the T-tubule of the muscle. It is thought to act as a calcium release channel, known as the ryanodine receptor (RYR), a postulated site of the MH defect. It was therefore of interest to study the effect of ryanodine in the tissue bath. Ryanodine has been shown to induce contractures of muscle, MH susceptible muscle being more sensitive than MH normal muscle. It appears to be a more sensitive test than caffeine but less sensitive than halothane. It is a useful addition to the standard IVCT and the use of a third test may help to increase the confidence and therefore the accuracy of phenotyping (Hopkins *et al.*, 1991). As with the other contracture tests ryanodine is not specific for MH and abnormal contractures have been reported in other neuromuscular disorders (Hopkins *et al.*, 1993).

Other invasive muscle tests

Skinned fibre technique

Muscle fibres can be chemically 'skinned' of their sarcolemma thus exposing the 'inside' of the muscle for studies on the sarcoplasmic reticulum. These samples can be prepared from needle biopsy specimens and can be stored for several weeks, a clear advantage over the IVCT technique that requires living tissue. The method was originally described by Endo *et al.* (1970) who used both halothane and caffeine to enhance calcium-induced calcium release from the sarcoplasmic reticulum, so eliciting contractures in MH susceptible patients compared with normals. Wood (1978) developed a technique for observing caffeine contractures on single fibres. This latter technique was evaluated by Britt *et al.* (1982) who found it to be a useful test, but unfortunately compared it with the combined halothane/caffeine test about which there are strong reservations (described above). This technique, therefore, has not been fully evaluated alongside the IVCT method but may be a valuable research tool for studies on the sarcoplasmic reticulum. It is a widely used screening method in Japan.

Histological examination of muscle

It might be expected that a muscle defect such as MH would be readily identified histologically. It was quickly apparent, however, that the majority of MH susceptible patients had entirely normal histopathology. Features that have been described in 'MH myopathy' are diffusely distributed internal nuclei, moth-eaten fibres and cores (Harriman, 1988). Thus histology is rarely used by most MH centres because it is too costly and unrewarding. It is valuable, however, as part of the routine investigation of the proband. Abnormal anaesthetic reactions can occur in most muscle disorders as well as MH and can be the first indication of a muscle disease in an asymptomatic or mildly affected patient. Histological examination will identify such patients who would be generally expected to have normal IVCT results. The exception is central core disease which is the only muscle disorder known to be clearly associated, although not invariably, with MH (Heytens *et al.*, 1992).

Calcium uptake technique

This method for determining the diagnosis of MH proved to be a salutary experience. The measurement of calcium uptake by the sarcoplasmic reticulum was claimed to demonstrate MH susceptibility and was used for some years by certain centres as the sole method of diagnosis. The main advantage was that frozen biopsy specimens could be used (Allen *et al.*, 1986). The incidence of MH susceptibility was found to be considerably higher than expected using this technique and thus its validity was questioned. Further studies comparing the Ca^{2+} uptake method with the IVCT result and also the clinical presentation of MH failed to show any correlation and therefore this technique has no significant predictive value in determining MH susceptibility (Nagarajan *et al.*, 1987).

Inositol 1,4,5 trisphosphate (IP₃)

Intracellular Ca^{2+} is also regulated by the phosphoinositide cycle involving inositol 1,4,5-trisphosphate (IP_3), a second messenger promoting the release of Ca^{2+} from intracellular stores. It has been reported that in MH swine the sarcoplasmic reticulum is deficient in inositol 1,4,5-trisphosphate phosphatase activity leading to high myoplasmic IP_3 and Ca^{2+}. Halothane inhibits the already depleted phosphatase activity leading to a further rise in myoplasmic IP_3 and Ca^{2+} resulting in an MH reaction. Thus IP_3 is suggested to play a primary role in the aetiology of MH (Foster *et al.*, 1989). Interestingly the putative IP_3 receptor located on the sarcoplasmic reticulum is reported to be partly homologous to the skeletal muscle ryanodine receptor (Mignery *et al.*, 1989). A further study has shown that the IP_3 content of human MHS muscle, measured by high performance liquid chromatography, is higher than in MH normal muscle with barely any overlap (Scholz *et al.*, 1991). These IP_3 measurements have yet to be evaluated fully so it is difficult to assess their potential role in the diagnosis of MH at this stage.

Non-invasive tests on muscle

Electromyographic studies

A promising electromyographic (EMG) study was reported by Eng *et al.*, (1984) several years ago but has never been followed up. Caffeine, halothane and suxamethonium were instilled separately into the thenar muscles under repetitive nerve stimulation and the EMG observed. A significantly greater decrease in the negative peaks of the motor unit potentials were seen in MHS patients compared to controls, correlating with 8 out of 9 *in vitro* studies.

Nuclear magnetic resonance spectroscopy (NMR-S)

NMR spectroscopy using ^{31}P follows the time course of the concentration changes in the phosphorylated metabolites such as creatine phosphate (PCr), inorganic phosphate (P_i), phosphodiesters (PDE), ATP and pH, during exercise (see Chapter 5 for description of the underlying principles). Studies carried out using exercise protocols have indicated evidence of a perturbed energy metabolism and probably increased anaerobic glycolysis in MH susceptible individuals and also in exercise hyperthermic individuals (Kozak-Reiss *et al.*, 1988; Olgin *et al.*, 1991). Higher P_i/PCr ratios at rest and slower post-exercise recovery of PCr/P_i ratio have been reported as well as a marked intracellular acidosis during effort in MH susceptible individuals (Payen *et al.*, 1991). Another study has found that the post-exercise rest period to be the more informative with the P_i/PCr ratio being the most useful indicator. A stepwise discriminative analysis of the two parameters P_i/PCr and PDE/PCr improved the predictive power of this method. Unfortunately the test is not specific as abnormalities can be detected in myopathic patients and after muscle injury. It cannot be used, therefore, for mass population screening of MH but it has been suggested that NMR studies could be used as a first step in the diagnosis prior to muscle biopsy in cases where there is a high chance of MH, e.g. family screening (Payen *et al.*, 1993).

Muscle relaxation rates

Lenmarken *et al.* (1987) reported a significantly greater rate of muscle relaxation in MHS subjects compared with controls; however, the population overlap rendered this test inappropriate for screening purposes. An attempt to repeat this work using refinements of temperature control on the thenar muscles subjected to tetanic stimulation was unable to confirm that relaxation rates in MH susceptible patients differed from MH normal patients and thus were of no value as a diagnostic test (Urwyler *et al.*, 1990).

Blood tests

Creatine Kinase (CK) estimations

CK was first suggested as a screening method for MH in 1970, the same year of publication as the caffeine IVCT (Isaacs & Barlow, 1970). Even today it is still frequently used by clinicians as an indication of MH susceptibility. Although CK measurements from a group of MH susceptible individuals are statistically significantly higher than a group of MH normal individuals the degree of overlap between the two groups makes this investigation useless at an individual level (Ellis *et al.*, 1986).

Membrane studies

While the molecular site of the MH defect remains unresolved there is still speculation as to whether MH is a generalised membrane disorder rather than a muscle membrane disorder. Assuming the former, tissues more easily accessible than muscle could be used as the basis of a screening test for MH.

Electron paramagnetic spin resonance

This is a method of determining the fluidity of a lipid membrane by the introduction of a spin label, in this instance 16-deoxystearic acid. It has been suggested that membranes from red blood cells are more fluid in MH susceptible subjects compared with normals on exposure to halothane, with a clear separation of the two groups MH susceptible and MH normal, predicting the IVCT MH diagnosis in 13 of 14 patients (Ohnishi *et al.*, 1988). This work has not been substantiated either in humans (Cooper & Meddings, 1991; Halsall *et al.*, 1992) or in pigs (Ervasti *et al.*, 1986), in the latter case looking at isolated sarcolemma, heavy sarcoplasmic reticulum and T-tubule membranes. Furthermore, there was no evidence to suggest a generalised membrane defect. The techniques used in these studies have been criticised and an improved study has claimed to identify differences between MH susceptible and MH normal membranes (Cooper *et al.*, 1992). This work still needs further study to resolve the two questions: is MH a generalised membrane disorder and can this method discriminate MH susceptible and MH normal patients without overlap to provide an alternative non-invasive screening test as originally claimed?

Calcium measurements

In 1985 it was reported (Lopez *et al.*, 1985) that the resting (i.e. without halothane exposure) intracellular ionised calcium concentration $[Ca^{2+}]$ in muscles was greater in MH susceptible humans compared with normals. This increase in the resting level of myoplasmic calcium was disputed by Iaizzo and colleagues who only found a difference with exposure to halothane (Iaizzo *et al.*, 1988). A specific calcium fluorescent chelator such as Fura-2 or Quin-2 is used as the calcium detector.

Similar techniques have been applied to blood mononuclear cells, where an increase in ionised calcium might be expected if MH were a generalised membrane disorder. Klip and colleagues have demonstrated a significant increase in cytoplasmic $[Ca^{2+}]$ following the addition of halothane in MH susceptible patients but not normals. Without the addition of halothane the $[Ca^{2+}]$ was the same for the two groups. The increase in $[Ca^{2+}]$ requires the presence of extracellular Ca^{2+} indicating a calcium ion influx at the plasma membrane (Klip *et al.*, 1987*a*). This study has been confirmed in pigs (Klip *et al.*, 1987*b*). Functional assays using lymphocytes are being assessed as potential replacements for the screening of IVCT (O'Brien *et al.*, 1990).

An improved technique using a new calcium fluorescent indicator, Indo-1, has also been described by the same group. Lower concentrations of the indicator can be used thereby decreasing the risk of cell damage and chelation of cytoplasmic Ca^{2+}, together with clinical concentrations of halothane. They found that the resting cytoplasmic $[Ca^{2+}]$ was slightly but significantly higher in MH susceptible humans but not MH susceptible pigs. Exposure to halothane produced a larger increase in cytoplasmic $[Ca^{2+}]$ in both MH susceptible humans and pigs compared with normals. Increasing the dose of halothane caused a further increase in cytoplasmic $[Ca^{2+}]$ in MH susceptible cases, a feature not seen in the previous studies, probably for technical reasons. It is, therefore, suggested that the higher dose of halothane should be used to differentiate MH susceptible and MH normal patients. A further difference from the original study was the response to extracellular Ca^{2+}. In this study removal of extracellular Ca^{2+} eliminated the halothane effect in normal patients only, a good but reduced response still being obtained from MH susceptible patients, thus giving conflicting evidence of the role of Ca^{2+} influx at the plasma membrane. These interesting findings need much further study and have yet to be confirmed by other groups working in the field before their role in the diagnosis of MH can be properly evaluated (Klip *et al.*, 1990).

DNA studies

The tremendous strides in DNA technology have opened the way for the possible identification of the MH defect and an alternative non-invasive screening test. Initial studies were encouraging, suggesting that chromosome 19, in particular the region close to the RYR1 gene (ryanodine receptor gene), 19q12-13.2, was a potential candidate area (McCarthy *et al.*, 1990; MacLennan *et al.*, 1990). Indeed one group has already proposed that MH diagnosis could be made on DNA linkage studies providing the family had already been extensively investigated by muscle biopsy (Healey *et al.*, 1991). This initial enthusiasm has been tempered by further studies on more families showing a significant degree of heterogeneity (Deufel *et al.*, 1992, 1991; Ball *et al.*, 1993), only one half of MH families showing evidence of linkage to chromosome 19. Other possible candidate genes have been studied including those of the β and γ subunits of the dihydropyridine receptor (a slow release calcium channel) located on chromosome 17 which showed no evidence of linkage (Iles *et al.*, 1993). It is envisaged that the next step will be a major European collaborative gene mapping study aimed at the localisation of new loci. A full account of the genetic aspects of MH and a review of the DNA studies can be found in Chapter 13.

Until the question of heterogeneity has been resolved DNA testing cannot supersede the muscle biopsy screening protocols which will probably remain the gold standard for MH screening for some time to come (Ball *et al.*, 1992; Ellis, 1992).

Whatever method of diagnosing MH eventually takes over from muscle biopsy, it will not merely involve the result of a laboratory test on a suspected individual but a continuing clinical commitment to the whole family.

References

Allen, P. D., Ryan, J. F., Jones, D. E., Mabuchi, K., Virga, Roberts, J. & Sreter F. (1986). Sarcoplasmic reticulum calcium uptake in cyrostat sections of skeletal muscle from malignant hyperthermia patients and controls. *Muscle and Nerve*, **9**, 475–9.

Ball, S. P., Dorkins, H. R., Ellis, F. R., Halsall, P. J., Hopkins, P. M., Mueller, R. F. & Stewart, A. D. (1993). Genetic linkage analysis of chromosome 19 markers in malignant hyperthermia. *British Journal of Anaesthesia*, **70**, 70–5.

Ball, S. P., Dorkins, H. R., Ellis, F. R., Hall, J. L., Halsall, P. J., Hopkins, P. M. & Stewart, A. D. (1992). Is muscle biopsy for malignant hyperthermia still necessary? *British Journal of Anaesthesia*, **69**, 222P–223P.

Britt, B. A., Frodis, W., Scott, E., Clements, M.-J. & Endrenyi, L. (1982). Comparison of the caffeine skinned fibre tension (CSFT) test with the caffeine-halothane contracture (CHC) test in the diagnosis of malignant hyperthermia. *Canadian Anaesthetists Society Journal*, **29**, 550–62.

Brownell, A. K. W. (1988). Malignant hyperthermia: relationship to other diseases. *British Journal of Anaesthesia*, **60**, 303–8.

Cooper, P., Kudynska, J., Buckmaster, H. A. & Kudynki, R. (1992). An EPR investigation of spin-labelled erythrocytes as a diagnostic technique for malignant hyperthermia. *Biochemica et Biophysica Acta*, **1139**, 70–6.

Cooper, P. & Meddings, J. B. (1991). Erythrocyte membrane fluidity in malignant hyperthermia. *Biochemica et Biophysica Acta*, **1069**, 151–6.

Denborough M. A. & Lovell, R. R. H. (1960). Anaesthetic deaths in a family. *Lancet*, **2**, 45.

Deufel, T., Golla, A., Iles, D. E., Meindl, A. Meitinger, T. Schindelhauer, D., DeVries, A., Pongratz D., MacLellan, D. H., Johnson, K. J. & Lehmann-Horn, F. (1992). Evidence for genetic heterogeneity of malignant hyperthermia susceptibility. *American Journal of Human Genetics*, **50**, 1151–61.

Ellis, F. R. (1992). Detecting susceptibility to malignant hyperthermia. *British Medical Journal*, **304**, 791–2.

Ellis, F. R., Halsall, P. J. & Christian, A. S. (1990). Clinical presentation of suspected malignant hyperthermia during anaesthesia in 402 probands. *Anaesthesia*, **45**, 838–41.

Ellis, F. R., Halsall, P. J. & Harriman, D. G. F. (1986). The work of the Leeds Malignant Hyperthermia Investigation Unit, 1971–84. *Anaesthesia*, **46**, 806–15.

Ellis, F. R., Halsall, P. J. & Hopkins, P. M. (1992). Is the 'k-type' caffeine/halothane responder susceptible to malignant hyperthermia? *British Journal of Anaesthesia*, **69**, 471–3.

Ellis, F. R., Harriman, D. G. F., Kearney, N. P., Kyei-Mensah, K. & Tyrell, J. H. (1971). Halothane-induced muscle contracture as a cause of hyperthermia. *British Journal of Anaesthesia*, **43**, 721–2.

Endo, M., Tanaka, M. & Ogawa, Y. (1970). Calcium induced release of calcium from the sarcoplasmic reticulum of skinned skeletal muscle fibres. *Nature*, **228**, 34–6.

Eng, G. D., Becker, M. J. & Muldoon, S. M. (1984). Electrodiagnostic tests in the detection of MH. *Muscle and Nerve*, **7**, 618–25.

European Malignant Hyperthermia Group (1984). A protocol for the investigation of malignant hyperthermia (MH) susceptibility. *British Journal of Anaesthesia*, **56**, 1267–9.

European Malignant Hyperthermia Group (1985). Laboratory diagnosis of malignant hyperthermia susceptibility (MHS). *British Journal of Anaesthesia*, **57**, 1038.

Ervasti, J. M., Mickelson, J. R., Lewis, S. M., Thomas, D. D. & Louis C. F. (1986). An electron paramagnetic resonance study of skeletal muscle membrane fluidity in malignant hyperthermia. *Biochemica et Biophysica Acta*, **986**, 70–4.

Foster, P. S., Gesini, E., Claudianos, C., Hopkinson, K. C. & Denborough, M. A. (1989). Inositol 1,4,5 trisphosphate phosphatase and malignant hyperthermia in swine. *Lancet*, **2**, 124–7.

Halsall, P. J., Ellis, F. R. & Knowles, P. F. (1992). Evaluation of spin resonance spectroscopy of red blood cell membranes to detect malignant hyperthermia susceptibility. *British Journal of Anaesthesia*, **69**, 471–3.

Harriman, D. G. F. (1988). Malignant hyperthermia myopathy: a critical review. *British Journal of Anaesthesia*, **60**, 309–16.

Healy, S. J. M., Heffron, J. J. A., Lehane, M., Bradley, D. G., Johnson, K. & McCarthy, T. V. (1991). Diagnosis of susceptibility to malignant hyperthermia with flanking DNA markers. *British Medical Journal*, **303**, 1225–8.

Heiman-Patterson, T., Rosenberg, H., Fletcher, J. E. & Tahmoush, A. J. (1988). Halothane-caffeine contracture testing in neuromuscular disease. *Muscle and Nerve*, **11**, 435–7.

Heytens, L., Martin, J. J., van der Kleft, E. & Bossaert, L. L. (1992). *In vitro* contracture tests in patients with various neuromuscular diseases. *British Journal of Anaesthesia*, **68**, 72–5.

Hopkins, P. M., Ellis, F. R. & Halsall, P. J. (1993). Comparison of *in vitro* contracture testing with halothane, caffeine and ryanodine in malignant hyperthermia and other neuromuscular disorders. *British Journal of Anaesthesia*, **70**, 397–401.

Hopkins, P. M., Ellis, F. R. & Halsall, P. J. (1991). Ryanodine contracture: a potentially specific *in vitro* diagnostic test for malignant hyperthermia. *British Journal of Anaesthesia* , **66**, 611–13.

Iaizzo, P. A., Klein, W. & Lehmann-Horn, F. (1988). Fura-2 detected myoplasmic calcium and its correlation with contracture force in skeletal muscle from normal and malignant hyperthermia susceptible pigs. *Pflügers Archiv*, **411**, 648–53.

Iles, D. E., Segers, B., Sengers, R. C. A., Monsieurs, K., Heytens, L., Halsall, P. J., Hopkins, P. M., Ellis, F. R., Hall-Curran, J. L., Stewart, A. D. & Wieringa, B. (1993). Genetic mapping of the β and δ subunits of the human skeletal muscle L-type voltage-dependent calcium channels on chromosome 17q and exclusion as candidate genes for malignant hyperthermia susceptibility. *Human Molecular Genetics*, **2**, 863–8.

Isaacs, H. & Barlow, M. B. (1970). Genetic background to malignant hyperpyrexia revealed by serum creatine phosphokinase estimates in asymptomatic relatives. *British Journal of Anaesthesia*, **42**, 1077–84.

Kalow, W., Britt, B. A., Terrau, M. E., & Haist, C. (1970). Metabolic error of muscle metabolism after recovery from malignant hyperthermia. *Lancet*, **2**, 895–8.

Klip, A., Britt, B. A., Elliott, M. E., Regg, W., Frodis, W. & Scott, E. (1987*a*). Anaesthetic-induced increase in ionised calcium in blood mononuclear cells from malignant hyperthermia patients. *Lancet*, **1**, 463–6.

Klip, A., Mills, G. B., Britt, B. A. & Elliott, M. E. (1990). Halothane-dependent release of intracellular Ca^{2+} in blood cells in malignant hyperthermia. *American Physiological Society*, C495–C503.

Klip, A., Ramlal, T., Walker, D., Britt, B. A & Elliott, M. E. (1987*b*). Selective increase in cytoplasmic calcium by anesthetics in lymphocytes from MH susceptible pigs. *Anesthesia and Analgesia*, **66**, 381–5.

Kozak-Reiss, G., Gascard, J. P., Herve, P. H., Jehenson, P. H. & Syrota, A. (1988). Malignant and exercise hyperthermia: investigation of 73 subjects by contracture tests and P31 NMR spectroscopy. *Anesthesiology*, **69**, 415 (abstract).

Larach, M. G. for the North American Malignant Hyperthermia Group (1989). Standardization of the caffeine halothane muscle contracture test. *Anaesthesia and Analgesia*, **69**, 511–5.

Larach, M. G., Landis, J. R., Bunn, J. S. & Diaz, M. (1992). The North American MH Registry. Prediction of MHS in low-risk subjects. *Anesthesiology*, **76**, 16–27.

Lehmann-Horn, F. & Iaizzo, P. A. (1990). Are myotonias and periodic paralysis associated with susceptibility to malignant hyperthermia? *British Journal of Anaesthesia*, **65**, 692–7.

Lenmarken, C., Rutberg, H. & Henriksson, K. G. (1987). Abnormal relaxation rates in subjects susceptible to malignant hyperthermia. *Acta Neurologica Scandinavica*, **75**, 81–3.

Lopez, J. R., Alamo, L., Caputo, C., Wikinsi, J. & Ledezma, D. (1985). Intracellular ionised calcium concentration in muscles from human with malignant hyperthermia. *Muscle and Nerve*, **8**, 355–8.

MacLennan, D. H., Duff, C., Zorzato, F., Fujii, J., Philips, M. S., Korneluk, R. G., Frodis, W., Britt, B. A. & Worton, R. G. (1990). Ryanodine receptor gene is a candidate for predisposition to malignant hyperthermia. *Nature*, **343**, 559–61.

McCarthy, T. V., Healy, J. M. S., Heffron, J. J. A., Lehane, M., Deufel, T., Lehmann-Horn, F., Farral, M. & Johnson, K. (1990). Localisation of the malignant hyperthermia susceptibility locus to human chromosome 19q 12-13.2. *Nature*, **343**, 562–4.

Melton, A. T., Martucci, R. W., Kien, N. D. & Gronert, G. A. (1989). Malignant hyperthermia in humans: standardisation of contracture testing protocol. *Anesthesia and Analgesia* **69**, 437–43.

Mignery, G. A., Sudhof, T. C., Takei, K & Camilli, P. D. (1989). Putative receptor for inositol 1,4,5 triphosphate similar to ryanodine receptor. *Nature*, **342**, 192–5.

Nagarajan, K., Fishbein, W. N., Muldoon, S. M. & Pezeshkpour, G. (1987). Calcium uptake in frozen muscle biopsy sections compared with other predictors of malignant hyperthermia susceptibility. *Anesthesiology*, **66**, 680–5.

Nelson, T. E., Flewellen, E. H. & Gloyna, D. F. (1983). Spectrum of susceptibility to malignant hyperthermia: diagnostic dilemma. *Anaesthesia and Analgesia*, **62**, 545–52.

O'Brien, P. J., Klip, A., Britt, B. A. & Kalow, B. I. (1990). MHS: biochemical basis for pathogenesis and diagnosis. *Canadian Journal of Veterinarian Research*, **54**, 83–92.

Ohnishi, S. T., Katagi, H., Ohnishi, T. & Brownell, A. K. W. (1988). Detection of malignant hyperthermia susceptibility using a spin-label technique on red blood cells. *British Journal of Anaesthesia*, **61**, 565–8.

Olgin, J., Rosenberg, H., Allen, G., Seestedt, R. & Chance, B. (1991). A blinded comparison of non-invasive, *in vivo* phosphorus nuclear magnetic resonance spectroscopy and the *in vitro* halothane/caffeine contracture test in the evaluation of malignant hyperthermia susceptibility. *Anesthesia and Analgesia*, **72**, 36–47.

Ørding, H. (1988). Diagnosis of susceptibility to malignant hyperthermia in man. *British Journal of Anaesthesia*, **60**, 287–302.

Payen, J. F., Bosson, J. L., Bourdon, L., Jacquot, C., le Bas, J. F., Stieglitz, P & Benabid A. L. (1993). Improved non-invasive diagnostic testing for malignant hyperthermia susceptibility from combination of metabolites determined *in vivo* with 31P magnetic resonance spectroscopy. *Anesthesiology*, **78**, 848–55.

Payen, J. F., Bourdon, L., Mezin, P., Jacquot, C., le Bas, J. F., Stieglitz, P. & Benabid, A. L. (1991). Susceptibility to malignant hyperthermia detected non-invasively. *Lancet*, **337**, 550–1.

Rosenberg, H. (1981). International workshop on MH. *Anesthesiology*, **54**, 530–1.

Rosenberg, H. (1989). Standards for the halothane/caffeine contracture test. *Anesthesia and Analgesia*, **69**, 429–30.

Scholz, R., Troll, U., Schute am Esch, J., Hartung, E., Pattern, M., Sundig, P. & Schmitz, W. (1991). Inositol 1,4,5-trisphosphate and malignant hyperthermia. *Lancet*, **1**, 1361.

Urywler, A., Ellis, F. R., Halsall, P. J. & Hopkins, P. M. (1990). Muscle relaxation rates in individuals susceptible to malignant hyperthermia. *British Journal of Anaesthesia*, **65**, 421–3.

Wood, D. S. (1978). Human skeletal muscle: analysis of Ca^{2+} regulation in skinned fibres using caffeine. *Experimental Neurology*, **58**, 218–30.

12

Skeletal muscle morphology

P. HARNDEN

Introduction

Since the first description of malignant hyperthermia (MH) in humans (Denborough & Lovell, 1960), there have been many reports of the changes seen in the muscle of susceptible patients, both after an episode of MH, when massive muscle necrosis may occur secondary to sustained contracture, and dissociated from an actual MH event (Gullotta & Helpap, 1975; Gullota, 1976; Gullotta & Spiez-Kiefer, 1983; Ranklev et al., 1986). Such descriptions have led some pathologists to put forward a case for a distinctive 'MH myopathy' (Harriman et al., 1973, 1978; Harriman, 1988), consisting of fibre hypertrophy, internal nuclei and moth-eaten and core fibres, whereas others highlight the lack of changes in MH susceptible muscle (Ranklev et al., 1986).

The association of MH susceptibility with myopathies is also well described (Harriman et al., 1973, 1978; Shuaib et al., 1987; Harriman, 1988; Heiman-Patterson et al., 1988; Peluso & Bianchini, 1992; Wedel, 1992). In the case of central core disease (CCD), there is both clinical and laboratory evidence of a linkage, including the proximity of the CCD gene to the ryanodine receptor gene on chromosome 19 (Kausch et al., 1991). There is also some evidence that clinical heat stroke and MH may be associated with similar (but not identical) inherited abnormalities of skeletal muscle (Hopkins et al., 1991). In other neuromuscular diseases, it may be that the primary muscle abnormality leads to an abnormal response to halothane or caffeine during the in vitro contracture test (IVCT). In one study (Heytens et al., 1992), 20% of patients investigated for a variety of neuromuscular disorders had either positive or equivocal results on IVCT.

These findings clearly indicate the necessity for vigilance in the interpretation of biopsies from individuals being screened for susceptibility, as the failure to diagnose a specific 'non-MH' myopathy may deprive individuals and families of the appropriate genetic counselling or treatment. The difficulty is compounded by the number of myopathies that are poorly defined both from a clinical and pathological point of view.

It is therefore important to delineate the changes in skeletal muscle morphology which can be attributed to MH susceptibility alone, from those that may represent an associated myopathy, in order to fully investigate that patient and his or her family.

Pathology of malignant hyperthermia susceptible muscle

Because of the variability in morphological descriptions of MH susceptible muscle (see above), only a large scale study of biopsies from a wide age range and both sexes would be definitive, if compared with MH negative controls of the same sex and age.

Study outline

A review of the files and patient records of the Leeds MH Investigation Unit identified individuals who were screened for susceptibility to MH (for details, see Ellis *et al.*, 1986) and who did not show any evidence of a systemic disease or a neuromuscular disorder. Morphometric analysis was then performed on the biopsies without knowledge of their age, sex or MH status. The cases were then divided into MH normal (296 cases) and MH susceptible (242 cases) groups on the basis of the test results. The MH susceptible group will include some cases that would currently be classified as equivocal (European Malignant Hyperpyrexia Group, 1985).

The muscle biopsy technique, histochemistry, morphometric analyses and statistical methods are described elsewhere (Harnden-Mayor, 1989), and only the key findings are presented here. The parameters investigated were mean fibre diameters and composition of types 1, 2A and 2B fibres, fibre size variability, and so-called 'myopathic' features, consisting of internal nuclei, regenerating or degenerating fibres, split fibres and core fibres.

Findings

Mean fibre diameters

Mean diameters are generally higher in MH susceptible than in MH normal biopsies for each fibre type (Table 12.1). There is much overlap, however, between the two groups, so that only a few values lie outside the upper limits.

Table 12.1. *Mean difference in diameters (μm) between MH susceptible and MH normal individuals*

Fibre type	1	2A	2B
Males			
Mean difference adjusted for age	6.8	6.5	4.2
Significance level (*p*)	<0.0001	<0.0001	<0.004
Females			
Mean difference adjusted for age	9.7	8.2	6.3
Significance level(*p*)	<0.0001	<0.0001	<0.0001

Histograms of the distribution of mean fibre diameters for all fibre types with the corresponding 95% prediction limits for MH normal biopsies are shown in Figure 12.1 for females as an example. Little relationship was found with age in females, so no adjustment was made for age.

Fibre size variability

There is often, but not always, higher variability in MH susceptible biopsies. This supports the contention that there is low-grade ongoing damage in MH susceptible muscle in some individuals, as increases in fibre size variability are taken to reflect such damage, with the coexistence of normal or even hypertrophied fibres and damaged, atrophic fibres within a given fibre type (Dubowitz & Brooke, 1973). This may of course vary over time in any one MH susceptible individual depending on recent activities or events, although only a longitudinal study could address this.

Fibre type composition

There is no consistent significant difference in composition from MH normal and MH susceptible biopsies.

There has been much discussion in the literature about the increased sensitivity of type 1 fibres to caffeine (Mitsumoto *et al.*, 1990; Adnet *et al.*, 1993), but given that there is no demonstrable preponderance of type 1 fibres in MH susceptible biopsies, this is not an issue in terms of MH susceptibility.

'Myopathic' features

Histograms of the relative frequency of these features in MH susceptible versus MH normal biopsies are presented in Figures 12.2 to 12.5. Rather than a distinct peak representing individuals with a myopathy, there is an overall wider spread of values in the MH susceptible population. Only 0.4% of MH

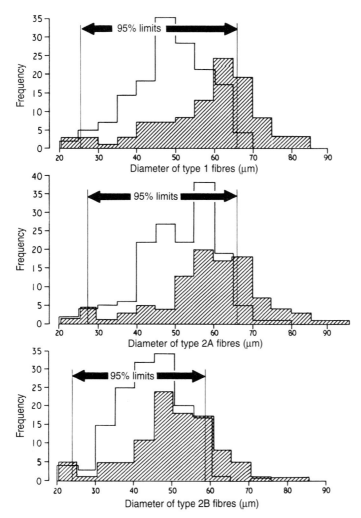

Figure 12.1. Distribution of mean fibre diameters in malignant hyperthermia susceptible (▨) and normal (☐) females.

susceptible biopsies had values for all four parameters outside the normal range. None of the MH susceptible individuals with values outside the normal range in this series had any clinical evidence of a myopathy.

The relative frequency of all features except core fibres generally increases with advancing age in both MH susceptible and MH normal subjects, but more obviously with increasing diameters, particularly in the MH susceptible group. For example in females the relationship between the percentage of internal nuclei and age fails to reach statistical significance (Figure 12.6)

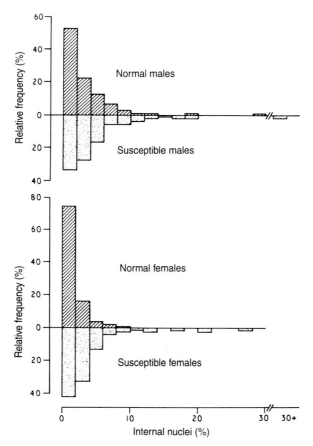

Figure 12.2. Percentage of internal nuclei in malignant hyperthermia normal versus malignant hyperthermia susceptible males and females.

whereas there is a clear relationship with diameters (Figure 12.7, $r = 0.42$, $p < 0.001$).

Malignant hyperthermia myopathy: a distinctive entity?

Many of the descriptions of this entity were based on case reports (Harriman *et al.*, 1973), and on cases where susceptibility to MH had not been confirmed by muscle contracture tests (Gullotta & Helpap, 1975; Gullotta, 1976; Gullotta & Spiez-Kiefer, 1983). In later reviews (Harriman *et al.*, 1978; Harriman, 1988), there was no systematic comparisons with MH normal biopsies, and biopsies were always interpreted in the knowledge of the MH status, which

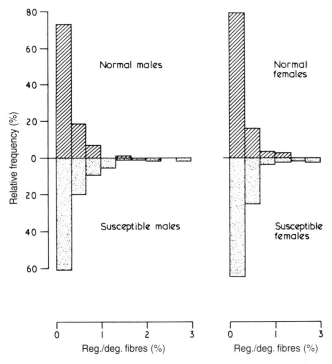

Figure 12.3. Percentage of regenerating(reg.)/degenerating(deg.) fibres in malignant hyperthermia normal versus malignant hyperthermia susceptible males and females.

may have led to bias. The only, albeit small scale, systematic analysis (Ranklev *et al.*, 1986) of MH susceptible biopsies failed to support the contention of a distinctive myopathy, either pathologically or clinically.

As seen above, changes are undoubtedly seen in MH susceptible muscle more frequently than in MH normal biopsies, but there should be some hesitation in calling these features 'myopathic' given that they are seen in biopsies from individuals who are not susceptible to MH and have no evidence of any other disease. These features probably represent non-specific damage occurring as a normal phenomenon in the ageing muscle or as a result of use. There is no evidence of a distinctive myopathy in MH susceptible muscle that would allow pathological recognition of susceptibility. The key event in MH susceptible muscle is a general increase in size, which is recognisable at a statistical rather than individual biopsy level, the other features being correlated more or less closely with fibre diameters. How this increase in fibre sizes relates to an inherent muscle defect and particularly to the putative abnormality in the ryanodine gene receptor is unclear (Hopkins *et al.*, 1992).

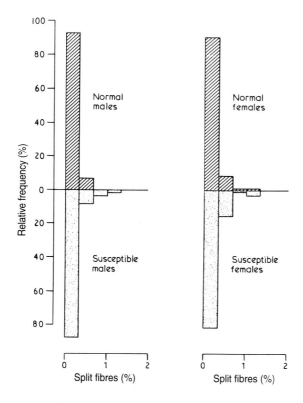

Figure 12.4. Percentage of split fibres in malignant hyperthermia normal versus malignant hyperthermia susceptible males and females.

Conclusion

While the boundaries of our knowledge of muscle disorders are constantly being extended, a proportion of patients remain difficult to categorise on clinical and pathological grounds if the biopsy findings fail to pattern a specific, well recognised entity. A proportion of individuals screened for MH will fall into this category, and their IVCT may be positive either because of genuine susceptibility to MH or as a non-specific reaction (Heytens *et al.*, 1992). It is important to recognise the limits of morphological changes attributable to MH susceptibility per se, so that the group of patients whose biopsy findings exceed those limits are correctly identified and reviewed regularly in the light of subsequent advances in knowledge and diagnostic modalities, both in the determination of genuine MH susceptibility and in the characterisation of new clinicopathological entities. This review may lead to genetic counselling

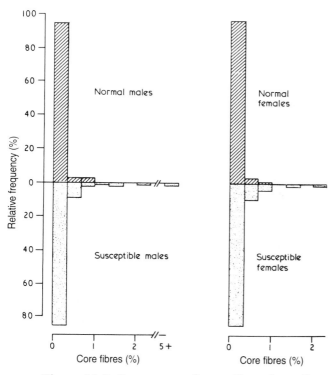

Figure 12.5. Percentage of core fibres in malignant hyperthermia normal versus malignant hyperthermia susceptible males and females.

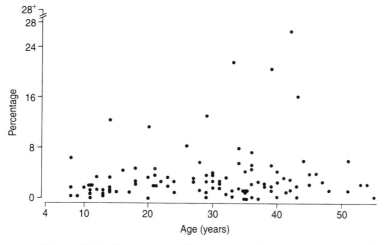

Figure 12.6. Percentage of internal nuclei versus age in malignant hyperthermia susceptible females.

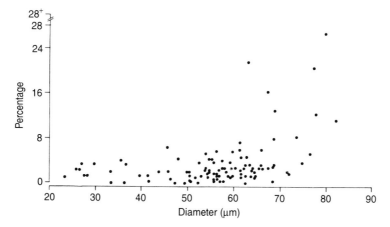

Figure 12.7. Percentage of internal nuclei versus mean diameters (all types pooled) in malignant hyperthermia susceptible females.

or therapeutic measures different from those associated with MH susceptibility. To fail to institute such procedures would be a disservice both to patients and progress.

References

Adnet, P. J., Bromberg, N. L., Haudecoeur, G., Krivosic, I., Adamantidis, M. M., Reyford, H., Bello, N. & Krivosic Horber, R. M. (1993). Fibre-type caffeine sensitivities in skinned muscle fibers from humans susceptible to malignant hyperthermia. *Anesthesiology*, **78**, 168–77.

Denborough, M. A. & Lovell, R. R. H. (1960). Anaesthetic deaths in a family. *Lancet*, **2**, 45.

Dubowitz, V. & Brooke, M. H. (1973). *Muscle Biopsy: A Modern Approach*. London, W. B. Saunders.

Ellis, F. R., Halsall, P. J. & Harriman, D. G. F. (1986). The work of the Leeds Malignant Hyperpyrexia Unit, 1971–84. *Anaesthesia*, **41**, 809–10.

European Malignant Hyperpyrexia Group. (1985). Laboratory diagnosis of malignant hyperpyrexia susceptibility. *British Journal of Anaesthesia*, **57**, 1038.

Gullotta, F. (1976). Reperi morphologici, istochimici ed ultrastrutturali nell' ipertermia maligna. *Acta Neurologica (Napoli)*, **31**, 56–7.

Gullotta, F. & Helpap, B. (1975). Histologische, Histochemische und elektronenmikroscopische Befunde bei maligner Hyperthermie. *Virchows Archiv–A, Pathological Anatomy and Histopathology*, **367**, 181–94.

Gullotta, F. & Spiez-Kiefer, C. (1983). Muskelbioptische Untersuchungen bei maligner Hyperthermie. *Anasthesie, Intensivtherapie und Notfallmedizin*, **18**, 21–7.

Haberer, J. P., Fabre, F. & Rose, E. (1989). Malignant hyperthermia and myotonia congenita (Thomsen's disease). *Anaesthesia*, **44**, 166 (letter).

Harnden-Mayor, P. (1989). *Quantitative studies in the human of normal, ageing and malignant hyperthermia susceptible muscle*, PhD Thesis, University of Leeds, Leeds.

Harriman, D. G. F. (1988). Malignant hyperthermia myopathy: a critical review. *British Journal of Anaesthesia*, **60**, 309–16.

Harriman, D. G. F., Ellis, F. R., Franks, A. J. & Sumner, D. W. (1978). Malignant hyperthermia myopathy in man: an investigation of 75 families. *Malignant Hyperthermia, The Second International Symposium on Malignant Hyperthermia*, ed. J. A. Aldrete & B. A. Britt, pp. 67–87. New York, Grune and Stratton.

Harriman, D. G. F., Sumner, D. W. & Ellis, F. R. (1973). Malignant hyperpyrexia myopathy. *Quarterly Journal of Medicine, New Series*, **168**, 639–64.

Heiman-Patterson, T., Martino, C., Rosenberg, H., Fletcher, J. & Tahmoush, A. (1988). Malignant hyperthermia in myotonia congenita. *Neurology*, **38**, 810–12.

Heytens, L., Martin, J. J., Van de Kelft, E. & Bossaert, L. L. (1992). *In vitro* contracture tests in patients with various neuromuscular diseases. *British Journal of Anaesthesia*, **68**, 72–5.

Hopkins, P. M., Ellis, F. R. & Halsall, P. J. (1991). Evidence for related myopathies in exertional heat stroke and malignant hyperthermia. *Lancet*, **338**, 1491–2.

Hopkins, P. M., Ellis, F. R. & Halsall, P. J. (1992). Inconsistency of data linking the ryanodine receptor and malignant hyperthermia genes (comment). *Anesthesiology*, **76**, 659–61 (letter).

Kausch, K., Lehmann-Horn, F., Janka, M., Wieringa, B., Grimm, T. & Muller, C. R. (1991). Evidence for linkage of the central core disease locus to the proximal long arm of human chromosome 19. *Genomics*, **10**, 765–9.

Mitsumoto, H., DeBoer, G. E., Bunge, G., Andrish, J. T., Tetzlaff, J. E. & Cruse, R. P. (1990). Fiber-type specific caffeine sensitivities in normal human skinned muscle fibers. *Anesthesiology*, **72**, 50–4.

Mortier, W. (1990). Malignant hyperthermia: relation to other diseases. *Acta Anaesthesiologica Belgica*, **41**, 119–26.

Peluso, A. & Bianchini, A. (1992). Malignant hyperthermia susceptibility in patients with Duchenne's muscular dystrophy. *Canadian Journal of Anaesthesia*, **39**, 1117–18 (letter).

Ranklev, E., Henriksson, K. G., Fletcher, R., Germundsson, J., Oldfors, A. & Kalimo, H. (1986). Clinical and muscle biopsy findings in malignant hyperthermia susceptibility. *Acta Neurologica Scandinavica*, **74**, 452–9.

Shuaib, A., Paasuke, R. T. & Brownell, K. W. (1987). Central core disease. Clinical features in 13 patients. *Medicine*, **66**, 389–96.

Wedel, D. J. (1992). Malignant hyperthermia and neuromuscular disease. *Neuromuscular Disorders*, **2**, 157–64.

13

Genetics of malignant hyperthermia

S. P. WEST

Introduction

The inheritable nature of malignant hyperthermia (MH) susceptibility was first proposed by Denborough *et al.* (1962) following their observations on a family in which ten otherwise unexplainable deaths had occurred as a result of general anaesthesia. In three of these cases elevated body temperatures had been recorded after the administration of the anaesthetic. The pattern of predisposition to MH in this pedigree was compatible with an autosomal dominant mode of inheritance with incomplete penetrance. That is, a single gene was segregating through the family, passed from parent to offspring, which predisposed an individual who had inherited this gene to MH. One individual in this pedigree, however, was believed to have transmitted the predisposing gene but she herself had not experienced an MH crisis when exposed to triggering anaesthetic agents. The penetrance, therefore, is less than 100%, meaning that the MH phenotype may not always be revealed in MH susceptible individuals on exposure to the triggering environment.

Definition and phenotype of malignant hyperthermia

In different patients MH episodes may assume different patterns but in all cases the episode results from exposure of a genetically susceptible individual to a triggering agent. Characteristically an early sign of an MH episode is muscle rigidity, the onset of which may be abrupt. This rigidity reflects an accelerated metabolic rate in the skeletal muscle that results in excessive heat generation causing the rise in body temperature characteristic of an MH crisis. The various patterns and possible reasons for these differences are described and discussed in Chapter 8.

In addition, similar clinical reactions during anaesthesia and surgery may arise in patients with other neuromuscular disorders. These conditions include myotonia congenita, myotonic dystrophy, Duchenne and Becker muscular dystrophies and central core disease (CCD). With the exception of CCD and MH these conditions are clinically and genetically distinct from one another. The locus encoding the gene defect in CCD has been localised on the human gene map to chromosome 19q13.1 and it has been proposed that CCD is allelic to MH on the basis of their coexistence in families and genetic linkage and mutation data (Mulley *et al.*, 1993; Zhang *et al.*, 1993; Quane *et al.*, 1993, 1994*b*; Keating *et al.*, 1994).

Since the presentation of MH can be so variable and non-specific it is necessary to seek physiological evidence that an MH episode has occurred. Conclusive diagnosis of MH is sought by means of *in vitro* contracture tests (IVCT) on living muscle biopsies from the surviving patient or from the parents of a patient who has not survived an MH crisis. If the MH diagnosis is confirmed it is obviously of great importance to identify other MH susceptible relatives in order to prevent avoidable MH reactions in the future.

Presymptomatic diagnosis of malignant hyperthermia

As a result of the demonstration of the inherited nature of susceptibility to MH (Denborough *et al.*, 1962) the need to be able to detect MH susceptible relatives of patients who have experienced an MH crisis has arisen (Ellis *et al.*, 1971). Several approaches to presymptomatic diagnostic testing for MH susceptibility have been proposed but currently the most reliable of these involves the *in vitro* exposure of living muscle fibres to halothane and caffeine (Ellis *et al.*, 1972) as discussed in Chapter 11.

A standard protocol for IVCT for MH susceptibility has been in use since 1984 by all members of the European Malignant Hyperthermia Group (EMHG; 1984). This test is used to confirm the diagnosis of MH in patients who have survived a possible MH crisis, or in their parents, if available, if the patient has not survived. If the diagnosis of MH is confirmed then IVCT of the relatives of the proband may be offered. IVCT of families in Europe has confirmed the autosomal dominant mode of inheritance of the MH susceptible phenotype and has also indicated that there is a virtually negligible rate of non-familial cases of MH that suggests a low rate of new mutations in this condition.

The nature of the IVCT is highly invasive and the highly specialised laboratory and intensive staffing required means that it is not feasible to test people not already known to be at risk of MH. In addition, IVCT of young children is seldom performed not only because it is undesirable to take muscle biopsies from children but also because immature muscle tissue frequently gives erratic responses in this test (Ellis *et al.*, 1986). MH, however, remains a common cause of avoidable deaths and serious morbidity as a result of general anaesthesia. There is a need, therefore, for reliable, cheap and non-invasive diagnostic testing for MH susceptibility.

Identification of the defective gene causing MH susceptibility in a family would permit presymptomatic diagnosis by a simple, non-invasive genetic test involving a small blood sample or even a mouth wash to provide material for testing from family members. Healy *et al.*, (1991) reported the use of genetic diagnosis of MH susceptibility in five individuals from a single large pedigree. At the present time, although highly desirable, genetic testing is not appropriate for presymptomatic diagnosis for the vast majority of MH susceptible families and not as a general screen of patients prior to general anaesthesia.

A possible animal model for malignant hyperthermia

Porcine stress syndrome (PSS) is an inherited condition in pigs that may be similar to malignant hyperthermia in humans. Pigs homozygous for the PSS abnormality respond to stress in a manner similar to a fulminant MH crisis. They show muscle rigidity and hypermetabolism resulting in excessive heat production and death. The meat of an animal that has died as a result of PSS reaction has very little commercial value because it has undergone extensive degradation and is described as pale, soft, exudative pork (PSEP). Therefore PSS has serious economic consequences for breeders of the six breeds of pigs in which this disorder occurs and as a result PSS has been the subject of intensive research in the agriculture industry.

The PSS reaction in sensitive animals may be triggered by normal stresses such as separation, weaning, fighting, coitus or slaughter. The animal exhibits shortness of breath, a rapid rise in body temperature, patches of blanching and flushing on the skin, collapse and rapid death followed by immediate *rigor mortis*. Unlike MH susceptibility in humans which is autosomal dominantly inherited PSS is considered to be transmitted by a single autosomal recessive gene, called the halothane sensitivity gene, *Hal*.

Sensitivity to halothane is determined by a 'barnyard' test in which a face mask is placed over the pig's snout and increasing amounts of halothane administered. If the pig exhibits limb rigidity as a result of this halothane challenge it is classified as halothane positive, if it does not exhibit limb rigidity it is classified as halothane negative. The halothane positive phenotype determined by this test corresponds with homozygosity for the *Hal* mutation. The apparent difference in the mode of inheritance between these two conditions in humans and pigs may, however, arise from differences in the sensitivities in the tests used.

Genetics of halothane sensitivity in pigs and humans

Owing to its commercial implications for breeders PSS has received considerable attention not only in terms of its physiology but also in terms of its genetics. Genetic linkage studies in pigs revealed that *Hal*, the halothane sensitivity locus responsible for PSS is closely linked to the locus encoding phosphohexose isomerase, *Phi*, also known as glucose phosphate isomerase, *Gpi* (Andresen & Jensen, 1977). These two loci were included in a linkage group with four other loci including two blood group loci, *H* and *S*, which is considered to be the porcine equivalent to the human secretor status locus *SE*. Also in the porcine linkage group were the locus encoding the $\alpha_1 B$ glycoprotein (*A1BG*), previously known as postalbumin-2, *Po2*, and the locus encoding the enzyme phosphogluconate dehydrogenase, *Pgd*. This porcine linkage group was predicted to span no more than 10 cM and the probable gene order was deduced to be *Gpi- Hal- S- H- A1BG- Pgd* (Juneja *et al.*, 1983; Archibald & Imlah, 1985). This linkage group was subsequently assigned to porcine chromosome 6 (Davies *et al.*, 1988) in the region of 6p11-q21 (Harbitz *et al.*, 1990).

Comparisons of the gene maps of various mammals including humans have shown that regions of their gene maps have been conserved through evolution. The region in which the porcine *Hal* locus is located was known to have homology with two regions of the human gene map. Previously *GPI* and *SE* had been assigned to the long arm (q) of human chromosome 19 while *PGD* has been assigned to the short arm (p) of human chromosome 1. The demonstration of linkage in humans between *A1BG* and *LU* (Eiberg *et al.*, 1989) and the consequent assignment of *A1BG* to chromosome 19q indicated that the probable location of the human *MHS* locus was also on chromosome 19q.

Linkage studies were undertaken in human MH families using polymorphic markers from this region of chromosome 19q. Evidence for linkage to this region was found in three large Irish families (McCarthy *et al.*, 1990). Simultaneously a gene encoding a strong candidate for the physiological defect underlying MH susceptibility, the skeletal muscle sarcoplasmic reticulum calcium release channel, also known as the ryanodine receptor, *RYR1*, was localised to the 19q13.1 region (MacKenzie *et al.*, 1990) and also showed complete segregation with MH susceptibility in nine small Canadian families (MacLennan *et al.*, 1990).

In pigs very tight linkage between *Hal* and this calcium release channel locus has been demonstrated (Harbitz *et al.*, 1990; Otsu *et al.*, 1991; Bolt *et al.*, 1992). Comparison of the molecular sequence of this calcium release channel gene in halothane sensitive and normal pigs revealed 18 nucleotide substitutions of which only one caused a different amino acid to be incorporated into the protein product of the mutant gene. This single base substitution of a T for a C in the normal sequence at nucleotide 1843 causes substitution of arginine for cysteine at residue 615 in the protein sequence (Fujii *et al.*, 1991). This same mutation has been detected in all the 450 halothane sensitive pigs examined from the six breeds in which this condition occurs and in no pigs that are not susceptible (Otsu *et al.*, 1992). On the basis of these findings it would seem wholly reasonable to deduce that mutations in the porcine ryanodine receptor gene, and in particular the 1843C → T substitution underlie malignant hyperthermia.

The equivalent mutation in the human ryanodine receptor gene sequence (Zorzato *et al.*, 1990), causing a C to T substitution at nucleotide 1840 and replacement of arginine 614 by cysteine in the protein product, has been detected in a few North American MH susceptible families (Gillard *et al.*, 1991; Hogan *et al.*,1992). In a survey of contributors to the EMHG Genetics Section meeting in December 1993, 16 out of 333 unrelated MH susceptible individuals tested, classified according to the European protocol for IVCT carried the *RYR1 1840T* → C mutation. This indicates that this mutation may account for around 5% of MH cases in the European population, although in a survey of 100 unrelated MH susceptible individuals from the UK this mutation was not detected (Hall-Curran *et al.*, 1993).

More recently further *RYR1* mutations have been described in MH patients and also in patients with the allelic myopathy CCD. Gillard *et al.* (1992) identified 21 single base substitutions in the *RYR1* gene, the majority of these were shown to be normal variants of *RYR1* gene sequence observed in the general population. One of these G742 → A, causes an amino acid substitution and cosegregates with MH susceptibility in a single family and was concluded to be a causative mutation. Zhang *et al.* (1993) reported a mutation, G7301 → A in a single family in which CCD occurred together with MH susceptibility. Quane *et al.* (1993) found a mutation G487 → T that occurred in two apparently unrelated small families in one of which MH susceptibility segregated as an isolated entity and in the other CCD occurred as well. In a third family with MH susceptibility and CCD another mutation, C1209 → G, was characterised. A single mutation, G1021 → A, which may account for 10% of MH susceptibility and is not detected in families also segregating for CCD was reported by Quane *et al* (1994*a*). The mutation A1565 → C was detected in a single MH susceptible/CCD pedigree (Quane *et al.*, 1994*b*) and

Table 13.1. *Mutations detected in the* RYR1 *gene in malignant hyperthermia susceptible individuals*

Nucleotide change	Codon and amino acid change	Comments	Reference
C487→T	Arg163→Cys	MH and CCD	Quane *et al.* (1993)
G742→A	Gly248→Arg	Single MH family	Gillard *et al.* (1992)
G1021→A	Gly341→Arg	~10% of MH families	Quane *et al.* (1994*a*)
C1209→G	Ile403→Met	Single CCD family	Quane *et al.* (1993)
A1565→C	Tyr522→Ser	Single CCD family	Quane *et al.* (1994*b*)
C1840→T	Arg614→Cys	Pig mutation ~5% of MH families	Gillard *et al.* (1991)
G7297→A	Gly2433→Arg	MH and CCD	Keating *et al.* (1994)
G7301→A	Arg2434→His	Single CCD family	Zhang *et al.* (1993)

CCD, central core disease; MH, malignant hyperthermia.

the G7297 → A mutation has been detected in four families also segregating for CCD (Keating *et al.*, 1994). These variants in the *RYR1* gene are summarised in Table 13.1 together with details concerning the amino acid changes they cause.

Each of these mutations causes a single amino acid in the protein product of the *RYR1* gene to be substituted by another amino acid and so they are called missense mutations. They are believed to be pathological because they have not been detected in the DNA of MH normal individuals, where the whole *RYR1* gene has been screened for mutations no other mutation has been detected and where the family structure has permitted these mutations segregate completely with MH susceptibility, although the same would be expected· of a normal genetic variant within the defective gene. More convincing evidence for the pathological nature of mutations in *RYR1* would be the observation of mutations causing more drastic disruption of the RYR1 protein. These more drastic mutations could cause premature truncation of the protein product as a result of a nucleotide substitution creating a novel protein translation stop signal; these would be nonsense mutations. Alternatively, the sequence of amino acids in the protein product may be changed, for example by deletion or insertion of a few nucleotides in the gene sequence; these are known as frameshift mutations. In other genetic conditions where the molecular pathology is well understood nonsense and frameshift mutations are usually detected in addition to missense mutations (Strachan, 1992). The reasons for the lack of frameshift or nonsense mutations in MH are unclear and may become apparent as the molecular events underlying this condition are revealed.

Taken together the linkage data and mutation data seem to confirm that molecular lesions in the *RYR1* gene underlie MH in humans in at least some families and for a brief period the prospects appeared to be good for the development of valuable, non-invasive presymptomatic tests for MH susceptibility, at least in families where the diagnosis of MH in the index case (proband) had been confirmed by IVCT.

Genetic heterogeneity

Subsequent studies soon revealed that in many other MH susceptible families the causative gene could not possibly be the ryanodine receptor or any other gene lying in the 19q12-q13.2 region. The evidence for this is that in these families MH susceptibility is not inherited together with alleles from polymorphic genetic markers either within the *RYR1* gene itself or lying very close to it. Between MH susceptibility and markers in 19q13.1-q13.2 levels of genetic recombination are being observed that could not occur within such a short region of a chromosome. There must be at least one other gene located elsewhere on the human gene map in which defects can occur to give rise to MH. The term genetic heterogeneity is used to describe this situation where at least two genes at different gene map locations apparently cause the same clinical phenotype. Evidence for genetic heterogeneity in MH was provided by families of UK, German, Scandinavian, Belgian, Dutch and North American origin (Deufel *et al.*, 1992: Fagerlund *et al.*, 1992; Iles *et al.*, 1992, 1993; Levitt *et al.*, 1991; Ball *et al.*, 1993). Of the families investigated for linkage with chromosome 19q13.1-q13.2 markers by members of the EMHG Genetics Section in approximately 50% mutations in *RYR1* or a closely-linked gene can be excluded as the cause of the MH (Ball & Johnson, 1993). Presymptomatic diagnosis by genetic testing is only appropriate for members of families where there is strong statistical evidence of linkage to 19q13.1-q13.2 markers with individuals previously typed by the IVCT. In practice very few families are likely to fulfil these criteria because of the large pedigree size and the large number of IVCT individuals required to provide the statistical evidence to verify linkage to 19q13.1-q13.2. The genetic markers used by the EMHG Genetics Section to establish linkage to 19q13.1 are shown with their locations on the chromosome 19 map in Figure 13.1.

Mapping of other candidate genes in malignant hyperthermia

The skeletal muscle sarcoplasmic reticulum calcium release channel does not hold all the answers to MH susceptibility so it is important to identify gene

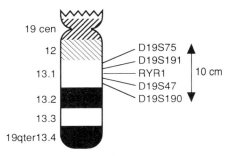

Figure 13.1. Locations of the genetic markers used by the European Malignant Hyperthermia Group Genetics Section to establish linkage between malignant hyperthermia and 19q13.1.

defects underlying MH in these non-19 linked families. The search for other defective genes in MH could follow two different strategies. One would be to investigate linkage between MH and genes encoding various plausible candidates for the defect underlying MH on the basis of knowledge of the physiology and pharmacology. Suitable candidate genes would be those encoding proteins involved in regulating Ca^{2+} levels and membrane stability by regulating fatty acid metabolism or inositol 1,4,5-trisphosphate (IP_3) levels in skeletal muscle (Chapter 10).

The second approach would be to launch a genome search, i.e. to investigate the linkage relationships of MH with polymorphic markers distributed throughout the entire human genome. Although at first glance this approach would appear to present the needle in the haystack problem recent developments in the technologies of human molecular genetic analysis mean that this is not an impossible task. For example the gene responsible for the dominantly inherited neurodegenerative disorder Huntington's disease was localised and eventually characterised by this method (Gusella *et al.*, 1983; The Huntington's Disease Collaborative Research Group, 1993) and the gene causing the recessively inherited disease cystic fibrosis was mapped and identified by means of an extensive genome search (Riordan *et al.*, 1989).

The prerequisite to be able to undertake either of these approaches is the availability of large families whose MH susceptibility follows a clear pattern of autosomal dominant inheritance, is not linked to the 19q13.1 region and where the majority of family members have had their MH status determined using a reliable protocol. In collaboration members of the EMHG can provide a large number of families which satisfy these stringent criteria and have been typed by a standardised IVCT protocol. To gain the maximum benefit from this invaluable resource the EMHG, Genetics Section, was formed in 1991 to collaborate in the identification of further MH-causing genes and to evaluate

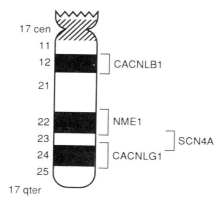

Figure 13.2. Locations of proposed candidate genes for malignant hyperthermia on chromosome 17q.

the reliability and practicability of novel genetic diagnostic methods as they are proposed.

A putative malignant hyperthermia locus on chromosome 17

Recently there has been a report of linkage between MH and markers on chromosome 17q11.2-q24 from a study on five small families from North America and South Africa (Levitt *et al.*, 1992) and a second locus for malignant hyperthermia, *MHS2*, proposed. The loci encoding several candidate genes are located in this region. These are the *β*-1 and *γ*-1 subunit genes of the skeletal muscle isoforms of the slow L-type calcium release channel of the transverse tubule also known as the dihydropyridine receptor, *CACNLB1* in 17q12 and *CACNLG1* in 17q24, respectively, and a subunit gene of the adult skeletal muscle sodium channel *SCN4A*, mutations in which are known to underlie myotonia congenita, myotonia fluctuans and hyperkalaemic periodic paralysis (Iaizzo & Lehmann-Horn, 1995), localised to 17q23. The locations of these loci are shown in Figure 13.2.

In 19 large MH families where linkage to *RYR1* had been excluded and in which MH status had been established by the European protocol there is no evidence for linkage to markers on chromosome 17q including these three candidate genes (Sudbrak *et al.*, 1993; Iles *et al.*, 1993; T. Fagerlund, personal communication). Until conclusive evidence for linkage between MH and markers on 17q can be established from a single large family then the validity of this tentative *MHS2* locus on chromosome 17q must remain in question (Johnson, 1993). If the *MHS2* locus on chromosome 17q can be confirmed to cause MH then the negative linkage data with both *MHS1* and *MHS2* regions on chromosomes 19q and 17q, respectively, from these European families must indicate that the level of heterogeneity in MH is very high with at least three genes at different genetic locations underlying this single disorder.

Private mutation on chromosome 7q

As part of a study to investigate the linkage relationships between MH and candidate genes Iles *et al.* (1994) found strong evidence for a defect in the gene encoding the $\alpha_2/\ \delta$-subunit of the L-type voltage dependent calcium channel (*CACNLA2*) or a gene very close by causing MH in a single large family in which linkage to *RYR1* has been excluded previously. The *CACNLA2* gene is located on chromosome 7 in the region 7q11.23-q21.1. Five more large MH families that had also been shown previously not to show linkage with chromosome 19q markers did not show linkage with 7q11.23-q21.1 markers either. This suggests that although a mutation in *CACNLA2* is highly likely to cause MH in one family and therefore could be described as a private mutation this is not the site of mutations in further non-19 linked MH families.

Other candidate gene loci

The 1,4-dihydropyridine sensitive calcium channel of the skeletal muscle transverse tubule is a heteropentameric protein with skeletal muscle specific isoforms of each subunit. The possibility that mutations in the genes encoding further skeletal muscle specific subunits of this calcium channel may cause MH has been investigated by genetic linkage analysis. Linkage between malignant hyperthermia and the locus encoding the α-1 subunit, *CACNL1A3* on chromosome 1 in the region 1q13-q32 has been excluded in nine European MH families in which there was also no evidence for linkage to 19q and 17q (Sudbrak *et al.*, 1993; D. Iles personal communication; J. Hall-Curran, personal communication).

In addition to the skeletal muscle expressed ryanodine receptor gene (*RYR1*) two further ryanodine receptor genes have been identified. One of these, *RYR2*, is expressed in brain and cardiac muscle but not in skeletal muscle and so is not considered to be a potential candidate for gene defects in MH. The third ryanodine receptor calcium release channel, *RYR3*, has been shown to be expressed in a wide range of tissues including skeletal muscle (Giannini *et al.*, 1992) and therefore could be considered as a candidate gene for the defect underlying MH. The *RYR3* gene has been localised recently to chromosome 15 in the region 15q14-q15 (Sorrentino *et al.*, 1993). Two further plausible candidate genes have also been mapped to chromosome 15q in the region 15q11.2-q12. These encode the β3- and the α5- subunits of the type A γ-aminobutyric acid (GABA$_A$) receptor, *GABRB3* and *GABRA5* (Sinnett *et al.*, 1993). The GABA$_A$ receptors are a heterogeneous family of oligomeric ligand-gated chloride channels that represent the major inhibitory neurotransmitter receptors in the nervous system. Linkage studies have been performed on non-19q, non-17q linked MH families using chromosome 15q markers spanning the 15q11.2-q21 region where these candidate loci are located. In three German and nine UK families there is no evidence for linkage between MH and this region of chromosome 15q (Sudbrak *et al.*, 1994; J. Hall-Curran, personal communication). This evidence suggests that mutations in *RYR3*, *GABRB3* and *GABRA5* are also unlikely to underlie MH susceptibility, at least in these 12 families.

Linkage studies investigating many other candidate genes are in progress to identify further MH loci. This approach, however, while excluding certain chromosomal regions of the genome has provided only one convincing MH susceptible locus identification and this has only been observed in a single family and dubious evidence for a further locus. The alternative approach involving a search of the entire genome appears to be the more rewarding course to take. Towards this end a collaborative project is being undertaken by members of the EMHG Genetics Section investigating the largest non-19 linked MH families from Europe with markers from the entire genome via the Généthon project in Paris.

Anonymous locus on chromosome 3q

Ten large families segregating for MH susceptibility, from various regions of Europe, typed according to the EMHG's IVCT protocol have been included in this genomic screen linkage project. Highly polymorphic markers covering approximately 40% of the human genome have been analysed so far. One further MH susceptibility locus has been identified through this study in a single German family MH009 (Sudbrak *et al.*, 1995). Cosegregation of markers from the region 3q13.1 is seen with MH susceptibility in part of this family and provides strong evidence for an, as yet unidentified, MH susceptibility locus in this region. The interpretation of the linkage data for this pedigree is complicated by the occurrence of two susceptibility alleles segregating in different branches of the family.

The salient message from these linkage studies identifying so many *MHS* loci is that MH susceptibility is genetically far more heterogeneous than had been anticipated. Furthermore, these results suggest that MH may have a more complex genetic basis than the straightforward Mendelian genetic model of an autosomal dominant disorder with reduced penetrance.

Prospects for genetic diagnosis of malignant hyperthermia

Genetic diagnostic testing for inherited disorders offers many advantages over classical diagnostic techniques in that these tests can be performed presymptomatically and in the case of severe genetic diseases may be used prenatally. Genetic tests usually analyse the DNA of individuals and this resource can be obtained relatively non-invasively often from a simple mouthwash or from a small blood sample. The tests are inexpensive to perform compared with many other diagnostic procedures and have a high level of accuracy to the point where they may be used to confirm an ambiguous clinical diagnosis.

Genetic diagnostic testing can be carried out by either direct or indirect analysis. Direct analysis is possible when the precise mutation known to cause the disease phenotype is revealed by the diagnostic test. Direct mutational analysis is available for many genetic disorders including cystic fibrosis, Duchenne muscular dystrophy and myotonic dystrophy. Direct mutational analysis for genetic diagnosis can be conducted in situations where there is little or no information regarding the genetic status of other family members of the individual being tested.

Indirect genetic analysis is the only means of genetic diagnosis available if the specific DNA mutation causing the disease phenotype is not known but where the gene map location of the genetic lesion has been established. Indirect genetic diagnosis involves analysis of the inheritance from parents to offspring of common genetic variants (markers) at genetic locations (loci) very close on the chromosome map to the genetic location of the disease gene. In an indirect test the flanking polymorphic markers are typed and the genetic (haplotype) data assembled to characterise the region of the chromosome surrounding the defective gene in the close relatives of the individual being tested. From these characteristic chromosome marker patterns the chromosome carrying the mutated copy of the disease gene can be distinguished from chromosomes carrying normal copies of the gene. Thus the segregation of the defective gene can be traced through the family and the presence of the mutation-bearing chromosome in an individual used to predict their disease status. In this way indirect analysis is used for prenatal diagnosis of severe genetic disorders and presymptomatically to determine susceptibility to late onset diseases or susceptibility to conditions with cryptic phenotypes triggered by environmental stresses. Inevitably indirect analysis is less powerful than direct analysis because of the need to identify the chromosome carrying the mutated gene by investigation of the relatives of the individual being tested. Often there is insufficient pedigree information for indirect tests to be conclusive. Furthermore, inaccuracy can arise in the test because of genetic recombination which causes segregation of genes on the same chromosome. If the marker genes being used to identify the chromosome carrying the mutated disease gene are at a distance from the disease gene itself then the chance of a genetic recombination event is increased so it is necessary for the sake of accuracy to have genetic markers as close as possible to the gene under investigation.

In the case of MH susceptibility indirect diagnosis is likely to be the exception rather than generally applicable. This is because of the high level of genetic heterogeneity already demonstrated with at least two, if not three, genes in which mutations can arise to cause this apparently uniform phenotype. Indirect diagnosis would only ever be applicable in families where the MH status of sufficient individuals had been established by the IVCT and an autosomal dominant mode of inheritance observed and where a genetic linkage study had verified the gene map location of the defective gene. These three stringent criteria were fulfilled in a single large Irish family and genetic presymptomatic diagnosis could be performed for five individuals (Healy *et al.*, 1991). The majority of MH families are not sufficiently large to generate conclusive evidence for genetic linkage with a candidate gene and so then the indirect approach to genetic diagnosis cannot be applied.

At present there is no direct molecular genetic test appropriate for presymptomatic diagnosis of MH susceptibility. The *RYR1* 1840C → T mutation has been proposed as a causative mutation and is readily detected using a rapid PCR-RFLP molecular genetic test (Gillard *et al.*, 1991) and this mutation is detected in approximately 5% of MH susceptible individuals in the European population. Data presented at the April 1994 meeting of the EMHG indicated inconsistencies between the MH susceptible phenotype and the presence of the 1840C → T mutation (Deufel *et al.*, 1995) and more recently inconsistency in segregation of the 1021G → A mutation with MH susceptibility has been observed (A. M. Adeokun *et al.*, unpublished data). Until a genetically acceptable explanation for these discrepancies is put forward and there is conclusive evidence to confirm the causative nature of mutations, genetic diagnostic tests are, therefore, wholly unreliable and irresponsible in view of the existence of the accepted IVCT.

The explanations given by both groups of authors for these unexpected observations challenge the simple Mendelian inheritance model of MH susceptibility involving rare autosomal dominant alleles. Such discussions question the causative role of identified *RYR1* mutations in MH susceptibility, at least in some families. Alternatively, MH susceptibility alleles may be far more common in the general population than the current estimates or that IVCT MH susceptibility status is a multigenic phenotype requiring the interaction of several genes possibly including *RYR1* mutations.

Despite these reservations the search for a reliable, cheap and non-invasive diagnostic test for MH susceptibility is ongoing. Experiments are underway in may of the MH investigation units to search for the precise DNA alterations causative of MH in families in which MH susceptibility is known to be linked to the 19q13.1-q13.2 region. The gene mapping project initiated collaboratively by members of the EMHG, Genetics Section to search for further genes causing MH is likely to identify new MH loci in the near future. Once new MH loci are identified the identification of causative mutations within these genes will have high priority. If their causative nature can be verified then knowledge of the specific molecular lesions causing MH can be used not only to perform simple and precise molecular genetic tests for predicting MH status but will also be of great value in advancing our understanding of the physiological mechanisms controlling skeletal muscle metabolism and contraction and in our understanding of the pharmacology of inhalation anaesthetics.

References

Andresen, E. & Jensen, P. (1977). Close linkage established between the *HAL* locus for halothane sensitivity and the *PHI* (phosphohexose isomerase) locus in pigs of the Danish Landrace breed. *Nordisk Veterinaire Medicin*, **29**, 502–4.

Archibald, A. L. & Imlah, P. (1985). The halothane sensitivity locus and its linkage relationship. *Animal Blood Groups and Biochemical Genetics*, **16**, 253–63.

Ball, S. P. & Johnson, K. J. (1993). The genetics of malignant hyperthermia. *Journal of Medical Genetics*, **30**, 89–93.

Ball, S. P., Dorkins, H. R., Ellis, F. R., Hall, J. L., Halsall, P. J., Hopkins, P. M., Mueller, R. F. & Stewart, A. D. (1993). Genetic linkage analysis of chromosome 19 markers in malignant hyperthermia. *British Journal of Anaesthesia*, **70**, 70–5.

Bolt, R., Davies, W. & Fries, R. (1992). A polymorphic microsatellite in the porcine calcium release channel gene is closely linked to the malignant hyperthermia locus. *Cytogenetics Cell Genetics*, **58**, 2017.

Davies, W., Harbitz I., Fries, R. Stranzinger, G. & Hauge, J. G. (1988). Porcine malignant hyperthermia carrier detection and chromosomal assignment using a linked probe. *Animal Genetics*, **19**, 203–12.

Denborough, M. A., Forster, J. F. A., Lovell, R. R. H., Maplestone, P. A. & Villiers, J. D. (1962). Anaesthetic deaths in a family. *British Journal of Anaesthesia*, **34**, 395–6.

Deufel, T., Golla, A., Iles, D., Meindl, A., Meitinger, T., Schindelhauer, D., De Vries, A., Pongratz, D.,MacLennan, D. H., Johnson, K. J. & Lehmann-Horn, F. (1992), Evidence for genetic heterogeneity of malignant hyperthermia susceptibility. *American Journal of Human Genetics*, **50**, 1151–61.

Deufel, T., Sudbrak, R., Feist, Y., Rubsam, B., Du Chesne, I., Schafer, K. L., Roewer, N., Grimm, T., Lehmann-Horn, F., Hartung, E. J. & Muller, C. R. (1995). Discordance in a malignant hyperthermia pedigree, between *in vitro* contracture test phenotypes and haplotypes for the MHS1 region of chromosome 19q12-13.2, comprising the C1840T transition in the *RYR1* gene. *American Journal of Human Genetics*, **56**, 1334–42.

Eiberg, H., Nielsen, L. S., Gahne, B., Juneja, J. K. & Mohr, J. (1989). Exclusion data for the α_1-B glycoprotein (GA1B) polymorphism. *Cytogenetics and Cell Genetics*, **51**, 994.

Ellis, F. R., Halsall, P. J. & Harriman, D. G. F. (1986). The work of the Leeds Malignant Hyperpyrexia Investigation Unit, 1971–84. *Anaesthesia*, **41**, 809–15.

Ellis, F. R., Harriman, D. G. F., Keaney, N. P., Kyei-Mensah, K. & Tyrell, J. H. (1971). Halothane-induced muscle contracture as a cause of hyperpyrexia, *British Journal of Anaesthesia*, **43**, 721–2.

Ellis, F. R., Keaney, N. P., Harriman, D. G. F., Sumner, D. W., Kyei-Mensah, K., Tyrell, J. H., Hargraves, J. B., Parikh, R. K. & Mulrooney, P. L. (1972). Screening for malignant hyperthermia. *British Medical Journal*, **3**, 559–61.

European Malignant Hyperpyrexia Group (1984). A protocol for the investigation of malignant hyperthermia (MH) susceptibility. *British Journal of Anaesthesia*, **56**, 1267–9.

Fagerlund, T., Islander, G., Ranklev, E., Harbitz, I., Hauge, J. G., Mokleby, E. & Berg, K. (1992). Genetic recombination between malignant hyperthermia and calcium release channel in skeletal muscle. *Clinical Genetics*, **5**, 270–2.

Fujii, J., Otsu, K. Zorzato, F., de Leon, S., Khanna, V. K., Weiler, J., O'Brien, P. J. & MacLennan, D. H. (1991). Identification of a mutation in the porcine ryanodine receptor that is associated with malignant hyperthermia. *Science*, **253**, 448–51.

Giannini, G., Clementi, E., Ceci, R., Marziali, G. & Sorrentino, V. (1992). Expression of a ryanodine receptor-Ca^{2+} channel that is regulated by TGF-β. *Science*, **257**, 91–4.

Gillard, E. F., Otsu, K., Fujii, J., Duff, C., de Leon, S., Khanna, V. K., Britt, B. A., Worton, R. G. & MacLennan, D. H. (1992). Polymorphisms and deduced amino acid substitutions in the coding sequence of the ryanodine receptor (*RYR1*) gene in individuals with malignant hyperthermia. *Genomics*, **13**, 1247–54.

Gillard, E. F., Otsu, K., Fujii, J., Khanna, V. K., de Leon, S., Derdemezi, J., Britt, B. A., Duff, C., Worton, R. G. & MacLennan, D. H. (1991). Substitution of cysteine for arginine 614 in the ryanodine receptor is potentially causative of human malignant hyperthermia. *Genomics*, **11**, 751–5.

Gusella, J. F., Wexler, N. S., Conneally, P. M., Naylor, S. L., Anderson, M. A., Tanzi, R. F., Watkins, P. C., Ottina, K., Wallace, M. R., Sakaguchi, A. Y., Young, A. B., Shoulson, I., Bonilla, E. & Martin, J. B. (1983). A polymorphic DNA marker genetically linked to Huntington's disease. *Nature*, **306**, 234–8.

Hall-Curran, J. L., Stewart, A. D., Ball, S. P., Halsall, P. J., Hopkins, P. M. & Ellis, F. R. (1993). No C1840 to T mutation in RYR1 in malignant hyperthermia. *Human Mutation*, **2**, 330.

Harbitz, I., Chowdhary, B., Thomsen, P. D., Davies, W., Kaufmann, U., Kran, S., Gustavsson, I., Christensen, K. & Hauge, J. G. (1990). Assignment of the porcine calcium release channel gene, a candidate for the malignant hyperthermia locus, to the 6p11-q21 segment of chromosome 6. *Genomics*, **8**, 243–8.

Healy, J. M. S., Heffron, J. J. A., Lehane, M., Bradley, D. G., Johnson, K. &

McCarthy, T. V. (1991). Diagnosis of susceptibility to malignant hyperthermia with flanking DNA markers. *British Medical Journal*, **303**, 1225–8.

Hogan, K., Couch, F., Powers, P. A. & Gregg, R. G. (1992). A cysteine-for-arginine substitution (R614C) in the human skeletal muscle calcium release channel cosegregates with malignant hyperthermia. *Anesthesia and Analgesia*, **75**, 441–8.

Huntington's Disease Collaborative Research Group. (1993). A novel gene containing a trinucleotide repeat that is expanded and unstable in Huntington's disease chromosomes. *Cell*, **72**, 1–20.

Iaizzo, P. A. & Lehmann-Horn, F. (1995). Anesthetic complications in muscle disorder. *Anesthesiology*, **82**, 1093–6.

Iles, D. E., Lehmann-Horn, F., Scherer, S. W., Tsui, L.-C., Olde Weghuis, D., Suijkerbuijk, R. F.,Heytens, L., Mikala, G., Schwartz, A., Ellis, F. R., Stewart, A. D., Deufel, T. & Wieringa, B. (1994). Localization of the gene encoding the $\alpha_2/$ δ-subunits of the L-type voltage-dependent calcium channel to chromosome 7q and analysis of the segregation of flanking markers in malignant hyperthermia susceptible families. *Human Molecular Genetics*, **3**, 969–75.

Iles, D., Segers, B., Heytens, L., Sengers, R. C. A. & Wieringa, B. (1992). High-resolution physical mapping of four microsatellite repeat markers near the *RYR1* locus on chromosome 19q13.1 and apparent exclusion of the MHS locus from this region in two malignant hyperthermia susceptible families. *Genomics*, **14**, 749–54.

Iles, D. E., Segers, B., Sengers, R. C. A., Monsieurs, K., Heytens, L., Halsall, P. J., Hopkins, P. M., Ellis, F. R., Hall-Curran, J. L., Stewart, A. D. & Wieringa, B. (1993). Genetic mapping of the beta- and gamma-subunits of the human skeletal muscle voltage dependent calcium channel on chromosome 17q, and exclusion as candidate genes for malignant hyperthermia susceptibility. *Human Molecular Genetics*, **2**, 863–868.

Johnson, K. J. (1993). Malignant hyperthermia hots up! *Human Molecular Genetics*, **2**, 849.

Juneja, R. K., Gahne, B., Edfors-Lilja, I. & Andresen, E. (1983). Genetic variation at a pig serum protein locus, *Po-2* and its assignment to the *Phi, Hal, S, H,Pgd* linkage group. *Animal Blood Groups Biochemical Genetics*, **14**, 27–36.

Keating, K. E., Quane, K. A., Manning, B. M., Lehane, M., Hartung, E., Censier, K., Urwyler, A., Klausnitzer, M., Müller, C. R., Heffron, J. J. A. & McCarthy, T. V. (1994). Detection of a novel RYR1 mutation in four malignant hyperthermia families. *Human Molecular Genetics*, **3**, 1885–8.

Levitt, R. C., Nouri, N., Jedlicka, A. E., McKusick, V. A., Marks, A. R., Shutack, J. G., Fletcher, J. E., Rosenberg, H. & Meyers, D. A. (1991). Evidence for genetic heterogeneity in malignant hyperthermia susceptibility. *Genomics*, **11**, 543–7.

Levitt, R. C., Olckers, A., Meyers, S., Fletcher, J. E., Rosenberg, H., Isaacs, H. & Meyers, D. A. (1992). Evidence for the localisation of a malignant hyperthermia susceptibility locus (MHS2) to human chromosome 17q. *Genomics*, **14**, 562–6.

McCarthy, T. V., Healy, J. M. S., Heffron, J. J. A., Lehane, M., Deufel, T., Lehmann-Horn, F., Farrall, M. & Johnson, K. (1990). Localisation of the malignant hyperthermia susceptibility locus to human chromosome 19q12-13.2. *Nature*, **343**, 562–4.

MacKenzie, A. E., Korneluk, R. G., Zorzato, F., Fujii, J., Phillips, M., Iles, D., Wieringa, B., Leblond, S., Bailly, J., Willard, H. F., Duff, C., Worton, R. G. & MacLennan, D. H. (1990). The human ryanodine receptor gene: its mapping to 19q13.1, placement in a chromosome 19 linkage group, and exclusion as the gene causing myotonic dystrophy. *American Journal of Human Genetics*, **46**, 1082–9.

MacLennan, D. H., Duff, C., Zorzato, R., Fujii, J., Phillips, M., Korneluk, R. G., Frodis, W., Britt, B. A. & Worton, R. G. (1990). Ryanodine receptor gene is a candidate for predisposition to malignant hyperthermia. *Nature*, **343**, 559–61.

Mulley, J. C., Kozman, H. M., Phillips, H. A., Gedeon, A. K., McCure, J. A., Iles, D. E., Gregg, R. G., Hogan, K., Couch, F. J., MacLennan, D. H. & Haan, E. A. (1993). Refined genetic localisation for central core disease. *American Journal of Human Genetics*, **52**, 398–405.

Otsu, K., Khanna, V. K., Archibald, A. L. & MacLennan, D. H. (1991). Cosegregation of porcine malignant hyperthermia and a probable causal mutation in the skeletal muscle ryanodine receptor gene in backcross families. *Genomics*, **11**, 744–50.

Otsu, K., Phillips, M. S., Khanna, V. K., de Leon, S. & MacLennan, D. H. (1992). Refinement of diagnostic assays for a probable causal mutation for porcine and human malignant hyperthermia. *Genomics*, **13**, 835–7.

Quane, K. A., Healy, J. M. S., Keating, K. E., Manning, B. M., Couch, F. J., Palmucci, L. M., Doriguzzi, C., Fagerlund, T. H., Berg, K., Ording, H., Bendixen D., Mortier, W., Linz, U., Müller, C. R. & McCarthy, T. V. (1993). Mutations in the ryanodine receptor gene in central core disease and malignant hyperthermia. *Nature Genetics*, **5**, 51–5.

Quane, K. A., Keating, K. E., Healy, J. M.S., Manning, B. M., Krivosic-Horber, R., Monnier, N., Lunardi, J. & MacCarthy, T. V. (1994 *b*). Mutation screening of the *RYR1* gene in malignant hyperthermia: detection of a novel Tyr to Ser mutation in a pedigree with associated central cores. *Genomics*, **23**, 236–9.

Quane, K. A., Keating, K. E., Manning, B. M., Healy, J. M. S. Monsieurs, K., Heffron, J. J. A.,Lehane, M., Heytens, L., Krivosic-Horber, R., Adnet, P., Ellis, F. R., Monnier, N., Lunardi, J. & McCarthy, T. V. (1994 *a*). Detection of a novel common mutation in the ryanodine receptor gene in malignant hyperthermia: implications for diagnosis and heterogeneity studies. *Human Molecular Genetics* **3**, 471–6.

Riordan, J. R., Rommens, J. M., Kerem, B., Alon, N., Rozmahel, R., Grzelczak, Z., Zielenski, J., Lok, S., Plavsic, N., Chou, J.-L., Drumm, M. L., Iannuzzi, M. C., Collins, F. S. & Tsui, L.-C. (1989). Identification of the cystic fibrosis gene: cloning and characterisation of complementary DNA. *Science*, **245**, 1966–73.

Sinnett, D., Wagstaff, J., Glatt, K., Woolf, E., Kirkness, E. J. & Lalande, M. (1993). High resolution mapping of the gamma-aminobutyric acid receptor subunit β and α-5 gene cluster on chromosome 15q11-q13 and localisation of breakpoints in two Angelman syndrome patients. *American Journal of Human Genetics*, **52**, 1216–29.

Sorrentino, V., Giannini, G., Malzac, P. & Mattei, M. G. (1993). Localisation of a novel ryanodine receptor gene (*RYR3*) to human chromosome 15q14-q15 by *in situ* hybridisation. *Genomics*, **18**, 163–5.

Strachan, T. (1992). *The Human Genome*. Oxford, BIOS Scientific Publishers.

Sudbrak, R., Golla, A., Lehmann-Horn, F., Sorrentino, V. & Deufel, T. (1994). Exclusion of a ubiquitously expressed ryanodine receptor calcium channel (RYR3) gene as a candidate for malignant hyperthermia susceptibility (MHS). *Muscle and Nerve*, S89 (suppl.1), A3-1-9.

Sudbrak, R., Golla, A., Hogan, K., Powers, P., Gregg, R., DuChesne, I., Lehmann-Horn, F. & Deufel, T. (1993). Exclusion of malignant hyperthermia susceptibility (MHS) from a putative *MHS2* locus on chromosome 17q and of the α-, β1-, and γ- subunits of the dihydropyridine receptor calcium release channel as candidates for the molecular defect. *Human Molecular Genetics*, **2**, 857–62.

Sudbrak, R., Procaccio, V., Klausnitzer, M., Curran, J. L., Monsieurs, K., Van Broekhaven, C., Ellis, R., Heytens, L., Hartung, E. J., Kozak-Ribbens, G., Heilinger, D., Weissenbach, J., Lehmann-Horn, F., Muller, C. R., Deufel, T., Stewart, A. D. & Lunardi, J. (1995). Mapping of a further malignant hyperthermia locus to chromosome 3q13.1. *American Journal of Human Genetics*, **56**, 684–91.

Zhang, Y., Chen, H. S., Khanna, V. K., de Leon, S., Phillips, M. S., Schappert, K., Britt, B. A., Brownell, A. K. W. & MacLennan, D. H. (1993). A mutation in the human ryanodine receptor gene associated with central core disease. *Nature Genetics*, **5**, 46–50.

Zorzato, F., Fujii, J., Otsu, K., Phillips, M., Green, N. M., Lai, F. A., Meissner, G. & MacLennen, D. H. (1990). Molecular cloning of cDNA encoding human and rabbit forms of Ca^{2+} release channel (ryanodine receptor) of skeletal muscle sarcoplasmic reticulum. *Journal of Biological Chemistry*, **265**, 2244–56.

14

Porcine stress syndrome

J. DINSMORE and G. M. HALL

Introduction

There has been an increasing body of research into the porcine stress syndrome (PSS) since the first description by Topel *et al.* (1968). Prior to this, Hall *et al.* (1966) described a case of suxamethonium and halothane-induced malignant hyperthermia (MH) in pigs. The PSS is a potentially fatal, hypermetabolic disorder induced by natural stressors such as severe exercise, high ambient temperatures or transportation in susceptible swine. The clinical manifestations, changes in vital signs, muscle activity and metabolism are almost identical to those described in human MH. As the PSS can also be triggered by anaesthesia, the two syndromes have been thought to be manifestations of the same disorder. In humans MH is rare and susceptible individuals appear completely normal until expression of the disorder is triggered by anaesthesia. The PSS, therefore, has provided a valuable model for the investigation, diagnosis, pathophysiology and treatment of susceptible individuals.

Another stimulus for research into PSS is the huge economic cost of the stress-induced deaths to the meat industry. In addition, stress susceptible pigs produce a poor quality meat that is pale, soft and exudative (PSE) meat. PSE meat is brought about as a consequence of the combined effects of an elevated muscle temperature and a rapid reduction in pH of susceptible muscle. This causes the soluble and structural proteins to denature, changing the translucency of the meat and decreasing its water holding capacity. The result is the characteristic paleness and the loss of free fluid (Mitchell & Heffron, 1982).

Certain breeds of pig, for example Pietrain and Belgian Landrace, appear to be more susceptible to the effects of stress, while others, for example Large White or Yorkshire, are almost completely resistant. Susceptible pigs tend to have a similar body morphology being lean, with heavy body musculature and rapid growth rates. The incidence of both PSE meat and the PSS has increased with breeding patterns designed to produce these improvements in carcass yield. It was estimated that between 1972 and 1981 the incidence of PSE meat had doubled (Chadwick & Kempster, 1983).

Finally it has been realised that stress syndromes occur in other species, for example capture myopathy in wild animals (Harthoorn *et al.*, 1974) and the canine stress syndrome (O'Brien *et al.*, 1990). This knowledge, along with the fact that the PSS could be consistently triggered in susceptible swine in the absence of anaesthesia, has led to interest in stress syndromes in general.

The syndrome

The clinical syndromes of PSS and established human MH are remarkably similar. There is little evidence, however, that either the triggering mechanisms or the integral intracellular or membrane defects are identical. The earliest detectable changes are the result of increases in skeletal muscle metabolism, both aerobic and anaerobic. There is a rise in oxygen consumption with an even greater rise in carbon dioxide production. An increase in both lactate and heat production results in a gross metabolic and respiratory acidosis. Clinically this hypermetabolic state manifests itself with muscle rigidity, increased body temperature, tachycardia, hypertension and intense peripheral vasoconstriction. In spontaneously breathing animals there is tachypnoea. Membrane permeability increases as a result of depletion of creatine phosphate and ATP and the fall in pH (Heffron, 1988). This leads to gross electrolyte changes with haemoconcentration and, later, to rises in creatine kinase and myoglobin. The PSS unless quickly recognised and treated by terminating the triggering agents and giving dantrolene is usually fatal. In susceptible pigs rigor mortis develops almost immediately after death and affected muscle shows similar biochemical changes to those of PSE meat due to the high temperature and low pH of the muscle before death (Mitchell & Heffron, 1982; Hall & Lucke, 1985). PSE meat is thought, therefore, to be a postmorten manifestation of the PSS or MH syndromes.

Mechanisms

Muscle metabolism

Research has generally focused on skeletal muscle as the site of the primary defect in the PSS, as this is where the major biochemical abnormalities occur. Experimental findings have confirmed a defect in Ca^{2+} regulation (Allen *et al.*, 1985) with elevated myoplasmic Ca^{2+} concentrations found during the acute episode (Lopez *et al.*, 1988). This rise in Ca^{2+} precedes the development of the clinical signs (Ryan *et al.*, 1994). Muscle contraction, relaxation and energy metabolism are all regulated by the intracellular Ca^{2+} concentration and a defect in Ca^{2+} regulation could account for all the signs found. Sustained muscle contraction results in rigidity and augmented glycolytic metabolism with increased production of heat and lactate. Sarcoplasmic Ca^{2+} concentration is regulated by a variety of pumps and channels located in the sarcoplasmic reticulum, the sarcolemma and transverse tubules, and the mitochondria.

Sarcoplasmic reticulum

The focus of most interest has been the sarcoplasmic reticulum: 80% of all skeletal muscle Ca^{2+} is stored here and it is the major regulator of sarcoplasmic Ca^{2+} levels (Endo, 1977). Ca^{2+} is pumped by a Ca^{2+}-dependent ATPase pump from the sarcoplasm into the sarcoplasmic reticulum initiating relaxation. The Ca^{2+} is then stored in the junctional terminal cisternae until release is triggered through a Ca^{2+} release channel to initiate contraction. Opening of the Ca^{2+} release channels during excitation-contraction coupling is the end result of a wave of depolarisation moving from nerve, to muscle, and then transverse tubular membrane. Here, the voltage sensitive Ca^{2+} channels of the transverse tubular junctional membrane, or dihydropyridine (DHP) receptors, sense the change in surface membrane potential and transduce this signal into one for Ca^{2+} release from the sarcoplasmic reticulum. The exact nature of the link between the Ca^{2+} release channel and the DHP receptor is still not known (for a review, see Joffe *et al.*, 1992). Ca^{2+} release can also be induced by inositol (1,4,5) trisphosphate (IP_3) and by a Ca^{2+}-induced release mechanism (Foster, 1990; Joffe *et al.*, 1992). Again the exact mechanisms of release are unknown but appear to involve direct interaction with the Ca^{2+} release channel independent of depolarisation.

The Ca^{2+} release channel itself has been isolated and characterised by virtue of its high affinity binding to the plant alkaloid ryanodine. This portion of the release channel has been termed the ryanodine receptor and corresponds to the junctional foot structure that spans the transverse tubule–sarcoplasmic reticulum junction (Inui *et al.*, 1987; Lai *et al.*, 1988). The ryanodine receptor consists of a 30S homotetrameric complex with a subunit molecular weight of 450 000. Four transmembrane sequences are located near the carboxy terminus of each subunit and the remainder protrudes into the cytoplasm to form the foot structure which is in close proximity to the DHP receptor (Figure 14.1). The transmembrane sequences from each subunit combine to enclose four radial channels that extend from the central transmembrane channel and exit in peripheral vestibules.

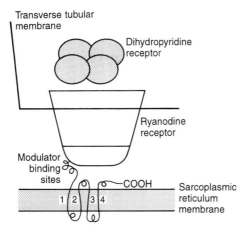

Figure 14.1. Ryanodine receptor at the triad junction of skeletal muscle. The large foot structure and its close relationship to the dihydropyridine receptor are shown schematically. The transmembrane sequences (1–4) and putative modulator binding sites are also shown.

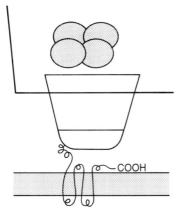

Figure 14.2. Schematic representation of the quatrefoil structure of the ryanodine receptor. This comprises a dense central mass divided into four radial channels connected to a central channel (Ca^{2+} release channel). The central mass is enclosed within an outer frame displaying a pinwheel appearance.

Detailed morphology reveals a homotetrameric complex displaying a four-leaf clover or quatrefoil three-dimensional architecture. This comprises a dense central mass enclosed within an outer frame that consists of four vestibules (Figure 14.2).

The Ca^{2+} release channel appears to contain binding sites for modulators.

Ca^{2+} release is stimulated by micromolar levels of Ca^{2+} and millimolar levels of adenine nucleotides and is inhibited by millimolar levels of Mg^{2+} and Ca^{2+}, micromolar calmodulin and ruthenium red (Lai *et al.*, 1988).

Defective calcium regulation in the sarcoplasmic reticulum could therefore result from abnormalities of the Ca^{2+} ATPase pump, the Ca^{2+} release channel or an abnormality of one of the proteins involved in the sequence of events leading to Ca^{2+} release described above.

Studies of the Ca^{2+} ATPase in MH susceptible pigs have yielded conflicting results but, when membrane purity and intactness are considered, the majority point to Ca^{2+} uptake being normal (Mickelson *et al.*, 1986; Louis *et al.*, 1992). Most research has focused on the Ca^{2+} release channel and both membrane bound and purified ryanodine binding protein have been reconstituted to produce Ca^{2+} release channels with characteristic properties. In porcine MH there is an increased affinity for ryanodine binding with greater rates and amounts of Ca^{2+} release (Mickelson *et al.*, 1988). The Ca^{2+} gating mechanism is abnormal. The Ca^{2+} release channel is hypersensitive to stimuli, with decreased luminal thresholds for induction of Ca^{2+} release, and is less than normally sensitive to inhibitory stimuli (Fill *et al.*, 1990; Mickelson *et al.*, 1990). This results in the channel remaining open for longer than normal (Fill *et al.*, 1990). From these results it was suggested that there was an abnormality of the ryanodine receptor in the region regulating the gating mechanism (Mickelson *et al.*, 1990).

To identify the molecular basis for the abnormality, the amino acid sequence of both the normal and the MH susceptible ryanodine receptor were compared. The deduced amino acid sequences differed by a single amino acid in the MH susceptible pig, cysteine was substituted for arginine at position 615 (Fujii *et al.*, 1991). A structural alteration in the ryanodine receptor protein was also suggested when immunopeptide maps showed distinct differences between the MH susceptible and normal pig (Knudson *et al.*, 1990). This mutation at residue 615 causes a detectable alteration in ryanodine receptor/Ca^{2+} channel activity (Shomer *et al.*, 1993).

Louis *et al.* (1992) demonstrated that halothane, enflurane and isoflurane in clinically appropriate concentrations interacted with the Ca^{2+} release channel to stimulate Ca^{2+} release from the MH susceptible, but not the normal, porcine sarcoplasmic reticulum. The interaction was such that the Ca^{2+} release channels from abnormal pigs could be activated at Ca^{2+} concentrations and pH values that would normally be expected to maintain the channel in a closed state. They were unable, however, to demonstrate inhibition of Ca^{2+} release by dantrolene. This substantiated earlier studies which also showed no evidence that dantrolene had any effect on the Ca^{2+} release channel (van Winkle, 1976;

Nelson, 1984). The site of action of this important therapeutic agent in skeletal muscle would, however, help to explain the nature of the defect. It was suggested that it might act by inhibiting charge movement at the DHP receptor in the transverse tubule (Morgan & Bryant, 1977). This would result in an altered association between the DHP receptor and the Ca^{2+} release channel and would cause abnormal functioning of the ryanodine receptor (Ervasti *et al.*, 1989*a*).

Other efforts to explain the defect in Ca^{2+} regulation include suggestions that the function of the Ca^{2+} release channel might be regulated by phosphorylation of certain proteins of the sarcoplasmic reticulum (Foster, 1990; Joffe *et al.*, 1991). Kim *et al.* (1988) proposed that the MH ryanodine receptor displays a higher rate of Ca^{2+} release because of a lower than normal level of calcium–calmodulin dependent phosphorylation of a 60 kDa protein, which they had previously shown to be involved in the normal inhibition of sarcoplasmic reticulum Ca^{2+} release.

There has been increasing interest in the role of IP_3 metabolism and its action as a second messenger in excitation-contraction coupling and Ca^{2+} mobilisation from the sarcoplasmic reticulum. Recent work has found that the IP_3 receptor is homologous with the ryanodine receptor (Mignery & Südhof, 1990) and this will increase this interest still further. Foster *et al.* (1989*a*) demonstrated that there was a deficiency in inositol 1,4,5 trisphosphate phosphatase (IP_35ase) activity in the sarcoplasmic reticulum of MH susceptible swine resulting in increased levels of IP_3 and increased Ca^{2+} release. Furthermore, they found that halothane inhibited IP_35ase activity still further, producing even greater Ca^{2+} concentrations that could result in the abnormal contractile responses of MH.

Mitochondria

The proposal for mitochrondrial involvement in the pathogenesis of MH arose from the suggestion that the uncoupling of oxidative phosphorylation was responsible for the thermogenesis, but this was shown not to be the case. Since then attention has turned to the role of the mitochondria in Ca^{2+} homeostasis (for reviews, see Gronert *et al.*, 1988; Foster, 1990). Ca^{2+} uptake by MH susceptible porcine mitochondria was investigated with conflicting results. It was reported to be decreased by some investigators, but found to be normal by others. Cheah & Cheah (1976) found enhanced porcine mitochondrial Ca^{2+} efflux under conditions of anaerobiosis with marked breed variations. This was considered to be sufficient to activate myofibrillar ATPase and phosphorylase kinase and to induce accelerated glycolysis. Furthermore, halothane increased efflux from MH susceptible mitochondria only. Although

Ca^{2+} efflux from mitochondria may be involved in the perpetuation of the syndrome, it does not offer a complete explanation.

Cheah & Cheah (1981) also suggested that mitochondrial phospholipase A_2 activity was abnormal, resulting in the liberation of fatty acids, which in turn inhibited the function of the sarcoplasmic reticulum. This finding has not been confirmed (Fletcher *et al.*, 1988) and, as the release of phospholipase A_2 is calcium dependent, it is difficult to determine which is the primary alteration as elevated Ca^{2+} concentrations are inevitable in MH. During acute MH, mitochondria appear to actively sequester Ca^{2+} resulting in restrictive functions. This has been proposed as an explanation for the less than expected whole body oxygen consumption during MH (Gronert *et al.*, 1988).

Sarcolemma

Studies are few in comparison with those of the sarcoplasmic reticulum and mitochondria, but the MH susceptible sarcolemma does seem to respond to stimuli abnormally. Porcine MH susceptible muscle fibres have a lower mechanical threshold and a lesser degree of depolarisation produces a contracture. Halothane depolarises the membrane and electrical stimuli result in exaggerated responses. It is difficult to know if these are simply abnormal responses of the internal sarcoplasmic structures responding to the transferred signal, rather than a direct membrane effect (Gronert *et al.*, 1988; Ervasti *et al.*, 1989*b*).

Other reports of altered sarcolemmal function include increased acetylcholinesterase activity and decreased accumulation of Ca^{2+} by MH susceptible sarcolemmal vesicles (Ervasti *et al.*, 1989*b*). A potentially important finding has been the observation that the content, or the activity, of the DHP receptor is decreased in MH susceptible skeletal muscle. In view of its critical role in the regulation of excitation-contraction coupling this may have significant implications for either the onset or maintenance of MH (Ervasti *et al.*, 1989*b*; Lamb *et al.*, 1989).

Although skeletal muscle undoubtedly carries the defect, other tissues and organisms have been implicated. These include the liver, cerebral tissue and cardiac muscle. In a study of cardiac sarcoplasmic reticulum of both normal and MH susceptible pigs, Ervasti *et al.* (1991) demonstrated identical [^{3}H] ryanodine binding properties. They concluded that despite the fact that the abnormal Ca^{2+} release channel of MH sarcoplasmic reticulum was expressed in both fast and slow twitch skeletal muscle, it was not expressed in cardiac muscle. Roewer *et al.* (1995) have recently demonstrated, however, that halothane produces alterations in the dynamic electrical properties of the ventricular excitable membrane of MH susceptible swine. They have suggested that there is a latent defect in the myocardium of susceptible pigs that becomes apparent in the presence of triggering agents. Reviews do not support the involvement of either liver or cerebral tissue (Mitchell & Heffron 1982; Gronert *et al.*, 1988).

A generalised membrane defect has been proposed with evidence of increased porcine red blood cell fragility and decreased lipid mobility (Cheah & Cheah 1985; Fletcher *et al.*, 1990) but again these suggestions have been disputed (Gronert *et al.*, 1988; Fletcher *et al.*, 1988, 1990; Ervasti *et al.*, 1989*b*). Further work has also demonstrated defects in lipid metabolism with suggestions that fatty acids are involved in effecting sarcoplasmic reticulum Ca^{2+} release. Cheah & Cheah (1981) and Fletcher *et al.* (1990) proposed that an altered lipase activity in MH susceptible pigs resulted in abnormal skeletal muscle calcium regulation. A mutation in the gene for hormone-dependent lipase (LIPE) has been proposed by Levitt *et al.* (1990). The LIPE gene is located on the same chromosome as, and close to, the ryanodine receptor gene. These proposals have yet to be substantiated.

Sympathetic nervous system

Catecholamine levels rise as a result of stress and therefore it is not surprising that increased levels are found in both normal pigs undergoing stress and in susceptible pigs during acute MH. Plasma catecholamine levels, however, increase up to 50-fold during the terminal stages of MH and are undoubtedly involved in the initiation and perpetuation of many of the signs. This, in combination with the fact that the PSS can be triggered by stress alone, suggests a primary role for catecholamines. This is much disputed.

The evidence to suggest a primary role includes the use of catecholamines to cause MH in susceptible swine and the prevention of MH in triggered animals by α-adrenergic blockade, epidural anaesthesia, depletion of catecholamines by reserpine and a combination of adrenalectomy and bretyllium pretreatment (for reviews, see Mitchell & Heffron 1982; Hall & Lucke 1985; Gronert *et al.*, 1988). Other workers have not found that MH can be caused by catecholamine infusions. Also, total spinal blockade prevents the changes in catecholamine levels without influencing the course of active MH, and neither α- or β-adrenergic antagonists can prevent or reverse established MH (Mitchell & Heffron 1982; Gronert *et al.*, 1988). Further evidence against a primary role for catecholamines or the sympathetic nervous system is that the clinical signs and metabolic effects of MH precede the increases in circulating catecholamines (Häggendal *et al.*, 1990). More recently, Adeola *et al.* (1993) found regional differences in neurotransmitter concentrations between the brains of susceptible and resistant pigs, leading them to suggest central nervous system involvement in the PSS.

There is no doubt that catecholamines and the sympathetic nervous system play a contributory role in the development of, and may well be integral to, porcine MH. The protective effects of chronic adrenalectomy found by Lucke *et al.* (1978) could be explained by prolonged activation of the sympathetic nervous system in MH susceptible pigs resulting in abnormal calcium regulation within the cell. Other possible methods of involvement of the sympathetic nervous system include enhanced adrenergic activity secondary to stimulation of inositol phosphate-lipid metabolism with higher basal concentrations of IP_3 in both skeletal and cardiac muscle of MH susceptible swine (Scholz *et al.*, 1991, 1993); also abnormal activity of peripheral sympathetic neurones secondary to defective calcium turnover (Häggendal *et al.*, 1988).

Identification

Accurate identification of susceptible swine is of great importance, but has not been straightforward. Until exposed to stress or triggering agents the animals appear normal. An accurate diagnostic test would provide a means of identifying susceptible animals prior to their exposure to potentially fatal triggering agents and would enable the elimination of the MH susceptible gene from the breeding stock. Also, as much of the research into human MH has been performed on swine which are assumed to be MH susceptible, it is obvious that results cannot be properly interpreted until accurate identification is possible.

Blood tests

Serum enzymes

Many serum enzymes have been proposed as potential diagnostic tests. These include aldolase, lactate dehydrogenase, glutamate oxalate and pyrophosphate (for a review, see Mitchell & Heffron, 1982) and more recently pyruvate kinase (Duthie *et al.*, 1989). None of these has been found to be accurate enough. Creatine kinase is the most studied. Values are elevated in virtually all susceptible swine or those undergoing MH. Its use as a predictive test has fallen into disrepute especially in human MH (Ørding, 1988) because of the variability and overlap of results between susceptible and normal subjects. Mitchell & Heffron (1975) clarified some of the causes of the variability and limitations of the test in swine and when combined with additional indicators it has proved a useful adjunct.

Red blood cells

These cells of MH susceptible swine showed greater osmotic fragility when compared with those of normal pigs and this was further increased during exposure to halothane. Susceptible pig red blood cells are also deficient in glutathione peroxidase making them more liable to haemolysis (Ørding, 1988; Duthie *et al.*, 1989). Chemiluminescence, a method of quantifying autooxidation in red blood cells, enabled Jones & Brady (1986) to distinguish between diagnostic groups of known MH genotypes before and after exposure to halothane.

Lymphocytes

When porcine MH susceptible lymphocytes were exposed to halothane their calcium concentration increased significantly. These findings have been disputed (Ørding, 1988; Gronert *et al.*, 1988).

Platelets

Platelets have many similar characteristics to muscle, so their metabolism has been investigated. Platelet aggregation and tests of nucleotide depletion in response to halothane have been used, but there is little evidence to suggest their reliability (Ellis & Heffron, 1985; Gronert *et al.*, 1988; Ørding, 1988). Miller *et al.* (1991) proposed that calcium handling was stimulated in a dose-dependent manner by caffeine and Basrur *et al.* (1988) suggested that MH susceptible platelets could be distinguished by electron microscopy on the basis of an open cannilicular system.

Nuclear magnetic resonance

Phosphorus nuclear magnetic resonance spectroscopy (^{31}P-NMR) is a non-invasive method of determining intracellular changes in high energy phosphates. Foster *et al.* (1989*b*) found that changes in the phosphate metabolite profile of MH susceptible porcine skeletal muscle occurred more readily under conditions of anoxia than did control muscle. Looking at skeletal muscle metabolism *in vivo*, Decanniere *et al.* (1993) demonstrated abnormal responses in MH susceptible piglets anaesthetised with halothane.

Muscle tests

The *in vitro* contracture test (IVCT) requires a muscle biopsy which is then exposed to halothane and caffeine. European and North American diagnostic criteria have been developed on the basis of the results obtained. Although the procedures have been standardised, and the test is the most specific available to date, it is invasive, expensive and time-consuming. Also there is a tendency to err on the side of false positive results (Ellis & Heffron, 1985; Ørding, 1988). For these reasons, and because there tended to be greater variability in the contracture responses of susceptible swine, the test has not been widely used in PSS. The most widely accepted test for animals is the 'halothane test'. This is quick, cheap, provides an immediate result and can be performed in farmyard conditions. To determine MH susceptibility, pigs usually of 8–12 weeks of age are anaesthetised with halothane. The Animal Breeding Research Organisation has adopted a standard three-minute test in which the amounts of halothane and oxygen are regulated so that the pig becomes anaesthetised within the first minute. Anaesthesia is then maintained for two minutes. Reactor pigs develop characteristic signs within these three minutes and anaesthesia is immediately terminated allowing the pig to recover, although some of the pigs will die (Webb, 1981).

There is, however, a wide spectrum of MH sensitivity that can also be modified by factors such as exercise or stress. Van den Hende *et al* . (1976) was able to change pigs from 42% susceptibility to 100% susceptibility after 60 minutes of gentle exercise. The differentiation between reactors and non-reactors is not always clear cut. Webb (1981) estimated the probability of misclassification as about 5%.

Genetics

The problems of accurately identifying susceptible swine and humans have resulted in numerous opinions on the exact modes of inheritance. It is presently assumed that human MH is inherited in an autosomal dominant manner. For porcine MH the most recent suggestion is of an autosomal recessive gene (Hogan *et al.*, 1992).

There have been a huge number of studies on the genetics of porcine MH in the past few years and linkage has been established between its inheritance (the *HAL* gene) and polymorphic markers. A linkage group consisting of HAL, glucose phosphate isomerase (GPI), 6 phosphogluconate dehydrogenase (PGD), alpha-IB glycoprotein (AIBG) genes, the H blood group locus and the loci controlling the expression of the A–O blood groups was localised near the centromere of pig chromosome 6 (MacLennan & Phillips, 1992). This corresponds to a region on the proximal long arm of human chromosome 19, and by virtue of this mapping, the gene encoding the ryanodine receptor protein became a candidate for the MH mutation (Harbitz *et al.*, 1990).

Both genetic and biochemical data pointed to a structural abnormality of this receptor protein, and (Fujii *et al.* (1991) investigated the amino acid sequencing of normal and MH susceptible swine. A single sequence difference was observed and this was localised to amino acid 615 where arginine was replaced by a cysteine residue. Linkage of the mutation to phenotypic porcine MH was then established by a combination of halothane challenge testing, GPI and PGD haplotyping and DNA amplification with testing for mutations. This combination provided precise evaluation of the MH status. Subsequent analysis of the appropriate nucleotide sequence determined the existence of the mutation (MacLennan & Phillips, 1992).

The same mutation was found to be present in five major breeds of lean, heavily muscled pigs, suggesting that leanness and muscling may be manifestations of the gene itself (Fujii *et al.*, 1991). These characteristics are thought of as desirable traits by breeders, and so the increase in incidence of the gene and MH could possibly be explained, despite its apparently deleterious effects. It also suggests that all porcine MH may be derived from a common ancestor.

These discoveries have made it possible to develop a diagnostic test for susceptible swine that is simple, non-invasive and which eliminates the 5% diagnostic error associated with the halothane challenge test (Rempel *et al.*, 1993; Vogeli *et al.*, 1994). Assuming that this mutation is the cause of MH, it would also allow breeders to either eliminate the gene or allow for its controlled inclusion in breeding programmes (MacLennan & Phillips, 1992). In order to estimate the frequency of the mutation O'Brien *et al.* (1993) tested 10 245 swine of various breeds in England and North America. They showed that the PSS mutation was present in a large proportion of the English and US swine. They rated the accuracy of genetic testing at more than 99% with a cost of less than $20 per animal.

Stress and heat stroke

Stress, such as exercise and extremes of temperature, can undoubtedly initiate MH in susceptible swine, but the role of stress in initiating human MH is more controversial. Is there a human 'stress syndrome' and is heat stroke a manifestation of this?

The role of exercise prior to exposure to triggering agents has been investigated. In swine it has been documented to worsen outcome and in humans it has been suggested that more severe episodes of MH occur if anaesthesia follows exercise or trauma (Gronert *et al.*, 1988). Abnormalities of MH susceptible human skeletal muscle during exercise have been demonstrated with delayed recovery of muscle pH after short duration, high intensity exercise (Allsop *et al.*, 1991). Also studies looking at the response of MH susceptible individuals to progressively severe exercise showed small, but consistent, results compatible with increased activity of the sympathetic nervous systems (Ellis *et al.*, 1991).

Wingard (1974) proposed a human 'stress syndrome' and produced an account of several families with a history of MH in whom there was a definite increase in unexpected deaths and unexplained fevers. Mogensen *et al.* (1974) proposed that MH was more common in those suffering from preoperative anxiety. Isolated case reports have also occurred. Pollock *et al.* (1992) reported the case of an 18-year-old who had survived an episode of MH at the age of 16. He underwent non triggering anaesthesia but developed MH after the operation. They proposed that MH had been triggered by physiological and psychological stress. Other cases have appeared in the literature (Hall & Lucke, 1985) but satisfactory documentation is scant and there is little consensus as to their significance.

There are strong similarities between the PSS and capture myopathy of wild animals. The stress of chasing a wild animal, for example a zebra, over long distances is associated with considerable mortality. The animals develop muscular rigidity, tachycardia and severe metabolic acidosis. It has been suggested that this is the manifestation of a stress syndrome but whether these animals would develop MH has not been established. O'Brien *et al.* (1990) reported a case of an exercise-induced canine stress syndrome which they claimed was analogous to PSS.

Heatstroke is induced by either excessive muscular exertion or high ambient temperatures in combination with dehydration. Exercise-induced heat stroke does have similarities to acute MH. The signs include raised body temperature, metabolic acidosis and rhabdomyolysis and it can respond dramatically to treatment with dantrolene. There is no evidence, however, to link its cause with that of PSS (Ellis & Heffron, 1985). Hopkins *et al.* (1991) investigated two young men who had developed heat stroke, and their immediate families with IVCT. Both men developed abnormal responses to halothane but had normal responses to caffeine. Both fathers had abnormal results: one to halothane and one to ryanodine. The results supported the theory that heat stroke may well be an inheritable muscular disorder but it does not seem to be identical to MH or PSS.

Conclusions

Biochemical and physiological studies in MH susceptible swine have implicated a structural and functional abnormality in the Ca^{2+} release channel, or ryanodine receptor, as the cause of the defect in Ca^{2+} regulation that occurs in porcine MH. Abnormal regulation of calcium could explain all the features found in MH. Genetic analysis of the ryanodine receptor confirms the presence of a structural abnormality. The deduced amino acid sequences of the MH susceptible ryanodine receptor shows a substitution of cysteine for arginine at position 615. The same mutation has subsequently been found in all breeds of pig investigated.

Exactly how volatile agents might trigger MH is not yet known, but Louis *et al.* (1992) have shown that in MH susceptible swine they result in increased opening of the Ca^{2+} release channel by interacting with the abnormal ryanodine receptor. The volatile agents are also able to activate the channel at Ca^{2+} concentrations and pH values that would normally maintain the channel in a closed state. The role of stress in triggering the MH response is still sought. Fujii *et al.* (1991) suggested that the neuroendocrine response to stress or anaesthesia was able to increase the levels of physiological channel gating agents to the point where the abnormal Ca^{2+} release channel was activated. Once opened, the channel was resistant to the normal stimuli that close the channel and so the rise in Ca^{2+} was perpetuated resulting in the MH syndrome. There is no doubt of the involvement of the sympathetic nervous system and catecholamines in the perpetuation of the disorder but the evidence suggests a secondary role.

The aetiology of human MH is less certain; almost all the experimental work has been performed on pigs. The common causal feature seems to be a defect in Ca^{2+} regulation in skeletal muscle cells. The only persuasive biochemical evidence for a defect in the ryanodine receptor has been obtained in swine and there is some evidence for a different function in human and porcine ryanodine receptors (Levitt *et al.*, 1991).

This mutation has appeared in humans but not in all families examined, compared with swine where the same mutation has appeared in five breeds of susceptible animal. This means that although mutations in the ryanodine receptor gene may be responsible for some forms of human MH, there may be more than one mutation involved and other entirely different mechanisms may be implicated. For example, proteins involved in calcium regulation of skeletal muscle may be altered or there may be an altered second messenger system such as IP_3 or fatty acids. MH in humans appears to be a more heterogeneous disorder and this, combined with the lack of evidence linking human MH to 'awake' triggering, suggests that PSS and human MH are indeed different disorders. At best PSS only corresponds to one small subgroup of human MH. This deduction also calls into question the justification for using the PSS as a screening method or model for humans MH.

Knowledge of the molecular alteration associated with the PSS has led to the development of a diagnostic test for susceptible swine that can distinguish between the normal, the heterozygote and homozygote for the MH gene. Assuming that this is the causal mutation there is now the potential to eliminate the gene from the breeding stock. Breeders need to choose between alternative breeding programmes. Do they eliminate the PSS gene with the resultant substantial savings to the meat industry resulting from a reduction in PSE meat and the prevention of PSS deaths? This strategy, however, has the disadvantage of potentially eliminating or decreasing the associated beneficial traits of leanness and heavy musculature.

Certainly, the presence of the MH gene (or an abnormal Ca^{2+} release channel) appears to be essential for the syndrome in swine. Additional or modulating mechanisms must also be involved to explain the variable expression of the syndrome and how it is triggered by stress (see Chapter 10).

References

Adeola, O., Ball, R. O., House, J. D. & O'Brien, P. J. (1993). Regional brain neurotransmitters concentrations in stress-susceptible pigs. *Journal of Animal Science*, **71**, 968–74.

Allen, P., Lopez, J. R., Jones, D., Alamo, L., Papp, L. & Sreter, F. S. (1985). Measurements of $[Ca^{2+}]$ in skeletal muscle of malignant hyperthermic swine. *Anesthesiology*, **63**, A268 (abstract).

Allsop, P., Jorfeldt, L., Rutberg, H., Lennmarken, C. & Hall, G. M. (1991). Delayed recovery of muscle pH after short duration, high intensity exercise in malignant hyperthermia susceptible subjects. *British Journal of Anaesthesia*, **66**, 541–5.

Basrur, P. K., Bouvet, A. & McDonnel, W. N. (1988). Open canicular system of platelets in the porcine stress syndrome. *Canadian Journal of Veterinary Research*, **52**, 380–5.

Chadwick, J. P. & Kempster, A. J. (1983). A repeat national survey (ten years on) of muscle pH values in commercial bacon carcasses. *Meat Science*, **9**, 101-11.

Cheah, K. S. & Cheah, A. M. (1976). The trigger for PSE condition in stress susceptible pigs. *Journal of Science and Food Agriculture*, **27**, 1137–44.

Cheah, K. S. & Cheah, A. M. (1981). Mitochondrial calcium transport and calcium activated phospholipase in porcine malignant hyperthermia. *Biochimica Biophysica Acta*, **634**, 70–84.

Cheah, K. S. & Cheah, A. M. (1985). Malignant hyperthermia: molecular defects in membrane permeability. *Experientia*, **41**, 656–61.

Decanniere, C., van Hecke, P., Vanstapel, F., Ville, H. & Geers, R. (1993). Metabolic response to halothane in piglets susceptible to malignant hyperthermia: an *in vivo* ^{31}P-NMR study. *Journal of Applied Physiology*, **75**, 955–62.

Duthie, G. G., Arthur, J. R., Bremner, P., Kikuchi, Y. & Nicol, F. (1989). Increased peroxidation of erythrocytes of stress susceptible pigs: an improved diagnostic test for porcine stress syndrome. *American Journal of Veterinary Research*, **50**, 84–87.

Ellis, F. R. & Heffron, J. J. A. (1985). Clinical and biochemical aspects of malignant hyperthermia. In *Recent Advances in Anaesthesia and Analgesia*, Ed, R. S. Atkinson & A. P. Adams, **15**, 173–207. Edinburgh, Churchill Livingstone.

Ellis, F. R., Green, J. H. & Campbell I. T. (1991). Muscle activity, pH and malignant hyperthermia. *British Journal of Anaesthesia*, **66**, 535–7.

Endo, M. (1977). Calcium release from sarcoplasmic reticulum. *Physiological Review*, **57**, 71–108.

Ervasti, J. M., Claessens, M. T., Michelson, J. R. & Louis, C. F. (1989*a*). Altered transverse tubule DHP receptor binding in malignant hyperthermia. *Journal of Biological Chemistry* **264**, 2711–17.

Ervasti, J. M., Mickelson, J. R., Lewis, S. M., Thomas, D. D. & Louis, C. F. (1989*b*). An electron paramagnetic resonance study of skeletal muscle membrane fluidity in malignant hyperthermia. *Biochimica et Biophysica Acta*, **986**, 70–4.

Ervasti, J. M., Strand, M. A., Hanson, T. P., Mickelson, J. R., & Louis C. F. (1991). Ryanodine receptor in different malignant hyperthermia susceptible muscles. *American Journal of Physiology*, **260**, C58–66.

Fill, M., Coronada, R., Mickelson, J. R., Vilven, J., Jacobson, B. A. & Louis, C. F. (1990). Abnormal ryanodine receptor channels in malignant hyperthermia. *Biophysical Journal*, **50**, 471–5.

Fletcher, J. E., Rosenberg, H., Michaux, K., Cheah, K. S. & Cheah, A. M. (1988). Lipid analysis of skeletal muscle from pigs susceptible to malignant hyperthermia. *Biochemistry Cell Biology*, **66**, 917–21.

Fletcher, J. E., Tripolitis, L., Erwin, K., Hanson, S, Rosenberg, H., Conti, P. A. & Beech, J. (1990). Fatty acids modulate calcium-induced calcium release from skeletal muscle heavy sarcoplasmic reticulum fractions: implications for malignant hyperthermia. *Biochemistry Cell Biology*, **68**, 1195–201.

Foster, P. S. (1990). Minireview. Malignant hyperpyrexia. *International Journal of Biochemistry*, **22**, 1271–22.

Foster, P. S., Gesini, E., Claudianos, C., Hopkinson, K. C. & Denborough, M. A. (1989*a*). Inositol 1,4,5-triphosphate phosphatase deficiency and malignant hyperpyrexia in swine. *Lancet*, **2**, 124–7.

Foster, P. S., Hopkinson, K. C. & Denborough, M. A. (1989*b*). ^{31}P-NMR spectroscopy: the metabolic profile of malignant hyperpyrexic porcine skeletal muscle. *Muscle and Nerve*, **12**, 390–6.

Fujii, J.,Otsu, K., Zorzato, F., de Leon, S., Khanna, V. K., Wiler, J. E., O'Brien, P. J. & MacLennan, D. H. (1991). Identification of a mutation in porcine ryanodine receptor associated with malignant hyperthermia. *Science*, **253**, 448–51.

Gronert, G. A., Mott, J. & Lee, J. (1988). Aetiology of malignant hyperthermia. *British Journal of Anaesthesia*, **6**, 253–67.

Häggendal, J., Jönsson, L. & Carlsten, J. (1990). A role of sympathetic activity in initiating malignant hyperthermia. *Acta Anaesthesiologica Scandinavica*, **34**, 677–82.

Häggendal, J., Jönsson, L., Johansson, G., Bjurstrom, S. & Carlsten, J. (1988). Disordered catecholamine release in pigs susceptible to malignant hyperthermia. *Pharmacology and Toxicology*, **63**, 257–61.

Hall, G. M. & Lucke, J. N. (1985). Of man and pigs: is malignant hyperthermia a stress-related disorder? *Stress Medicine*, **1**, 47–53.

Hall, L. W., Woolf, N., Bradley, J. W. P. & Jolly, D. W. (1966). Unusual reaction to suxamethonium chloride. *British Medical Journal*, **2**, 1305.

Harbitz, I., Chowdhary, B., Thomsen, P. D., Davies, W., Kaufman, U., Krans, S., Gustavsson, I., Christensen, K. & Hauge, J. G. (1990). Assignment of the porcine calcium-release channel gene, a candidate for the malignant hyperthermia locus, to the 6p11-q21 segment of chromosome 6. *Genomics*, **8**, 243–8.

Harthoorn, A. M., van der Walt, K. & Young, E. (1974). Possible therapy for capture myopathy in captured wild animals. *Nature*, **247**, 577.

Heffron, J. J. A. (1988). Malignant hyperthermia: biochemical aspects of the acute episode. *British Journal of Anaesthesia*, **60**, 274–8.

Hogan, K., Couch, F., Powers, P. A. & Gregg, R. G. (1992). A cysteine-for-arginine substitution (R614C) in the human skeletal muscle calcium release channel cosegregates with malignant hyperthermia. *Anesthesia and Analgesia*, **75**, 441–8.

Hopkins, P. M., Ellis, F. R. & Halsall, P. J. (1991). Evidence for related myopathies in exertional heat stroke and malignant hyperthermia. *Lancet*, **338**, 1491–92.

Inui, M., Saito, A. & Fleischer, S. (1987). Purification of the ryanodine receptor and identity with feet structures of junctional terminal cisternae of sarcoplasmic reticulum from fast skeletal muscle. *Journal of Biological Chemistry*, **262**, 1740–7.

Joffe, M., Savage, N., Du Sayutoy, C., Mitchell, G. & Isaacs, H. (1991). Kinase activity and protein phosphorylation in control and malignant hyperthermic skeletal muscle. *International Journal of Biochemistry*, **23**, 443–53.

Joffe, M., Savage, N. & Silove, M. (1992). Minireview. The biochemistry of malignant hyperthermia: recent concepts. *International Journal of Biochemistry*, **24**, 387–98.

Jones, J. & Bready, L. L. (1986). Evaluation of a simplified chemiluminescent blood test in malignant hyperthermia susceptible pigs. *Anesthesiology*, **65**, 240 (abstract).

Kim, D. H., Sreter, F. A. & Ikemoto N. (1988). Involvement of the 60 kDa phosphoprotein in the regulation of Ca^{2+} release from sarcoplasmic reticulum of normal and malignant hyperthermia susceptible pig muscles. *Biochimica et Biophysica Acta*, **945**, 246–52.

Knudson, C. M., Mickelson, J. R., Louis, C. F. & Campbell, K. P. (1990). Distinct immunopeptide maps of the sarcoplasmic reticulum Ca^{2+} release channel in malignant hyperthermia. *Journal of Biological Chemistry*, **265**, 2421–4.

Lai, F. A., Erickson, H. P., Rousseau, E., Liu, Q. Y. & Meissner, G. (1988). Purification and reconstitution of calcium release channel from skeletal muscle. *Nature*, **333**, 315–19.

Lamb, G. D., Hopkinson, K. C. & Denborough, M. A. (1989). Calcium currents and asymmetric charge movement in malignant hyperthermia. *Muscle and Nerve*, **12**, 135–40.

Levitt, R. C., McKusick, V. A., Fletcher, J. E. & Rosenberg, H. (1990). Gene candidate. *Nature*, **345**, 297–8.

Levitt, R. C., Meyers, D., Fletcher, J. E. & Rosenberg, H. (1991). Molecular genetics and malignant hyperthermia. *Anesthesiology*, **75**, 1–3.

Lopez, J. R., Allen, P. D., Alamo, L., Jones, D. & Sreter F. (1988). Myoplasmic free $[Ca^{2+}]$ during a malignant hyperthermia episode in swine. *Muscle and Nerve* **11**, 82–8.

Louis, C. F., Zualkerman, K., Roghair, T. & Mickelson, J. R. (1992). The effects of volatile anesthetics on calcium regulation by malignant hyperthermia-susceptible sarcoplasmic reticulum. *Anesthesiology*, **77**, 114–25.

Lucke, J. N., Denny, H., Hall, G. M., Lovell, R. & Lister, D. (1978). Porcine malignant hyperthermia. *VI:* The effects of bilateral adrenalectomy and pretreatment with bretylium on the halothane-induced response. *British Journal of Anaesthesia*, **50**, 241–6.

MacLennan, D. H. & Phillips, M. S. (1992). Malignant hyperthermia. *Science*, **256**, 789–94.

Mickelson, J. R., Gallant, E. M., Litterer, L. A, Johnson, K. M., Rempel, W. E. &

Louis, C. F. (1988). Abnormal sacroplasmic reticulum ryanodine receptor in malignant hyperthermia. *Journal of Biological Chemistry*, **263**, 9310–15.

Mickelson, J. R., Litterer, L. A., Jacobson, B. A. & Louis, C. F. (1990). Stimulation and inhibition of [3H] ryanodine binding to the sarcoplasmic reticulum from malignant hyperthermia susceptible pigs. *Archives of Biochemistry and Biophysics*, **278**, 251–7.

Mickelson, J. R., Ross, J. A., Reed, B. K. & Louis, C. F. (1986). Enhanced Ca^{2+} induced calcium release by isolated sarcoplasmic reticulum vesicles from malignant hyperthermia susceptible pig muscle. *Biochimica et Biophysica Acta*, **862**, 318–28.

Mignery, G. A. & Südhof, T. C. (1990). The ligand binding site and transduction mechanism in the inositol-1,4,5-triphosphate receptor. *EMBO Journal*, **9**, 3893–8.

Miller, K. E., Brooks, R. R., Bonk, K. R. & Carpenter, J. F. (1991). Calcium handling by platelets from normal and malignant hyperthermia susceptible pigs. *Life Sciences*, **48**, 471–6.

Mitchell, G. & Heffron, J. J. A. (1975). Factors affecting serum creatine phosphokinase activity in pigs. *Journal of the South African Veterinary Association*, **46**, 145–8.

Mitchell, G. & Heffron, J. J. A. (1982). Porcine stress syndromes. *Advances in Food Research*, **28**, 167–230.

Mogensen, J. V., Misfeldt, B. B. & Hanel, H. K. (1974). Preoperative excitement and malignant hyperthermia. *Lancet*, **1**, 461.

Morgan, K. G. & Bryant, S. H. (1977). The mechanism of action of dantrolene sodium. *Journal of Pharmacology and Experimental Therapeutics*, **201**, 138–47.

Nelson, T. E. (1984). Dantrolene does not block calcium pulse-induced calcium release from a putative calcium channel in sarcoplasmic reticulum from malignant hyperthermia and normal pig muscle. *FEBS Letters*, **167**, 123–6.

O'Brien, P. J., Pook, H. A., Klip, A., Britt, B. A., Kalow, B. I., McLaughlin, R. N., Scott, E. & Elliott, M. E. (1990). Canine stress syndrome/malignant hyperthermia susceptibility: calcium homeostasis defect in muscle and lymphocytes. *Research in Veterinary Science*, **48**, 124–8.

O'Brien, P. J., Shen, H., Cory, C. R. & Zhang, X. (1993). Use of a DNA-based test for the mutation associated with porcine stress syndrome (malignant hyperthermia) in 10 000 breeding swine. *Journal of the American Veterinary Medical Association*, **203**, 842–51.

Ørding, H. (1988). Diagnosis of susceptibility to malignant hyperthermia in man. *British Journal of Anaesthesia*, **60**, 287–302.

Pollock, N., Hodges, M. & Sendall, J. (1992). Prolonged malignant hyperthermia in the absence of triggering agents. *Anaesthesia and Intensive Care*, **20**, 520–3.

Rempel, W. E., Lu, M., el Kandelgy, S., Kennedy, C. F., Irvin, L. R., Mickelson, J. R. & Louis, C. F. (1993). Relative accuracy of the halothane challenge test and a molecular genetic test in detecting the gene for porcine stress syndrome. *Journal of Animal Science*, **71**, 1395–9.

Roewer, N., Greim, C., Rumberger, E. & Schulte am Esch, J. (1995). Abnormal action potential responses to halothane in heart muscle isolated from malignant hyperthermia-susceptible pigs. *Anesthesiology*, **82**, 947–53.

Ryan, J. F., Lopez, J. R., Sanchez, V. B., Sreter, F. A. & Allen, P. D. (1994). Myoplasmic calcium changes precede metabolic and clinical signs of porcine malignant hyperthermia. *Anesthesia and Analgesia*, **79**, 1007–11.

Scholz, J., Roewer, N., Rum, U., Schmitz, W., Scholz, H. & Schulte am Esch, J. (1991). Possible involvement of inositol-lipid metabolism in malignant hyperthermia. *British Journal of Anaesthesia*, **66**, 692–5.

Scholz, J., Steinfath, M., Roewer, N., Patten, M., Troll, U., Schmitz, W., Scholz, H. & Schulte am Esch, J. (1993). Biochemical changes in malignant hyperthermia susceptible swine: cyclic AMP, inositol phosphates, alpha 1, beta 1- and beta 2-adrenoceptors in skeletal and cardiac muscle. *Acta Anaesthesiologica Scandinavica*, **37**, 575–83.

Shomer, N. H., Louis, C. F., Fill, M., Litterer, L. A. & Mickelson, J. R. (1993). Reconstitution of abnormalities in the malignant hyperthermia-susceptible pig ryanodine receptor. *American Journal of Physiology*, **264**, C125–35.

Topel, D. G., Bicknell, E. J., Preston, K. S., Christian, L. L. & Matsuschima, C. Y. (1968). Porcine stress syndrome. *Modern Veterinary Practice*, **49**, 40–1, 59–60.

Van den Hende, A., Lister, D., Muylle, E., Ooms, L. & Oyaert, W. (1976). Malignant hyperthermia in Belgian Landrace pigs rested or exercised before exposure to halothane. *British Journal of Anaesthesia*, **48**, 421–9.

Van Winkle, W. B. (1976). Calcium release from skeletal muscle sarcoplasmic reticulum: site of action of dantrolene sodium? *Science*, **193**, 1130–1.

Vogeli, P., Bolt, R., Fries, R. & Stranzinger, G. (1994). Co-segregation of the malignant hyperthermia and the Arg 615-Cys 615 mutation in the skeletal muscle calcium release channel protein in five European Landrace and Pietrain pig breeds. *Animal Genetics*, **25**, 59–66.

Webb, A. J. (1981). The halothane sensitivity test. In *Porcine Stress and Meat Quality*, pp. 105–24, ed. T. Frøystein, E. Slinde & N. Standal. Norway, Agricultural Food Research Society.

Wingard, D. W. (1974). Malignant hyperthermia: a human stress syndrome? *Lancet*, **2**, 1450–1.

Section 3

Other hypermetabolic syndromes

15

Neuroleptic malignant syndrome

P. J. ADNET, H. REYFORD and
R. M. KRIVOSIC-HORBER

Introduction

The neuroleptic malignant syndrome (NMS) is a relatively rare but probably under recognised potentially fatal complication of the use of neuroleptic drugs. This syndrome was first described in the French medical literature with the introduction of neuroleptics in 1960, where it was referred to as 'akinetic hypertonic syndrome' (Delay et al., 1960). Over the last decade, almost 1000 cases of NMS have been reported (Davis et al., 1990), but many features of this syndrome remain controversial. Indeed, a grading scale of specific signs and symptoms for the diagnosis of NMS and a spectrum of clinical severity are two issues that await resolution (Guze & Baxter, 1985; Adityanjee et al., 1988). Many diagnostic criteria have been proposed, but no single set of criteria has been adopted for general use. Hence different presentations of this disorder could explain some contradictory findings associated with NMS: prospective studies have provided disparate estimates of the frequency of NMS, ranging from 0.07% (Gelenberg et al., 1988) to 2.20% (Hermesh et al., 1992) among patients receiving neuroleptic agents, risk factors for NMS vary in different patient populations (Keck et al., 1989) and the association between NMS and other potentially fatal syndromes such as malignant hyperthermia is unclear.

Pathogenesis of neuroleptic malignant syndrome

Two major but not necessarily competing theories to explain NMS are a neuroleptic-induced alteration of central neuroregulatory mechanisms and an abnormal reaction of predisposed skeletal muscle. This latter alternative hypothesis is based on similarities between NMS and malignant hyperthermia (MH) and suggests that neuroleptic medications induce abnormal calcium availability in muscle cells of susceptible individuals and thereby trigger muscle rigidity, rhabdomyolysis and hyperthermia. Alternatively, another hypothesis could be that in some circumstances neuroleptics may exert a direct toxic effect on normal skeletal muscle.

Central dopamine receptor blockade

Dopamine plays a role in the central thermoregulation of mammals. A dopamine injection into the preoptic anterior hypothalamus causes a reduction in core temperature (Cox *et al.*, 1978). Neuroleptic drugs block dopamine receptor sites, so the hyperthermia associated with NMS may result from a blockade of the hypothalamic dopamine site. This was first suggested by Henderson & Wooten (1981) reporting a patient with Parkinson's disease and chronic psychosis who developed NMS when dopaminergic agonists were withdrawn whereas haloperidol was continued. Burke *et al.* (1981) also observed the NMS in a patient with Huntington's chorea who was taking methyltyrosine, a cathecholamine synthesis inhibitor, and tetrabenazine which depletes central nervous system (CNS) catecholamines. This suggests that NMS is caused by dopamine depletion or blockade, leading to abnormal central thermoregulation. The dopamine blockade theory is also supported by a reported case in which NMS developed when L-dopa/carbidopa and amantadine were abruptly discontinued in a patient with Parkinson's disease who had never taken neuroleptics (Toru *et al.*, 1981). On the other hand some dopamine function-enhancing drugs, such as bromocriptine (Bond, 1984; Figa-Talamanca *et al.*, 1985) or amantadine (McCarron *et al.*, 1982) have shown efficacy in treating NMS.

The blockade of dopamine receptors in the hypothalamus is thought to lead to impaired heat dissipation. In addition, a blockade of dopamine receptors in the corpus striatum is thought to cause muscular rigidity with the generation of heat. Hence, the excess of heat production in association with a decrease in heat dissipation produce hyperthermia which is one of the main signs of the syndrome. The peripheral anticholinergic effects of neuroleptics which reduce sweating most probably do not play a major role in hyperthermia associated with NMS as most of the NMS patients (70%) are diaphoretic. It is unlikely that the blockade of dopamine receptors in the hypothalamus and corpus striatum could completely explain all the signs of NMS. Indeed, hypothalamic thermoregulation involves noradrenergic, serotonergic, cholinergic and central dopaminergic pathways (Blingh *et al.*, 1971). Many neuroleptics may have additional selective effects on peptides cotransmitting with dopamine in the striatum and other parts of the brain.

Primary skeletal muscle defect similar to malignant hyperthermia

The hypothesis regarding a common pathophysiology of NMS and MH has been suggested (Delacour *et al.*, 1981; Tollefson, 1982; Denborough *et al.*, 1985). This hypothesis is based mainly on three points: (1) NMS and MH have clinical features in common, including hyperthermia, rigidity, elevated creatinine phosphokinase (CK) level, and a mortality rate for both NMS and MH ranging from 10 to 30%; (2) sodium dantrolene, a peripheral muscle relaxant, has been used successfully in both syndromes, and (3) abnormal results have been found in the *in vitro* contracture tests (IVCT) in patients with either of these two disorders. These *in vitro* tests, with halothane and caffeine are at present the most reliable diagnostic measures for patients susceptible to MH (European Malignant Hyperpyrexia Group, 1984). The tests determine the sensitivity of muscle fibres to halothane or caffeine added to the bathing solution. Muscle fibres from patients susceptible to MH have a lower contracture threshold for these drugs than do those from normal patients (Chapter 11). Hence, to evaluate a possible association between NMS and MH, several investigators have used the halothane and caffeine tests on skeletal muscle fibres removed from patients with documented NMS episodes. Conflicting results, however, have been reported regarding the prevalence of MH susceptibility among NMS patients (Caroff *et al.*, 1987; Araki *et al.*, 1988; Adnet *et al.*, 1989). Three main series and some sporadic case reports have now been published. The first by Caroff *et al.* (1987) reported five of seven NMS patients as MH susceptible on the basis of the 3% halothane response. The second by Araki *et al.* (1988) reported abnormal contracture in six NMS patients similar to MH using a caffeine skinned fibre technique. The third by our laboratory (Krivosic-Horber *et al.*, 1987; Adnet *et al.*, 1989) found only one NMS patient as MH equivocal and 13 NMS patients as MH normal.

One possible explanation for these discrepancies is that patients diagnosed as having NMS may represent a heterogeneous group showing great variability in clinical presentation, response to treatment and, possibly, response to test drugs as well. In addition, some of the variations in the *in vitro* results from different centres may be attributed to variations in laboratory procedures. The tests used for MH diagnosis varied in their protocol: caffeine alone (Araki *et al.*, 1988), halothane and caffeine on separate muscle bundles (Denborough *et al.*, 1985; Krivosic-Horber *et al.*, 1987), halothane associated with cumulative concentrations of caffeine (Tollefson, 1982), caffeine on skinned muscle fibres (Araki *et al.*, 1988). The sensitivity of this latter method may be inadequate as the technique itself excludes any detection of a possible defect in the sarcolemma (Adnet *et al.*, 1991*a*). Differences were also observed in the IVCT

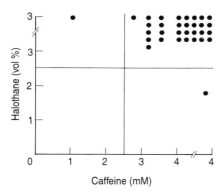

Figure 15.1. Threshold concentration of halothane and caffeine according to the criteria of the European Malignant Hyperthermia Group for 32 patients with neuroleptic malignant syndrome.

criteria for the diagnosis of MH. Caroff *et al.* (1987) used as the threshold, the development of a contracture of more than 0.5 g in response to 1% halothane or more than 0.7 g in response to 3% halothane. The European Malignant Hyperthermia Group (EMHG) (1984) required, for an abnormal response to halothane, a contracture of 0.2 g or more in response to 2% halothane or less. Protocol and diagnostic criteria from other sporadic case reports were not fully explained.

Delay between the adverse reaction to the neuroleptic drug and the biopsy was either not mentioned (Araki *et al.*, 1988) or was one month (Caroff *et al.*, 1987) or two to three weeks in our previous studies (Krivosic-Horber *et al.*, 1987; Adnet *et al.*, 1989). Caroff *et al.* (1987) found no correlation between the maximum halothane response and the time between normalisation of CK and the biopsy. Positive contracture test results in NMS patients, however, may be falsely positive and reflect coincidental changes in muscle resulting from NMS. For example, Gallant *et al.* (1986) reported that muscle fibre injury during biopsy and IVCT procedures enhances halothane sensitivity and could contribute to false positive IVCT results. Denborough *et al.* (1985) reported positive results in two patients who recovered from episodes of rhabdomyolysis not related to drugs. Adnet *et al.* (1991*b*) found that if cut fibre specimens depolarise with time after biopsy, these preparations become less sensitive to caffeine, thus leading to caution to be needed in the interpretation of the caffeine IVCT. This suggests that non-specific muscle damage secondary to metabolic factors, drug exposure, abnormalities in CNS activity or testing procedures may have contributed to abnormal responses observed *in vitro* in muscle obtained from survivors of NMS episodes. Since our previous reports, 18 additional patients have been investigated according to the EMHG protocol. None of these patients was MH susceptible, two patients were equivocal (Figure 15.1). On the basis of these negative results a statistical analysis for inferences can be calculated (Grayzel, 1989). The increase of our population from 14 to 32 patients decreases the possible rate of MH among NMS patients from 31% to less than 10% with 95% confidence. Our study alone, therefore, does not justify abandoning precautions against MH in NMS patients. According to the formula described by Grayzel (1989), a total number of 59 consecutive NMS patients should be tested negative with a similar *in vitro* protocol to statistically exclude any crossreactivity between MH and NMS. Until such results are available, we suggest that all patients with clinical NMS should be tested for MH susceptibility before being considered at no risk for MH during anaesthesia.

Direct toxic effect on skeletal muscle induced by neuroleptics

Muscle contracture has been produced *in vitro* by neuroleptic agents such as chlorpromazine (Kelkar & Jindal, 1974). The drug is reported to influence calcium ion transport across the sarcoplasmic reticulum and has been studied in various experimental muscle preparations. In a study on skinned fibres, chlorpromazine influenced both the contractile system and the function of the sarcoplasmic reticulum (Takagi, 1981). In a previous report by us, however, the drug induced contracture to the same extent in both NMS and normal muscle (Adnet *et al.*, 1989). Likewise, Caroff *et al.* (1987) also found no significant differences in the muscle response to another neuroleptic drug (fluphenazine) between NMS, MH susceptible and control patients.

To explore further a possible direct action of neuroleptic drugs on skeletal muscle, we analysed the *in vitro* muscle contracture response to four neuroleptic agents implicated in NMS episodes (Figures 15.2 and 15.3). No increase in sensitivity to neuroleptic drugs was found in muscle from NMS patients compared with muscle from normal patients (Reyford *et al.*, 1990). These negative findings may indicate that the *in vitro* contracture response to neuroleptic agents does not correlate with the clinical evidence of NMS. This may also show, however, that neuroleptics are potentially active on skeletal muscle. Thus, it is possible that in some circumstances such as exhaustion, psychomotor agitation or dehydration, which are not explored by the *in vitro* method, neuroleptics may exert a potent toxic effect on skeletal muscle leading to contracture and rhabdomyolysis. The neuroleptic contracture tests may, therefore, be inadequate to reproduce *in vivo* conditions. Many factors present *in vivo*, such as neuroleptic metabolites, central dopaminergic blockade and

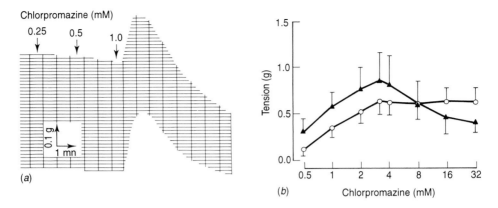

Figure 15.2. (a) Typical *in vitro* response of a muscle strip from an NMS patient to increasing concentrations of chlorpromazine. (b) Cumulative dose-response curve to chlorpromazine for contracture responses in muscle strips from NMS patients and controls. (▲), Neuroleptic malignant syndrome, *n* =10; ○, controls, n=10, where n=number of patients tested. NMS compared with controls : $p > 0.05$.

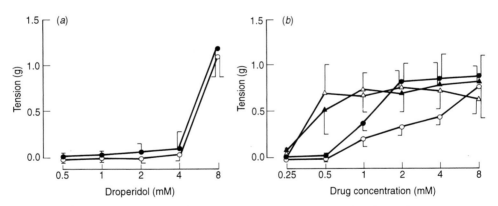

Figure 15.3. Cumulative dose–response curve to: (a) droperidol (●, NMS (neuroleptic malignant syndrome), *n*=7; ○, controls, *n*=5. (*b*) fluphenazine (▲), NMS, *n*=13; ○, controls, *n*=6) and levomepromazine (●, NMS, *n*=1); ○, controls, *n*=5) for contracture responses in muscle strips from NMS patients and controls. NMS compared with controls: $p > 0.05$. *n*=number of patients tested.

risk factors for NMS are important to take into consideration when developing more precise pharmacological models to explore possible interactions between neuroleptics and skeletal muscle function. Of particular interest is the fact that rechallenge with the original agent may not result in a recurrence of

NMS. This suggests that neuroleptics may be a necessary but not exclusive cause of the syndrome (Caroff, 1980; Levenson, 1985).

Clinical features

NMS typically develops over a period of 24–72 hours but many investigators have described a more insidious evolution of symptoms. It has been reported to last 10–20 days after oral neuroleptics were discontinued and even longer when associated with depot forms of the drugs. Consistent diagnostic criteria have been used only in some clinical studies (Levenson, 1985; Addonizio *et al.*, 1986; Pope *et al.*, 1986). Three major symptoms indicate a high probability of the presence of NMS: hyperthermia, rigidity and elevated CK level (Levenson, 1985). In the absence of these criteria, the diagnosis of NMS should be questioned because other symptoms of the disorder may be seen in patients taking neuroleptics without having NMS. Elevated temperature (38.5 °C or more) in the absence of other systemic illness is observed in most patients. Muscle rigidity consists of a generalised 'lead pipe' increase in tone that may result in decreased chest wall compliance with resulting tachypnoeic hypoventilation and secondary pulmonary infection. This increase in muscle tone may be accompanied by extrapyramidal symptoms including dyskinesia, dysarthria or Parkinsonism. The CK level is always elevated (more than 1000 IU/L) reflecting myonecrosis secondary to intense muscle contracture. This often results in acute myoglobinuric renal failure. Minor manifestations do not indicate by themselves a high probability of NMS. Diaphoresis, tachycardia and abnormal blood pressure are common signs of autonomic dysfunction. Altered consciousness ranges from agitation to stupor or coma. Many other clinical signs of lesser frequency were reported including opisthotonos, grand mal seizures, Babinski's sign, chorea and trismus.

Leucocytosis, ranging from slight elevation to as high as $30\,000/mm^3$, is the only frequent laboratory finding included in the minor manifestations of NMS. Other non-specific laboratory abnormalities have been reported, such as mildly elevated hepatic enzymes (transaminase, lactic dehydrogenase and alkaline phosphatase). The results of electroencephalograms (EEG) suggest non-specific encephalopathy or no abnormality. Lumbar puncture should be carried out for differential diagnosis but is usually normal in NMS. The results of cerebral CT scans are normal. Non-specific changes are usually observed in muscle biopsy or in postmortem histopathological studies of the brain.

Some authors are in favour of an approach that requires the presence of essential manifestations of the syndrome. For example, Levenson (1985) suggests that the presence of all three major, or two major and four minor manifestations indicate a high probability of the presence of NMS. These criteria for guidance in the diagnosis of NMS are commonly used in clinical research studies (Caroff *et al.*, 1987; Adnet *et al.*, 1989). Likewise Pope *et al.* (1986) have published 'definite' and 'probable' criteria for NMS. In contrast, others still prefer to think in terms of a spectrum of neuroleptic-related neurotoxicity with varying combinations that enhance the potential for inappropriate diagnosis or management (Levinson & Simpson, 1992).

A decrease in mortality from NMS has been reported in recent years. NMS resulted in a 76% mortality before 1970, a 22% mortality from 1970 to 1980, and a 15% mortality since 1980. Shalev *et al.* (1989) reported a significant decrease in mortality since 1984 (11%), that occurred independently of the treatment used: dopamine agonist or dantrolene. Renal failure is a strong predictor of mortality, representing a mortality risk of approximately 50%. A possible association between NMS and MH was discussed earlier in this chapter.

Medications and risk factors

A wide variety of antipsychotic agents are associated with this syndrome and includes phenothiazines, butyrophenones, thioxanthines, benzamides and miscellaneous antipsychotic agents such as loxapine. Other circumstances such as abrupt discontinuation of neuroleptic or antiparkinsonian agents, and the use of dopamine-depleting agents, have also been reported to produce NMS. The onset of the syndrome is not related to the duration of exposure to neuroleptics or to toxic overdoses. All ages, children included, and both sexes are affected in NMS but young adult males predominate among reported cases. Cases have been reported in both psychiatric and medical patients including after multiple trauma (Boorse & Rhodes, 1990) or the preoperative use of neuroleptic agents. Alcoholic patients are at greater risk of developing NMS during delirium treatment or its prevention by droperidol or tiapride (Adnet *et al.*, 1989). Abnormalities of muscle metabolism in alcoholic patients are caused by ethanol toxicity and nutritional stress (Bollaert *et al.*, 1989). This may predispose the muscle to the action of neuroleptics. In a psychiatric population, Keck *et al.* (1989) showed that patients with NMS displayed significantly greater psychomotor agitation, received significantly higher doses of neuroleptics at greater rates of dose increments, and received a greater number of intramuscular injections than other patients taking similar medications without evidence of NMS. Many authors have pointed out that most cases have occurred in patients taking haloperidol or, to a lesser extent, depot fluphenazine. These clinical observations do not necessarily mean that the two drugs carry a higher risk of causing NMS and one must consider the frequency with which the drug is prescribed; haloperidol is one of the most commonly used medications. Furthermore, patients who are more sick are more likely to receive haloperidol or fluphenazine than other neuroleptics. These sicker patients may also be at higher risk for NMS because of a higher rate of dehydration, exhaustion or malnutrition (Caroff, 1980; Levenson, 1985). Other suggested predisposing factors include infection and concurrent organic brain disease.

Differential diagnosis

Patients on neuroleptics who develop hyperthermia, muscle rigidity and autonomic dysfunction should have all psychotropic medications immediately withdrawn until rigorous diagnostic investigation reveals a specific cause. Disorders that can be mistaken for NMS include rhabdomyolysis from other causes, CNS infections or a cerebral mass, tetanus and lithium toxicity. Other specific illnesses should be considered in the differential diagnosis of NMS and include neuroleptic-related heat stroke, catatonia, drug interactions with monoamine oxidase inhibitors, the central anticholinergic syndrome and anaesthetic-induced MH. A possible association between NMS and MH is extensively discussed elsewhere. To assess a diagnosis, the physician who is evaluating a patient with suspected NMS should include the following procedures in addition to a careful history and physical examination: determination of CK level, white blood cell count, renal function, EEG, CT scan, lumbar puncture and determination of serum lithium level.

Neuroleptic-induced heat stroke

Classic heat stroke is a life-threatening condition where the heat gain from the metabolism and the environment exceeds the heat loss by evaporation and convection. Neuroleptics predispose the hyperthermia by their anticholinergic properties, which block sweating and heat dissipation, and by their antidopaminergic properties, which interfere with hypothalamic thermoregulation. Contributing factors include hot, humid weather and excessive agitation or exercise not accompanied by an adequate fluid intake. When an acutely catastrophic disorder associated with hyperthermia and altered consciousness develops in a patient taking neuroleptics, an early correct diagnosis between these two disorders is imperative if potentially life-saving treatment, which differs according to the condition, is to be given promptly.

Neuroleptic-induced heat stroke can be differentiated from NMS by its abrupt onset, often with seizures, the absence of extrapyramidal signs, absence of diaphoresis and a history of physical exercise or exposure to high ambient temperature (Lazarus, 1989). Heat stroke needs rapid effective cooling methods initiated as early as possible with continuous monitoring of the core temperature and vigorous fluid replacement for both rehydratation and a more rapid reduction in the temperature.

Acute lethal catatonia

Lethal catatonia is a very rare psychiatric syndrome that shares some features with NMS including hyperthermia, akinesia and muscle rigidity. Neuroleptics themselves may be the most common cause of catatonic states secondary to severe akinesia. Neither laboratory findings, CT scans, EEGs nor any other somatic data have so far proved to be of value in differentiating the two conditions, and therefore support must derive from careful reconstitution of the patient's condition in the preceding two to three week period (Fleischbacker *et al.*, 1990). The catatonic syndrome may be preceded by emotional withdrawal, depressive symptoms, neglect of previous hobbies, anxiety symptoms or acute agitation. These signs do not differ from those of other patients with schizophrenia but they seldom last for more than two weeks. The complete picture is more likely to involve choreiform stereotypy, primitive hyperkinesias, torsion spasms and rhythmic circling movements of the arms. Death may result from respiratory arrest or cardiovascular collapse.

Drug interactions with monoamine oxidase inhibitors

Agitation, delirium, hyperthermic reactions and death have been described as adverse effects of monoamine oxidase inhibitors in combination with narcotic drugs or tricyclic antidepressants. It has been suggested that the amine reuptake inhibitory properties of tricyclic antidepressants could interact dangerously with the sympathomimetic properties of monoamine oxidase inhibitors. Similar signs may be seen with overdoses of monoamine oxidase inhibitors. Patients taking neuroleptics may also be treated with monoamide oxidase inhibitors.

Central anticholinergic syndrome

Peripheral signs of atropine poisoning characterise the syndrome including dry skin, dry mouth, dilated pupils and urinary retention. The patient is usually confused and disoriented (anticholinergic delirium), the temperature is often elevated. Physostigmine may induce a resolution of symptoms that is not observed in NMS.

Treatment

Successful treatment of NMS depends on early clinical recognition and prompt withdrawal of the neuroleptic agents. Neuroleptics are not dialysable and blood levels will decline slowly. The use of general symptomatic treatment such as hydration, nutrition and reduction of fever is essential. Secondary complications such as hypoxia, acidosis and renal failure must be treated vigorously. Low-dose heparin seems to be indicated to prevent venous thrombosis in a patient who will usually be immobile. Other dopamine antagonists such as metaclopramide should be avoided. In Caroff's review of 60 cases (1980), supportive therapy was the predominant treatment modality. The benefit of adding specific therapies to supportive measures is still debated. Insufficient data are available to evaluate the efficacy of specific treatments reported in the literature. The potential benefits from their use cannot, therefore, be excluded.

The place of sodium dantrolene, the drug of choice for MH, is less well defined in the treatment of NMS. Sodium dantrolene inhibits calcium release from the sarcoplasmic reticulum decreasing available calcium for ongoing muscle contracture. The drug is a non-specific, direct acting muscle relaxant and the decrease in body temperature coincides with muscle relaxation. Oxygen consumption diminishes, heart rate and respiratory rate decrease correspondingly. It has been suggested that the initial dosage should be 2 mg/kg given intravenously (Delacour *et al.*, 1981). This dose may be repeated every 10 minutes, up to a total dose of 10 mg/kg/day. The oral dosage has ranged from 50 to 200 mg per day. Hepatic toxicity may occur with doses above 10 mg kg/day.

Bromocriptine mesylate, a dopamine agonist, is also used to treat NMS (Bond, 1984; Figa-Talamanca *et al.*, 1985). Bromocriptine doses have ranged from 2.5 to 10 mg four times a day. Hypotension is the most limiting side-effect and the drug seems to be well tolerated by psychotic patients despite it being a strong central dopamine agonist. Rigidity may begin to decrease during the first few hours followed by a decrease in temperature, along with normalisation of the blood pressure. This effect on rigidity and tremor supports the hypothesis of a dopamine-receptor blockade in NMS. Bromocriptine and dantrolene have been used together without complications (Rosenberg & Green, 1989).

Another dopamine agonist, amantadine hydrochloride, was used successfully in some cases (McCarron *et al.*, 1982). Levo-dopa, combined with the dopa decarboxylase inhibitor carbidopa, has also been reported to be effective in reversing hyperthermia (Henderson & Wooten, 1981). Treatment may need to be continued for several days. Anticholinergic drugs such as benzatropine, are usually ineffective for reversing the rigidity of NMS and they do not affect hyperthermia. Benzodiazepine derivatives, which enhance GABA-ergic function, have caused transient reductions of symptoms; in any case, these drugs are recommended to control 'agitated' NMS patients.

Electroconvulsive therapy reportedly improved some components of the syndrome, notably fever, sweating and level of consciousness (Hermesh *et al.*, 1987). This could be an alternative for patients in whom there is a significant risk of recurrence of NMS on restarting neuroleptics.

Only one study evaluated treatment options of NMS (Rosenberg & Green, 1989). In a series of 64 cases derived from an extensive review of the literature, 11 patients received only supportive therapy. The others received other therapies including dantrolene (14 patients), bromocriptine (22 patients), benzodiazepine (one patient) and combinations of the above (nine patients). Efficacy was evaluated in each case by determining the delay of clinical response as well as the time to complete recovery. Therapy with bromocriptine (5 mg orally or nasogastrically four times daily) was effective after approximately one day. This was significantly more rapid than that achieved by supportive therapy alone. Complete resolution was achieved more quickly with bromocriptine (ten days) or with dantrolene (nine days; 2–3 mg/kg/day intravenously without exceeding 10 mg/kg/day) than with supportive therapy (15 days).

Recurrence of neuroleptic malignant syndrome

Many patients with NMS are schizophrenic and may require further neuroleptic treatment in the course of their illness, often very soon after the onset of NMS. Rechallenge with drugs of the same potency as that which was causative resulted in recurrent NMS in five of six cases, two of which were fatal. Rechallenge with lower potency antipsychotics, such as thioridazine, was safe in nine of ten cases (Shalev & Munitz, 1986). McCarthy (1988) reported a fatal case of neuroleptic syndrome after a milder episode three months earlier. The safest approach for the prevention of recurrence is a regimen where doses of a low potency neuroleptic are increased very slowly. Substitute treatments, such as lithium carbonate or electroconvulsive therapy (ECT), may offer a safe alternative in those patients who respond to these treatments. Prevention of

NMS awaits a better understanding of the underlying pathophysiology. Of prime importance seems to be the avoidance of marked dehydration in patients treated with neuroleptics: this may reduce the prevalence and morbidity of the syndrome.

Electroconvulsive therapy in patients with a history of NMS

A common pathophysiology has been suggested between NMS and malignant hyperthermia (Tollefson, 1982; Denborough *et al.*, 1985); therefore, the possibility that patients with a history of NMS may be vulnerable to developing MH is an important factor when one considers general anaesthesia including suxamethonium (succinylcholine) administration for ECT. This procedure frequently involves the use of suxamethonium (succinylcholine) just before electrical stimulation. To date, there is no report in the literature of MH as a complication of ECT in NMS patients. A recent study by Hermesh *et al.* (1988) found that none of the patients who had NMS and underwent ECT or their relatives who also underwent ECT had any MH-like symptoms or other secondary effects despite the repeated use of suxamethonium (succinylcholine) in all cases. The authors reported a total of 147 intravenous administrations of suxamethonium (succinylcholine) in a dose range of 15–30 mg in 12 patients without any complication. These results are consistent with sporadic reports of the safe use of ECT for patients with NMS (for a review, see Hermesh *et al.*, 1988).

ECT with the use of suxamethonium, which is an effective and rapid mode of treatment for cases of NMS unresponsive to supportive medical therapy, should not, therefore, be contraindicated. Until the association, however, between NMS and MH is conclusively disproved, careful metabolic monitoring of general anaesthesia is obligatory.

References

Adityanjee, Singh, S., Singh, G. & Ong, S. (1988). Spectrum concept of neuroleptic malignant syndrome. *British Journal of Psychiatry*, **153**, 107–11.

Addonizio, G., Susman, V. L. & Roth, S. D. (1986). Symptoms of neuroleptic malignant syndrome in 82 consecutive inpatients. *American Journal of Psychiatry*, **143**, 1587–90.

Adnet, P. J., Krivosic-Horber, R. M., Adamantidis, M. M., Haudecoeur, G., Adnet-Bonte, C. A., Saulnier, F. & Dupuis, B. A. (1989). The association between the neuroleptic malignant syndrome and malignant hyperthermia. *Acta Anaesthesiologica Scandinavica*, **33**, 676–80.

Adnet, P. J., Krivosic-Horber, R. M., Adamantidis, M. M., Reyford, H., Cordonnier,

C. & Haudecoeur, G. (1991*a*). Effects of calcium-free solution, calcium antagonists and the calcium agonist BAY K 8644 on mechanical responses of skeletal muscle from patients susceptible to malignant hyperthermia. *Anesthesiology*, **75**, 413–19.

Adnet, P. J., Krivosic-Horber, R. M., Adamantidis, M. M., Haudecoeur, G., Reyford, H. G. & Dupuis, B. A. (1991*b*). Is resting membrane potential a possible indicator of viability of muscle bundles used in the *in vitro* caffeine contracture test? *Anaesthesia and Analgesia*, **74**, 195–11.

Araki, M., Takagi, A., Higuchi, I. & Sugita, H. (1988). Neuroleptic malignant syndrome: caffeine contracture of single muscle fibres and muscle pathology. *Neurology*, **38**, 297–301.

Blingh, J., Cottle, W. H. & Maskrey, M. (1971). Influence of ambient temperature on the thermoregulatory responses to 5-hydroxytryptamine, noradrenaline and acetylcholine injected into the lateral cerebral ventricles of sheep, goats and rabbits. *Journal of Physiology*, **212**, 377–392.

Bollaert, P. E., Robin-Lherbier, B., Escange, J. M., Bauer, Ph., Lambert, H., Robert, H. & Larcan, A. (1989). Phosphorus nuclear magnetic resonance: evidence of abnormal skeletal muscle metabolism in chronic alcoholics. *Neurology*, **39**, 821–24.

Bond, W. S. (1984). Detection and management of the neuroleptic malignant syndrome. *Clinical Pharmacology*, **3**, 302–7.

Boorse, R. C. & Rhodes, M. (1990). Neuroleptic malignant syndrome in a multiple trauma patient. *Archives of Surgery*, **125**, 274–75.

Burke, R. E., Fann, S., Mayeux, R., Weinberg, H., Louis, K. & Wilmer, J. H. (1981). Neuroleptic malignant syndrome caused by dopamine-depleting drugs in a patient with Huntingdon's disease. *Neurology*, **31**, 1022–5.

Caroff, S. N. (1980). The neuroleptic malignant syndrome. *Journal of Clinical Psychiatry*, **41**, 79–83.

Caroff, S. N., Rosenberg, H., Fletcher, J. E., Heiman-Patterson, T. D. & Mann, S. C. (1987). Malignant hyperthermia susceptibility in neuroleptic malignant syndrome. *Anesthesiology*, **67**, 20–5.

Cox, B., Kerwin, R. & Lee, T. E. (1978). Dopamine receptors in the central thermoregulatory pathways of the rat. *Journal of Physiology (Lond.)*, **282**, 471–83.

Davis, J. M., Janicak, P. & Sakkas, P. (1990). Neuroleptic syndrome: the first 1000 cases. *Biological Psychiatry*, **27**, 132 (abstract).

Delacour, J. L., Daoudal, P., Chapoutot, J. L. & Rocq, B. (1981). Traitement du syndrome malin des neuroleptiques par le dantrolène. *Nouvelle Presse Médicale*, **10**, 3572–73.

Delay, J., Pichot, P., Lemperiere, T., Blissalde, B. & Peigne, F. (1960). Un neuroleptique majeur non phenothiozinique et non réserpinique l'halopéridol, dans la traitement des psychoses. *Annales Médicine Psychologie*, **18**, 145–52.

Denborough, M. A., Collins, S. P. & Hopkinson, K. C. (1985). Rhabdomyolysis and malignant hyperpyrexia. *British Medical Journal*, **ii**, 1878.

European Malignant Hyperpyrexia Group. (1984). A protocol for the investigation of malignant hyperpyrexia susceptibility. *British Journal of Anaesthesia*, **56**, 1267–69.

Fleischbacker, W. W., Unterweger, B., Kane, J. M. & Hinterhuber, H. (1990). The neuroleptic malignant syndrome and its differentiation from lethal catatonia. *Acta Psychiatrica Scandinavica*, **81**, 3–5.

Figa-Talamanca, L., Gualandi, C., Dimeo, L., Dibattista, G., Neri, G. & Lorusso, F.

(1985). Hyperthermia after discontinuance of levodopa and bromocriptine therapy: impaired dopamine receptors a possible cause. *Neurology*, **35**, 258–61.

Gallant, E. M., Fletcher, T. F., Goettl, V. M. & Rempel, W. E. (1986). Porcine malignant hyperthermia: cell injury enhances halothane sensitivity of biopsies. *Muscle and Nerve*, **9**, 174–84.

Gelenberg, A. J., Bellinghausen, B., Wojcik, J. D., Falk, W. E. & Sachs, G. S. (1988). A prospective survey of neuroleptic malignant syndrome in a short-term psychiatric hospital. *American Journal of Psychiatry*, **145**, 517–18.

Grayzel, J. (1989). A statistic for inferences based upon negative results. *Anesthesiology*, **71**, 320–21.

Guze, B. H. & Baxter, C. R. Jr. (1985). Current concepts. Neuroleptic malignant syndrome. *New England Journal of Medicine*, **313**, 163–6.

Henderson, V. W. & Wooton, G. F. (1981). Neuroleptic malignant syndrome: a pathogenetic role for dopamine receptor blockade? *Neurology*, **31**, 132–7.

Hermesh, H., Aizenberg, D., Lapidot, M. & Munitz, H. (1988). Risk of malignant hyperthermia among patients with neuroleptic malignant syndrome and their families. *American Journal of Psychiatry*, **145**, 1431–4.

Hermesh, H., Aizenberg, D. & Weizman, A. (1987). A successful electroconvulsive treatment of neuroleptic malignant syndrome. *Acta Psychiatrica Scandinavica*, **75**, 236–9.

Hermesh, H., Aizenberg, D., Weizman, A., Lapidot, M., Mayer, C. & Munitz, H. (1992). *British Journal of Psychiatry*, **161**, 254–7.

Keck, P. E., Pope, H. G., Cohen, B. M., McElroy, S. L. & Nierenberg, A. A. (1989). Risk factors for neuroleptic malignant syndrome. *Archive of General Psychiatry*, **46**, 914–18.

Kelkar, V. V. & Jindal. M. N. (1974). Chlorpromazine-induced contracture of frog rectus abdominis muscle. *Pharmacology*, **12**, 32–8.

Krivosic-Horber, R., Adnet, P., Guevart, E., Theunynck, D. & Lestavel, P. (1987). Neuroleptic malignant syndrome and malignant hyperthermia. *British Journal of Anaesthesia*, **59**, 1554–6.

Lazarus, A. (1989). Differentiating neuroleptic-related heatstroke from neuroleptic malignant syndrome. *Psychosomatics*, **30**, 454–6.

Levenson, J. L. (1985). Neuroleptic malignant syndrome. *American Journal of Psychiatry*, **142**, 1137–45.

Levinson, D. F. & Simpson, G. M. (1992). The treatment and management of neuroleptic malignant syndrome. *Progress in Neuro Psychopharmacology and Biological Psychiatry*, **16**, 425–43.

McCarron, M. M., Boettger, M. L. & Peck, J. I. (1982). A case of neuroleptic malignant syndrome successfully treated with amantadine. *Journal of Clinical Psychiatry* **43**, 381–2.

McCarthy, A. (1988). Fatal recurrence of neuroleptic malignant syndrome. *British Journal of Psychiatry*, **152**, 558–9.

Pope, A. G., Keck, P. E. & McElroy, A. L. (1986). Frequency and presentation of neuroleptic malignant syndrome in a large psychiatric hospital. *American Journal of Psychiatry*, **143**, 1227–33.

Reyford, H. G., Cordonner, C., Adnet, P. J., Krivosic-Horber, R. M. & Bonte, C. A. (1990). The *in vitro* exposure of muscle strips from patients with neuroleptic malignant syndrome cannot be correlated with the clinical features. *Journal of Neurological Science*, **98S**, (suppl., 6.6), 527.

Rosenberg, M. R. & Green, M. (1989). Neuroleptic malignant syndrome: review of response to therapy. *Archives of Internal Medicine*, **149**, 1927–31.

Shalev, A., Hermesh, H. & Munitz, H. (1989). Mortality from neuroleptic malignant syndrome. *Journal of Clinical Psychiatry*, **50**, 18–25.

Shalev, A. & Munitz, H. (1986). The neuroleptic malignant syndrome: agent and host interaction. *Acta Psychiatrica Scandinavica*, **73**, 337–47.

Takagi, A. (1981). Chlorpromazine and skeletal muscle: a study of skinned single fibres of the guinea pig. *Experimental Neurology*, **734**, 477–86.

Tollefson, G. (1982). A case of neuroleptic malignant syndrome: *in vitro* muscle comparison with malignant hyperthermia. *Journal of Clinical Psychopharmacology*, **2**, 266–70.

Toru, M., Matsuda, O., Makigudin, K. & Sugano, K. (1981). Neuroleptic malignant syndrome-like state following a withdrawal of antiparkinsonian drugs. *Journal of Nervous and Mental Diseases*, **169**, 324–7.

16

Drug overdose, drugs of abuse and hypermetabolism

J. A. HENRY

Introduction

Although most poisons depress physiological and biochemical processes, and thus in general tend to cause hypometabolism, a small number of drugs and chemicals can cause hypermetabolism and may produce hyperthermia. Some of these cases occur as a result of exposure to natural or synthetic chemical agents. Some are an adverse effect on the therapeutic use of drugs or a result of drug overdose, while others are a consequence of illicit drug abuse. These are reviewed in this chapter.

Diagnosis and presentation of the hypermetabolic poisoned patient

The patient with a drug-induced hypermetabolic syndrome will sometimes give a clear history of exposure; in other cases this will be absent, and careful detective work may be required. There may be evidence of exercise or agitation following the administration of drugs such as atropine, amphetamines, phencyclidine or cocaine. Sympathomimetic and related agents in high dose lead to vasoconstriction, tremor and agitation; theophylline, caffeine and salbutamol may be associated with hypermetabolism and sometimes rhabdomyolysis. Other central stimulants such as camphor can cause agitation and seizures but have a less clearly defined modes of toxicity. Seizures induced by a wide range of substances may cause a lactic acidosis and a rise in body temperature. A general scheme of the causes and pathogenesis of toxic hypermetabolic states is given in Figure 16.1. The screening of plasma and urine samples in consultation with a toxicology laboratory may be helpful.

The clinical presentation varies greatly. The patient may be obviously pyrexial and sweating profusely, but in many cases, the skin may be dry, due to an anticholinergic agent or from established heat illness. Measurement of the

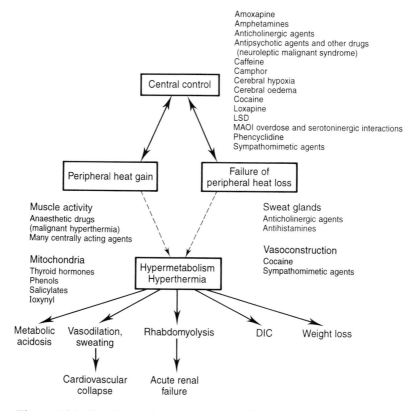

Figure 16.1. Outline of the main causes of hyperthermic and hypermetabolic syndromes and the resultant complications. DIC, disseminated intravascular coagulation; LSD, lysergic acid diethylamide; MAOI, monoamineoxidase inhibitors.

core temperature is essential. The axillary temperature is usually 2°C below the core temperature, so that a life-threatening hyperpyrexia may go undetected. Oral temperatures may also be unreliable: a doubling of carbon dioxide production because of hypermetabolism requires a doubling of alveolar ventilation, and the patient's breathlessness may mask the real body temperature. A rapid cardiovascular assessment is required as some hypermetabolic toxins can produce severe hypertension, and pyrexial states tend to cause severe volume depletion and cardiovascular collapse. Neurological assessment should include the mental state and the tone and degree of muscle activity; determining whether this is the result of agitation, hyperactivity, spasm or seizures is particularly important because it can help in diagnosis of the agent and indicate the source of heat production. Key laboratory investigations include arterial blood gas estimation, plasma biochemical parameters includ-

ing urea, creatinine and electrolytes, creatine phosphokinase, fibrin degradation products and investigations to exclude other causes of hypermetabolism
and pyrexia. Established heat illness is a final common pathway of many
hypermetabolic and hyperthermic syndromes, and the hyperthermic patient
may have tachycardia, tachypnoea, hypercapnia, hypoxaemia, mental
changes, stiff muscles, metabolic acidosis, hyperkalaemia and rhabdomyolysis. In severe cases the patient may develop disseminated intravascular coagulation (DIC), cardiac arrhythmias, acute tubular necrosis and non-cardiogenic
pulmonary oedema. Hypoxaemia is the commonest cause of death.

Secondary hypermetabolic states

Hypermetabolic states may occur secondary to hypoxic cerebral damage
following a variety of insults, most commonly a cerebrovascular accident or
following a cardiac arrest, but drug-induced respiratory or circulatory failure
or a cerebral haemorrhage may also be responsible. The mechanism involves
damage to the hypothalamic regulatory centres caused by oedema or haemorrhage. The outlook is usually grave as the hyperpyrexia is most commonly a
reflection of widespread cerebral damage.

Hypermetabolism may also occur following administration of a saline
emetic. Although this treatment is no longer recommended, cases still occur.
Cerebral oedema may affect central control of temperature regulation by the
hypothalamus, with a massive rise in body temperature. Plasma sodium may
be in the range 160–200 mmol/L and plasma chloride in the range of
120–160 mmol/L.

Thyroid hormones

Thyroxine (T_4) and triiodothyronine (T_3) are used as replacement therapy in
the management of hypothyroidism. Chronic overdosage with either can
produce a hypermetabolic syndrome similar to hyperthyroidism, with weight
loss (often despite a marked increase in appetite), tremor, sweating and heat
intolerance. In severe cases there may be fever, myopathy, diarrhoea or
cardiac failure. Acute overdosage with T_3 can produce symptoms within 4–12
hours while acute overdosage of T_4 can produce symptoms within 5–11 days.
Symptomatic cases are rare. Antithyroid drugs affect the synthesis of thyroid
hormones so the administration of these drugs is of no use in the management
of acute or chronic overdose; however, as the effects of thyroid hormones are
mediated by potentiating cellular sensitivity to circulating catecholamines, a
beta-adrenergic antagonist such as propranolol, orally or in critical cases
intravenously, may be used to modify the effects of overdose.

Antidepressants

Tricyclic antidepressants

The mechanisms involved in the pharmacological actions and the overdose toxicity of the tricyclic antidepressants are complex. Toxicity in overdose mainly results from the quinidine-like or membrane-stabilising effect of these drugs on the heart. Overdose with a tricyclic antidepressant, however, may occasionally lead to a hypermetabolic syndrome, probably from excessive heat generation caused by combination of the properties of these drugs, including their anticholinergic effect and central sympathomimetic effects from the inhibition of noradrenaline reuptake. The clinical presentation may be one of agitation and hallucinations, giving way to coma, with brisk tendon reflexes, convulsions and possibly hyperthermia. Death or permanent neurological damage may result (Rosenberg *et al.*, 1984); hypotension and cerebral hypoxia may contribute to a poor outcome.

Amoxapine

Amoxapine (nor-loxapine) is a tricyclic agent which blocks dopamine receptors and has neuroleptic as well as antidepressant activity. When taken in overdose, cardiovascular toxicity is usually mild, but there is a high incidence of convulsions, rhabdomyolysis and hyperthermia. Acute renal failure as a result of rhabdomyolysis may occur (Litovitz & Troutman, 1983; Jennings *et al.*, 1983). Management includes aggressive anticonvulsant therapy and early intubation. Diazepam or thiopentone may be used for the immediate control of seizures. There are insufficient case data to report on the usefulness or otherwise of curarisation.

Monoamine oxidase inhibitor overdose

Overdose of monoamine oxidase inhibitors does not usually produce a hypertensive crisis, which is typically precipitated by an interaction with foods containing tyramine. The syndrome following overdose consists of progressive muscle spasms and resembles the serotoninergic syndrome that is seen in animals. The mechanism may thus be accumulation of serotonin at synaptic sites in the central nervous system, possibly at a spinal level. There is little evidence of a peripheral effect, and the rapid response to curarisation supports this assumption.

Symptoms usually build up over 12–14 hours, with muscle twitching progressing to widespread muscle spasms, trismus and opisthotonus. The blood pressure may vary between hypotension and moderate hypertension; there is usually a sinus tachycardia and the skin is hot to the touch with the patient sweating profusely. The pupils are fixed and dilated. Heat generation resulting from continued muscle contraction exceeds heat loss, and the body temperature may rise to a point where hyperthermia is fatal, unless muscle relaxants are given. DIC, rhabdomyolysis and acute renal failure are recognised complications.

Management

Sedation with diazepam is unlikely to be of use. Central venous pressure should be measured and fluid losses replaced as a matter of urgency. If the rectal temperature rises above 39 °C, the patient should be electively paralysed with a muscle relaxant such as vecuronium or pancuronium and mechanically ventilated for up to 24 hours to correct hyperthermia and prevent rhabdomyolysis. The temperature usually falls rapidly without the need for any further measures because the body's thermoregulatory mechanisms should be able to reduce body temperature once the overproduction of heat has been controlled. Dantrolene has also been used successfully in a case of phenelzine overdose (Kaplan *et al.*, 1986).

Reversible inhibitors of monoamine oxidase A

Monoamine oxidase is found in two main forms: A and B. A new class of drug has recently become available, the reversible inhibitors of monoamine oxidase A (Amrein *et al.*, 1988; Haefely *et al.*, 1992). These drugs are less likely to provoke interactions with tyramine (Gieschke *et al.*, 1988) and the pattern of toxicity in overdose appears to be much less severe, with drowsiness and hypotension predominating (Hertzel, 1992). Although cases of muscle rigidity and hyperthermia have been described, they are unusual.

Serotoninergic interactions with monoamine oxidase inhibitors

A similar syndrome to monoamine oxidase inhibitor overdose may be precipitated by an interaction between a tricyclic antidepressant (particularly clomipramine) and a monoamine oxidase inhibitor (Tackley & Tregaskis, 1987; Richards *et al.*, 1987). In this case the onset is more rapid and follows within two to four hours of administration of the tricyclic drug. This interaction may result from the combined serotoninergic tendency of the monoamine oxidase inhibitor and serotonin reuptake inhibition by the tricyclic drug. Clinically, the syndrome is a serotonin syndrome. The same mechanism underlies the interaction between monoamine oxidase inhibitors and a number of other drugs, particularly pethidine (meperidine) which inhibits the reuptake of serotonin. This type of interaction can occur with both the older and the newer, reversible monoamine oxidase inhibitors.

Selective serotonin reuptake inhibitors

Interactions between selective serotonin reuptake inhibitors and other drugs, particularly monoamine oxidase inhibitors, may lead to a serotonin syndrome with muscle rigidity, hyperthermia and sweating. Overdose of the drugs is unlikely to produce a serotonergic syndrome, although a case has been reported in a child following accidental ingestion of sertraline (Kaminski *et al.*, 1994). The child had the typical symptoms of tachycardia, hypertension, hallucinations, coma, hyperthermia, tremors of the extremities and skin flushing.

Uncouplers of oxidative phosphorylation

Nitrophenols

Dinitrophenol, trinitrophenol, pentachlorophenol and many related agents are capable of uncoupling oxidative phosphorylation and stimulating mitochondrial heat production in interscapular adipose tissue. Large doses can lead to a pyrexial state with sweating, thirst, tachycardia and tachypnoea. Cardiorespiratory compensation may fail to keep pace with metabolic demand, leading to hypoxia and cardiovascular collapse. Severe weight loss can occur in chronic cases.

Salicylates

Although the use of aspirin (acetylsalicylic acid) as an analgesic is decreasing, the management of salicylate poisoning remains a major challenge. The potentially lethal dose in adults is about 500 mg/kg but death can occur in children under 18 months from as little as 300 mg. Most fatal poisonings occur in the elderly, largely because they lack the metabolic reserves to cope with salicylate poisoning. The toxic mechanisms involved are multiple and complex. The clinical features are mainly due to gastrointestinal irritation, stimulation of the respiratory centre causing respiratory alkalosis, and uncoupling of oxidative phosphorylation, leading to heat production and metabolic acidosis. The patient usually presents with nausea and vomiting, increased rate and depth of respiration, sweating, tinnitus and sometimes deafness. The patient is usually severely volume depleted because of vomiting, hyperventilation and sweating. In adults excess heat production is usually controlled by compensatory sweating but occasionally there may be hyperpyrexia, particularly in children (Segar, 1969). Whether increased production of organic acids accounts predominantly for uncoupling of oxidative phosphorylation remains unclear (Bartels & Lund-Jacobsen, 1986). The association between acidaemia and death has been documented; prognosis may be more closely related to an increased arterial hydrogen ion concentration than to the type of acid-base disturbance that has caused it (Chapman & Proudfoot, 1989).

Management of salicylate toxicity

Plasma salicylate should be measured on presentation, and at intervals of four to six hours thereafter until they have fallen below the toxic range. Salicylates are precipitated in an acidic environment and so may therefore be deposited in the stomach, with subsequent delayed absorption so that plasma concentration following a large overdose, may rise for many hours after presentation. Experience has shown that in most cases with a fatal outcome, plasma salicylate levels have demonstrated a progressive rise following admission to hospital. The hyperpyrexia rarely requires separate attention and tends to resolve once fluid losses have been replaced.

Ioxynil containing herbicides

Some chemicals used as herbicides are capable of uncoupling oxidative phosphorylation. Ioxynil (4-cyano-2,6-dinitrophenol benzonitrile) is typical of this group, and was shown as long ago as 1965 to be an uncoupler of oxidative phosphorylation (Parker, 1965). Ingestion of a few grams can cause severe and sometimes fatal consequences in humans. Typical symptoms include vomiting, agitation, muscle pain, coma, meiosis, tachycardia, tachypnoea, metabolic acidosis, cardiac arrhythmias, pulmonary oedema and hyperpyrexia. Management of clinical cases requires urgent gastrointestinal decontamination and correction of the metabolic disturbances.

Antipsychotic agents

Neuroleptic malignant syndrome

Although fully dealt with in Chapter 15, neuroleptic malignant syndrome (NMS) is mentioned here because it enters into the differential diagnosis of many toxic hyperthermic syndromes, and the term NMS is frequently applied incorrectly to a variety of drug and poison-induced hyperthermic syndromes in everyday speech and also in the medical literature, which can lead to confusion in diagnosis and management (Kellam, 1987).

Loxapine

Loxapine in overdose can cause a syndrome similar to amoxapine, with tachycardia,widespread muscle spasms and hyperthermia. Rhabdomyolysis is common. Treatment-resistant convulsions and cardiac toxicity have been reported (Peterson, 1981). Whether loxapine can precipitate NMS remains unresolved (Chong & Abbot, 1991). It is possible that in some case reports, severe muscle spasms may have been mistakenly described as convulsions.

Clozapine

It was thought that clozapine, being an atypical antipsychotic agent, may not cause NMS. It has remarkably few extrapyramidal effects and only a weak affinity for dopamine 1 and 2 receptors. Case reports have appeared, however, in sufficient numbers to indicate that NMS follows clozapine therapy in rare cases (Thornberg & Ereshefsky, 1993; Reddig *et al.*, 1993).

Lithium

Lithium toxicity may follow acute or chronic overdosage (Dyson *et al.*, 1987). Toxicity following chronic intoxication most commonly occurs with serum lithium concentrations over 2 mEq/L and occasionally below this, but the correlation between clinical features and serum concentrations is poor. Alterations in consciousness and neuromuscular abnormalities are the most common clinical presenting features of toxicity. There may be confusion, agitation, dysarthria and visual disturbances as well as coarse tremors, ataxia, nystagmus, hyperreflexia and extensor plantar responses. With increasing severity, there may be mutism, extrapyramidial signs, muscle rigidity, choreoathetosis, increasing stupor, convulsions and coma. Fatalities occur, and this type of toxicity has the risk of permanent sequelae if left untreated.

In some patients the muscle rigidity and tremor may be associated with hyperpyrexia and there is a danger of misdiagnosing lithium toxicity as NMS. Case reports of NMS in association with lithium alone or plus other drugs should be interpreted with caution.

Strychnine

Strychnine causes extensor spasms, opisthotonus and convulsions mainly because of its action at a spinal level. Glycine is an inhibitory neurotransmitter, and strychnine blocks its postsynaptic uptake at spinal cord and brain stem receptors. This leads to hyperexcitation of peripheral muscle groups because of the lack of normal inhibition by glycine. Strychnine is sometimes taken in suicide attempts, and may also be added to illicit heroin. The muscle contractions are often severe enough to lead to hyperthermia and lactic acidosis. Sedation and muscle relaxation with intravenous diazepam should be sufficient for the patient who is conscious and has mild to moderate symptoms (Boyd *et al.*, 1983). In severe cases, endotracheal intubation, mechanical ventilation and paralysis with a muscle relaxant such as vecuronium or pancuronium may be required to prevent hypoxic cerebral damage and also hyperthermia and rhabdomyolysis (O'Callaghan *et al.*, 1982).

Drugs of abuse

Amphetamines

It has long been known that amphetamine sulphate can cause hyperthermia, usually as a result of overdose. Although this may be partly due to the sympathomimetic effects of amphetamine sulphate, it has long been known that the effects of amphetamine are different when given to a single animal than when given to a group of animals together; the study of this phenomenon has been described as aggregation toxicology. The effects of amphetamine sulphate on a group of animals is to make them hyperactive and hyperthermic, while the behaviour of a single animal appears to be largely unaffected by administration of the drug. The degree of hyperthermia depends on the size of the group and their duration of cohabitation (Vargas-Rivera *et al.*, 1990). More recently it has been shown that the hallucinogenic amphetamine 3,4-methylenedioxymethamphetamine (MDMA) causes a rise in body temperature in rats, which is greater at high ambient temperatures (Gordon *et al.*, 1991). Although this drug was widely used in the USA during the 1980s, the few reports of serious adverse effects and fatalities from the use of MDMA indicated that the most serious problems were cardiovascular in nature. Then the drug began to be used as a dance drug in the UK, at clubs and parties where large numbers of young people, sometimes thousands in number, would dance continuously for several hours. Reports began to appear of deaths from heat stroke (Henry *et al.*, 1992). The pattern of these cases was remarkably

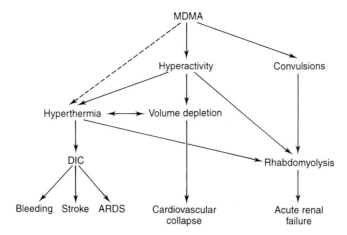

Figure 16.2. Mechanisms by which hallucinogenic amphetamines such as MDMA (3,4-methylenedioxymethamphetamine) may produce major complications. Hyperthermia is more commonly an indirect effect, mediated through hyperactivity, rather than a direct pharmacological effect. DIC, disseminated intravascular coagulation; ARDS, adult respiratory distress syndrome.

similar, with a history of collapse or convulsions occurring in a young person in their late teens or early twenties either at or just outside the venue. On arrival at hospital the clinical findings included hyperthermia (40–43 °C) and hypotension, with the development of DIC, rhabdomyolysis and acute renal failure. Death in most cases was secondary to DIC. High core temperature is more likely to be associated with a fatal outcome (O'Connor, 1994). A clinical pattern of toxicity can be established, with drug ingestion leading to prolonged hyperactivity, and hypovolaemia resulting from insufficient volume repletion, which are the main factors responsible for the development of hyperthermia which triggers DIC (Figure 16.2). It is possible that many of these deaths could have been prevented by fluid replacement while dancing, but the amphetamine-like effects of the drug may have led to diminished awareness of the body's fluid requirements. One patient who was admitted in a collapsed state after ingestion of MDMA required 3.5 litres of liquid in the first two hours (Woods & Henry, 1992). The continuous prolonged activity leading to hyperthermia in large groups of people may be a reflection of the hyperactivity and hyperthermia which occur in groups of animals but not in individual animals following amphetamine administration.

Management of amphetamine-induced hyperthermic crisis

The main priority is to facilitate thermoregulation and prevent the development of DIC. Full supportive care should be provided and an anticonvulsant such as intravenous diazepam should be given if necessary. The most urgent priority is to restore intravascular volume, as extracellular fluid volume may be grossly depleted. If the patient is not sweating and has established heat stroke, the use of dantrolene may be indicated. Estimation of serum creatinine phosphokinase and analysis of blood and urine for myoglobin will indicate whether rhabdomyolysis has occurred, and analysis of serum for fibrinogen degradation products will indicate whether DIC is present. Sometimes this diagnosis is clinically obvious because the patient bleeds profusely from needle puncture sites.

Narcotic analgesics

Abuse of opioids can cause a variety of serious medical complications but problems are commonest with heroin (diamorphine). Heroin abuse in the UK results in approximately 200 deaths per year, most of which are from respiratory depression following intravenous administration of the drug. Hypothermia may occur following overdose owing to immobility and exposure, but less commonly severe hyperthermia may be a sequel of hypoxic cerebral damage. The prognosis in such cases is poor. Pyrexia may also result from a chemical pneumonitis following aspiration of vomit, or the infective complications of intravenous drug abuse such as lung abscess, septicaemia and right-sided endocarditis.

Hypermetabolic syndrome resulting from 'chasing the dragon'

A heroin-induced hypermetabolic syndrome has been described in abusers who inhale heroin vapour from heated aluminium foil ('chasing the dragon'). In the early stages restlessness and cerebellar ataxia progress to spastic paresis. By two to four weeks, the syndrome may enter an irreversible phase, with extensor spasms, profuse sweating, central pyrexia, hypotonia, akinesia, widespread muscle rigidity and death. The characteristic pathology is a spongiform leucoencephalopathy. There is a high fatality rate; one series reported 11 deaths out of 47 cases (Wolters *et al.*, 1982). The cause of this syndrome is not clear but it may result from inhalation of a pyrolysis product of diamorphine or a contaminant of illicit heroin.

Cocaine

Hyperthermia is a complication of cocaine abuse, usually from excessively heavy use or from an overdose (Merigian & Roberts, 1987). The main nervous system effects of cocaine are to inhibit the reuptake of catecholamines at synapses in the central and peripheral nervous systems. Several mechanisms may be involved in the hypermetabolic effects of cocaine: dopaminergic hyperactivity and seizures that increase heat production, and sympathomimetic effects leading to vasoconstriction that decreases heat loss. A report of seven sudden deaths following overdose of cocaine attributed these deaths, however, to a variant of NMS that follows withdrawal of dopamine agonists (Kosten & Kleber, 1987). Rhabdomyolysis is also a common complication of heavy cocaine use that may result from a variety of effects including the hyperactivity, seizures, hyperthermia and sympathetic overactivity. Cocaine intoxication has been reported to be associated with a 5% incidence of rhabdomyolysis (Brody *et al.*, 1990).

Cocaine agitated delirium

Cocaine abuse also appears to be responsible for an unusual syndrome, cocaine agitated delirium, which consists of agitation, incoordination, sweating, excessive strength and hyperpyrexia. The person may exhibit paranoid behaviour, and may start to attack glass and mirrors, strip off all his clothing and run shouting through the streets until apprehended by the police. After a period of time the person becomes quiet with shallow breathing and hypotension, and death may occur within a few minutes (Wetli & Fishbain, 1985). Not surprisingly, the authorities may be blamed for causing death by exercising excessive restraint. At postmortem analysis, there is frequently a high concentration of cocaine metabolites such as benzoylecgonine which suggest that the syndrome may follow prolonged heavy use of cocaine; it is also possible that cocaine withdrawal may be a precipitating factor.

Lysergic acid diethylamide

Lysergic acid diethylamide (LSD) is a partial agonist at serotonin receptors. Ingestion of relatively small amounts (50–250 μg) may produce an hallucinogenic experience. The use of this drug, however, may be accompanied by signs of sympathetic activation with tachycardia, hypertension, dilated pupils and piloerection. These physiological changes are not well related to the size of the dose, and very large overdoses may be accompanied by mild effects. Temperature elevation is usually only mild or moderate but massive rises in temperature have been documented.

Ingestion of LSD has also been documented as precipitating NMS (Behan *et al.*, 1991). In one such case, a pathological description of muscle findings was used by authors to support the view that, in NMS, the muscle rigidity is caused by a central mechanism and is responsible for the hyperpyrexia.

Phenyclidine

Phencyclidine 1-(1-phenylcyclohexyl) piperidine (PCP) binds selectively and reversibly both to the active sites of cholinesterases and to the cholinergic receptor centrally. Together these effects produce mild anticholinergic activity. Phencylidine appears to have intracellular nicotinic binding sites, and blocks voltage dependent ion channels associated with nicotinic cholinoceptors. Nicotinic receptor blockade may affect neurotransmission in areas with large numbers of nicotinic receptors.

Phencyclidine, introduced in 1958 as a general anaesthetic, was noted to produce adverse psychiatric reactions including agitation, disorientation and hallucinations. Its human use was discontinued, although it remained available as a veterinary product for the production of a trance like analgesic state. Illicit use was first reported in 1967 and it obtained the street name 'angel dust'; fortunately its use remains confined almost entirely to the USA. It may be snorted, smoked, ingested or injected. Typical clinical features of toxicity include confusion, agitation, aggression, hallucinations and coma. The gait is usually ataxic, muscle tone is increased and severe dystonias may occur, with muscle rigidity and opisthotonus leading to hyperthermia, rhabdomyolysis and acute renal failure. There are many cases where the patient is virtually uncontrollable, with massive strength and total insensitivity to pain. Management is largely supportive and aimed at preventing self-injury. Acid diuresis can increase the elimination of phencyclidine (Aronow *et al.*, 1980).

Anticholinergic agents

Anticholinergic (antimuscarinic) drugs and chemicals antagonise the muscarinic actions of acetylcholine. They include many natural substances, particularly the belladonna alkaloids, atropine and scopolamine. Although *Atropa belladonna* (deadly nightshade) is widely regarded as highly toxic, deaths from ingestion of the berries are extremely rare, but have been recorded from ingestion of as few as three berries; however, small children are usually quite resistant to the anticholinergic effects. Many drugs with antimuscarinic effects are used mainly for the inhibition of secretions or in the prevention of motion sickness. The clinical features of toxicity include dry mouth, dry hot skin, urinary retention, and blurring of vision from spasm of the muscles of accommodation and photophobia. The pupils are usually fixed and dilated. There is mental confusion and sometimes hallucinations. Cardiac effects include tachycardia and cardiac arrhythmias. A rise in body temperature is common, and hyperpyrexia may result from the combination of hyperactivity and inhibition of sweating. A student mnemonic describes the syndrome in this way:

> blind as a bat
> dry as a bone
> red as a beet
> hot as a hare
> mad as a hatter.

In practice, hyperthermia is rarely life-threatening and usually self-limiting. The supportive management is to relax the patient and prevent hyperactivity. Physostigmine salicylate antagonises the central anticholinergic effects and neostigmine, which does not cross the blood–brain barrier, may be used to antagonise the peripheral effects. Physostigmine in a dose of 2–4 mg intravenously (adults) should cause a fall in body temperature.

Antihistamines

Overdosage with antihistamines tends to produce symptoms of the anticholinergic effects of these drugs, although some newer antihistamines such as astemizole and terfenadine are more likely to produce cardiac effects (Craft, 1986). Overdose with the older drugs, such as chlorpheniramine, will produce behaviourial changes, hallucinations, dilated pupils, flushing and fever. Hyperthermia usually occurs within two hours of exposure to antihistamines and temperatures of 41.8 °C have been reported (Wyngaarden & Seevers, 1951).

Umbilliferous plants

Many plants of the genus *Umbillifera* such as parsnips and carrots have culinary uses while others contain toxic agents and may cause severe poisoning. These toxic effects, although perhaps not leading to true hypermetabolic reactions, are included because they have several similar features.

Conium maculatum

Hemlock (*Conium maculatum*) contains alkaloids, including coniine, which cause muscular flaccidity and death from respiratory paralysis, although convulsions are also commonly reported to occur. Coniine is said to have a curare-like action on the neuromuscular junction and nicotinic effects at autonomic ganglia, with early stimulation causing increased secretions, meiosis and diarrhoea and later dry mucosae, hypotonia and mydriasis. Ingestion may lead to severe myalgia within hours, followed by rhabdomyolysis. In certain parts of Italy, where it is customary to shoot and eat small birds, there have been numerous cases of poisoning by coniine following ingestion of larks or chaffinches which eat the buds of *Conium maculatum* in the months of April and May (Rizzi *et al.* (1989). Epidemics of serious poisoning and numerous deaths have occurred from this source.

Oenanthe crocata *and* Cicuta virosa

Hemlock water dropwort (*Oenanthe crocata*) is an extremely poisonous plant. The active toxic principle is oenanthotoxin which is present in the roots in very high concentrations in the winter and early spring, and the stalk, leaves and flowers also contain the toxin. Vomiting is usually the earliest symptom which may be followed by hallucinations, convulsions, hyperventilation, trismus and muscle spasms. Rhabdomyolysis may occur and a fatal outcome is not uncommon. People have ingested the leaves by mistake for edible plants such as parsley or watercress and the roots been mistaken for wild parsnips (Mitchell & Rutledge, 1978). One case of water hemlock poisoning involved ingestion of a whole root. The chief symptoms were convulsions, unconsciousness, reddish tinted cyanosis, dilated pupils and marked metabolic acidosis. Treatment with haemodialysis, haemoperfusion, forced diuresis and artificial ventilation facilitated patient survival (Knutsen & Paszkowski, 1984).

A related toxin, cicutoxin, is found in similar plant, *Cicuta virosa* (water hemlock or cowbane) which has similar toxicity and although its effects are more strychnine-like it is even more likely than *Oenanthe crocata* to produce rhabdomyolysis (Carlton *et al.*, 1979).

Sympathomimetic agents and anorectic agents (fenfluramine diethylpropion)

All of these drugs can produce a rise in body temperature, probably because of a direct effect on mitochondrial heat production, although muscle tone is usually also increased and agitation may occur. Sympathomimetic drugs such as salbutamol and ritodrine tend to cause tachycardia and tremor; the hypermetabolism produced does not usually cause fever. Anorectic agents tend to be related to amphetamine, and may cause agitation, euphoria, widely dilated pupils and fever if taken in overdose.

Drug fevers and withdrawal syndromes

Many drugs have been associated with pyrexia. Sometimes this is accompanied by the systemic and cutaneous features of an adverse reaction to the drug, while more rarely it may be the only manifestation of a drug reaction. Antibiotics, cardiovascular drugs and centrally acting drugs are the most commonly implicated agents. The magnitude of the fever and its pattern of rise and fall are unhelpful in diagnosis. Patients with fever from drug hypersensitivity may appear generally well with a fever as high as 40 °C (Kumar & Reuler, 1986). Resolution occurs on withdrawal, and rechallenge may provoke the fever within hours, whereas the fever may have originally appeared after seven to ten days of drug administration. Some drug fevers result from interleukin 2 release, and a diagnostic trial of interleukin 2 blockade with indomethacin may be very revealing, with a rapid return to normal as long as indomethacin is continued.

Drug withdrawal reactions are most commonly associated with ethanol, sedatives, central nervous depressants and opiates. In general, to manifest such a reaction, tolerance and dependence must have developed. The withdrawal symptoms include agitation and hypermetabolism because of 'sympathetic overdrive' with the patient progressing to a self-limiting syndrome characterised by seizures, anxiety, agitation, fever, hypertension and cardiac arrhythmias. In alcohol withdrawal hallucinations are common. One drug that deserves special mention is levodopa. Sudden withdrawal in patients on regular high doses may lead to a state of severe muscle rigidity and hyperthermia which appear clinically to be similar to the NMS (Gibb & Griffith, 1986). This phenomenon has led to an improvement in the understanding of hyperthermia and hypermetabolism, and highlights the importance of dopamine blockade or withdrawal in the genesis of hyperthermic syndromes (Kornhuber & Weller, 1994).

Management of drug and chemical-induced hypermetabolism and related hyperthermia

It is evident that any triggering factors should be removed and that the patient should be cared for in a relatively cool environment. First aid workers and other staff should be prevented from administering antipyretic medication such as salicylates. Agitation and tremor causing muscle hyperactivity should be controlled: depending on the case, diazepam, propranolol, dantrolene and baclofen should be considered. The traditional method of treating acute hyperthermia is to attempt to accelerate heat loss by tepid sponging and fanning, although extracorporeal circulation such as cardiopulmonary bypass has also been used. Cooling blankets or iced saline gastric lavage may also be appropriate with profound hyperthermia. Excessive external cooling may lead to cutaneous vasoconstriction which could be counterproductive in the patient with massive overproduction of heat.

In many of the conditions described, there appears to be a sudden loss of control of intracellular ionised calcium when certain triggering agents are present, which leads to the formation of short and rigid actomyosin; the reaction can become self-sustaining because the heat produced eliminates the calcium requirement for actin–myosin interaction. The excess calcium may also be absorbed by mitochondria where it can uncouple oxidative phosphorylation, leading to further heat production. A pharmacological approach to decrease muscle spasm and heat production appears to be the best method of treatment for severe cases of drug-induced hyperthermia. Depending on the cause, this may be achieved by giving a specific relaxant drug such as dantrolene, or by curarisation and mechanical ventilation. Paralysis is indicated where the hyperthermia results from centrally generated muscle contraction. Early administration of dantrolene reduces mortality and morbidity in NMS and malignant hyperthermia (MH) and heat illness, and its use should be considered at an early stage in any hyperthermic syndrome. Once the core temperature has reached 39–40 °C, the decisions on management should be formulated as a matter of urgency. Other aspects of care deserve close attention. Rapid intravenous fluid replacement may be needed to correct volume depletion and facilitate thermoregulation. Acidosis and electrolyte imbalances should be corrected. Oxygen should be given in high concentration by face mask as the patient is being assessed, and an early decision should be made as to whether mechanical ventilation is needed.

Conclusion

This chapter has outlined some of the more dramatic hypermetabolic and hyperthermic syndromes that can be caused by drugs and toxins. If the cause is not known, the differential diagnosis is very wide, and as well as drug-induced toxicity, includes factitious fever, alcoholic hepatitis and a wide range of medical conditions such as infections and neoplastic, collagen–vascular, endocrine and metabolic disorders (POISINDEX, 1995).

In acute or severe cases, a careful clinical approach needs to be combined with rapid decision making and appropriate action in order to prevent a fatal outcome. Detailed documentation of cases and possibly phenotyping of survivors should in time enable the many causative factors and the syndromes they produce to be more clearly defined, and this should improve our understanding. In the meantime it is important that unexplained syndromes be described as hypermetabolic or hyperthermic rather than being labelled NMS or MH, when there is insufficient evidence to support a diagnosis of one of these clearly defined syndromes.

Acknowledgements

I thank Dr Gordon Taylor and Ursula Groening for their help with this manuscript.

References

Amrein, R., Allen, S. R., Guentert, T. W., Hootman, D., Lorscheid, T., Schoerlin, M. P. & Vranesic, D. (1988). The pharmacology of reversible monoamine oxidase inhibitors. *British Journal of Psychiatry*, **155**, 66–71 (suppl).

Aronow, R., Miceli, J. N. & Done, A. K. (1980). A therapeutic approach to the acutely overdosed PCP patients. *Journal of Psychedelic Drugs*, **12**, 259–67.

Bartels, P. D. & Lund-Jacobsen, H. (1986). Blood lactate and ketone body concentrations in salicylate intoxication. *Human Toxicology*, **5**, 363–6.

Behan, W. M., Bakheit, A. M., Behan, P. O. & Moore, I. A. (1991). The muscle findings in the neuroleptic malignant syndrome associated with lysergic acid diethylamide. *Journal of Neurology, Neurosurgery and Psychiatry*, **54**, 741–3.

Boyd, R. E., Brennan, P. T., Deng, J. F., Rochester, D. F. & Spyker, D. A. (1983). Strychnine poisoning. Recovery from profound lactic acidosis, hyperthermia and rhabdomyolysis. *American Journal of Medicine*, **74**, 507–12.

Brody, S. L., Wrenn, K. D., Wilber, M. M., Slovis, C. M. (1990). Predicting the severity of cocaine associated rhabdomyolysis. *Annals of Emergency Medicine*, **19**, 1137–43.

Carlton, B. E., Tufts, E. & Girard, D. E. (1979). Water hemlock poisoning complicated by rhabdomyolysis and renal failure. *Clinical Toxicology*, **14**, 87–93.

Chapman, B. J. & Proudfoot, A. T. (1989). Adult salicylate poisoning: deaths and outcome in patients with high plasma salicylate concentrations. *Quarterly Journal of Medicine*, **72**, 699–707.

Chong, L. S. & Abbott, P. M. (1991). Neuroleptic malignant syndrome secondary to loxapine. *British Journal of Psychiatry*, **159**, 572–3.

Craft, T. M. (1986). Torsade de pointes after astemizole overdose. *British Medical Journal*, **292**, 660.

Dyson, E. H., Simpson, D., Prescott, L. F. & Proudfoot, A. T. (1987). Self-poisoning and therapeutic intoxication with lithium. *Human Toxicology*, **6**, 325–9.

Gaudreault, E., Temple, A. R. & Lovejoy, F. H. (1982). The relative severity of acute versus chronic salicylate poisoning in children: a clinical comparison. *Paediatrics*, **70**, 566–9.

Gibb, W. R. & Griffith, D. N. (1986). Levodopa withdrawal syndrome identical to neuroleptic malignant syndrome. *Postgraduate Medical Journal*, **62**, 59–60.

Gieschke, R. Schmid-Burgk, W. & Amrein, R. (1988). Interaction of moclobemide, a new reversible monamine oxidase inhibitor with oral tyramine. *Journal of Neural Transmission*, **26**, 97–104.

Gordon, C. J., Watkinson, W. P., O'Callaghan, J. P. & Miller, D. B. (1991). Effects of 3,4-methlyenedioxymethamphetamine on autonomic thermoregulatory responses of the rat. *Pharmacology, Biochemistry and Behaviour*, **38**, 339–44.

Haefely, W., Burkard, W. P., Cesura, A. M., Kettler, R., Lorez, H. P., Martin, J. R., Richards, J. G., Scherschlicht, R. & DaPrada, M. (1992). Biochemistry and pharmacology of moclobemide, a prototype RIMA. *Psychopharmacology*, **106**, (Suppl.), S6–514.

Henry, J. A., Jeffreys, K. J. & Dawling, S. (1992). Toxicity and deaths from 3,4-methylenedioxymethamphetamine ('ecstasy'). *Lancet*, **2**, 384–7.

Hertzel, W. (1992). Safety of moclobemide taken in overdose for attempted suicide. *Psychopharmacology*, **106**, (suppl.) S127–S129.

Jennings, A. E., Levey, A. S. & Harrington, J. T. (1983). Amoxapine-associated acute renal failure. *Archives of Internal Medicine*, **143**, 1525–7.

Kaminski, C. A., Robbins, M. S. & Weibley, R. E. (1994). Sertraline intoxication in a child. *Annals of Emergency Medicine*, **23**, 1371–4.

Kaplan, R. F., Feinglass, N. G., Webster, W. & Mudra, S. (1986). Phenelzine overdose treated with dantrolene sodium. *Journal of the American Medical Association*, **255**, 642–9.

Kellam, A. M. (1987). The neuroleptic malignant syndrome, so-called. A survey of the world literature. *British Journal of Psychiatry*, **150**, 752–9.

Knutsen, O. H. & Paszkowski, P. (1984). New aspects in the treatment of water hemlock poisoning. *Journal of Toxicology – Clinical Toxicology*, **22**, 157–66.

Kornhuber, J. & Weller, M. (1994). Neuroleptic malignant syndrome. *Current Opinion in Neurology*, **7**, 353–7.

Kosten, T. R. & Kleber, H. D. (1987). Sudden death in cocaine abusers: relation to neuroleptic malignant syndrome. *Lancet*, **1**, 1198–9.

Kumar, L. & Reuuler, J. B. (1986). Drug fever. *Western Journal of Medicine*, **144**, 753–5.

Litovitz, T. L. & Troutman, W. G. (1983). Amoxapine overdose. Seizures and fatalities. *Journal of the American Medical Association*, **250**, 1069–71.

Merigian, K. S. & Roberts, J. R. (1987). Cocaine intoxication: hyperpyrexia, rhabdomyolysis and acute renal failure. *Journal of Toxicology – Clinical Toxicology*, **25**, 135–48.

Mitchell, M. I. & Rutledge, P. A. (1978). Hemlock water dropwort poisoning: a review. *Clinical Toxicology*, **12**, 417–26.

O'Callaghan, W. G., Joyce, N., Counihan, H. E., Ward, M., Lavelle, P. & O'Brien, E. (1982). Unusual strychnine poisoning and its treatment: report of eight cases. *British Medical Journal*, **285**, 478.

O'Connor, B. (1994). Hazards associated with the recreational drug 'ecstasy'. *British Journal of Hospital Medicine*, **52**, 507, 510–14.

Parker, V. H. (1965). Uncouplers of rat liver mitochondrial oxidative phosphorylation. *Biochemical Journal*, **97**, 658–62.

Peterson, C. D. (1981). Seizures induced by acute loxapine overdose. *American*

Journal of Psychiatry, **138**, 1089–91.

POISINDEX, *Micromedex*, Vol. 86, 1995.

Reddig, S., Minnema, A. M. & Tandon, R. (1993). Neuroleptic malignant syndrome and clozapine. *Annals of Clinical Psychiatry*, **5**, 25–7.

Richards, G. A., Fritz, V. U., Pincus, P. & Reyneke, J. (1987). Unusual drug interactions between monamine oxidase inhibitors and tricyclic antidepressants. *Journal of Neurology, Neurosurgery and Psychiatry*, **50**, 1240–1.

Rizzi, D., Basile, C., Di Maggio, A., Sebastio, A., Introna, F. Jr., Rizz, R., Bruno, S., Scohzzi, A. & DeMarlo, S. (1989). Rhabdomyolysis and acute tubular necrosis in coniine (hemlock) poisoning, *Lancet*, **2**, 1461–2.

Rosenberg, J., Pentel, P. R., Pond, S., Benowitz, N. & Olsen, K. (1984). Hyperthermia associated with drug intoxication. *Veterinary and Human Toxicology*, **26**, 413 (abstract).

Segar, W. E. (1969). The critically ill child: salicylate intoxication. *Pediatrics*, **44**, 440–4.

Tackley, R. M. & Tregaskis, B. (1987). Fatal disseminated intravascular coagulation following a monoamine oxidase inhibitor/tricyclic interaction. *Anaesthesia*, **42**, 760–3.

Tenenbein, M. & Dean, H. J. (1986). Benign course after massive levothyroxine ingestion. *Pediatric Emergency Care*, **2**, 15–17.

Thornberg, S. A. & Ereshefsky, L. (1993). Neuroleptic malignant syndrome associated with clozapine monotherapy. *Pharmacotherapy*, **13**, 510–14.

Todd, P. J., Sillis, J. A., Harris, F. & Cowan, J. M. (1981). Problems with overdose of sustained-release aspirin. *Lancet*, **1**, 777.

Vargas-Rivera, J., Ortega-Oronoa, B. G., Garcia-Pineda, J., Carranza, J., Salazar, L. A. & Villareal, J. (1990). Influence of previous housing history of the toxicity of amphetamine in aggregated mice. *Archivos de Investigacion Medica (Mexico)*, **21**, 65–9.

Wetli, C. V. & Fishbain, D. A. (1985). Cocaine-induced psychosis and sudden death in recreational cocaine users. *Journal of Forensic Sciences*, **30**, 873–80.

Wolters, E., van Wijngaarden, G. K., Stam, F. C., Renelink, H., Lonsberg, R. J., Schupper, M. E. & Verbeeten, B. (1982). Leucoencephalopahy after inhaling 'heroin' pyrolysate. *Lancet*, **2**, 1233–7.

Woods, J. D. & Henry, J. A. (1992). Hyperpyrexia induced by 3,4-methylenedioxymethamphetamine 'Eve'. *Lancet,*, 340.

Wyngaarden, J. B. & Seevers, M. H. (1951). The toxic effects of antihistamine drugs. *Journal of the American Medical Association*, **145**, 277–82.

17

Hypermetabolism in endocrine disorders

P. E. BELCHETZ

Introduction

The thyroid gland has long been recognised as a major regulator of metabolism. Indeed, measurement of the basal metabolic rate was one of the earliest methods of assessing thyroid status (Magnus-Levy, 1895; Gross *et al.*, 1952). Thyroid hormones influence many aspects of most cells in the body and our understanding has been greatly advanced by recent discoveries concerning the nature and action of the nuclear receptors for thyroid hormones. There is an exceedingly wide range in timescale over which the effects of thyroid hormone changes can be observed, stretching from within an hour when considering the fine-tuning that the hypothalamus exerts on pituitary thyroid stimulating hormone (TSH) secretion up to long-term, slow influences on cellular growth and differentiation. In general, as can be seen clinically when thyroid hormone levels are changed relatively abruptly, the biological responses are slow, taking place over weeks or even months.

The catecholamines, adrenaline and noradrenaline (the other major endocrine influences on metabolic rate), act much more rapidly by means of β-adrenergic receptors on cell membranes (Cryer, 1980). Recent years have added much relevant information on the structure and activation of adrenoreceptors as well as the second messenger systems conveying the effects downstream within the cell. It should also be noted that other hormones may also be involved in metabolic regulation, not only working in isolation, but also forming a network of dynamic relationships with thyroid hormone and catecholamine secretion. Major examples, among many of course, include insulin and growth hormone.

Synthesis and secretion of thyroid hormones

The thyroid gland is distinguished from other endocrine glands by the quantity of stored hormone that is usually retained within it. This is largely within the colloid inside the thyroid follicles where it is synthesised by the process of coupling of adjacent tyrosine moieties along the thyroglobulin molecules after they have been iodinated to form either mono-iodo or di-iodotyrosine. The ratio of mono-iodotyrosine (MIT) to di-iodotyrosine (DIT) determines how much l.thyroxine (T_4) and l.tri-iodothyronine (T_3) are synthesized and secreted. T_4 is produced in much greater molar concentrations than T_3 but in circumstances of reduced intrathyroidal iodine content, for example in areas of iodine deficiency or in circumstances of increased turnover within the thyroid there is enhancement of T_3 production (Rapaport & Ingbar, 1974). T_4 is now recognised to have relatively little intrinsic activity in most situations compared with T_3. It is, however, metabolised by various routes including deiodination to T_3. This is a regulated process catalysed by a series of deiodinases which differ in activity and biochemical properties and are differentially distributed among different tissues. Thus T_4 can be largely regarded as a pro-hormone, circulating in much greater concentrations than T_3 which is the metabolically active hormone. The great majority of T_3 is derived from T_4 by deiodination. Of the circulating T_3 only 20% is derived from direct thyroidal secretion although this fraction can change in various metabolic states. The circulating level of T_3 does not accurately reflect its metabolic role because in many tissues there is intracellular conversion of T_4 to T_3 which then exerts its physiological activity (Larsen *et al.*, 1981). This is seen most dramatically in the thyrotrophin cells of the anterior pituitary gland which possess a very powerful 5-deiodinase enzyme (type II) that converts virtually all T_4 entering the cell to T_3 within a very short time. In several tissues, particularly the liver, under a variety of metabolic stresses especially starvation, sepsis or other severe illness including cirrhosis, renal failure or surgery, the conversion of T_4 to T_3 is largely inhibited and frequently replaced by an alternative pathway leading to 3', 5', 3-tri-iodothyronine (reverse T_3) which is practically devoid of metabolic activity (Chopra *et al.*, 1975; Nomura *et al.*, 1975). The finding of a low serum T_3 is an almost constant finding in a state designated 'sick euthyroidism'. The mechanisms underlying these changes remain obscure but it is clear that they represent a prognostically poor situation especially in the context of patients on intensive care units (Slag *et al.*, 1981). It is also widely held that this may represent a compensatory response to hypercatabolic states and that treatment with exogenous T_3 is not beneficial.

Thyroid hormones in the circulation are very largely protein bound, especially T_4 that is approximately 99.95% protein bound. The binding proteins include the high affinity thyroxine binding globulin (TBG) that is synthesised in the liver and is responsive to a variety of genetic and hormonal influences. The most important clinically is oestrogen which in the high levels seen during pregnancy or when oral oestrogens are taken for contraception or hormone replacement therapy, raises the synthesis and secretion of TBG. Approximately three-quarters of T_4 is bound to TBG, one-fifth to thyroxine binding pre-albumin and 5% to albumin. The miniscule concentrations of non-protein bound T_4 and T_3 (so-called free hormones) are nevertheless largely responsible for most of the biological actions of thyroid hormones (Himsworth, 1992). This is presumably because the major site of thyroid hormone action is thought to be intranuclear. The direct measurement of these very tiny free hormone levels is therefore a desirable but difficult undertaking. In recent years several methodologies have been devised to achieve this aim but most are not direct measurements and some techniques are liable to distorted readings if there are abnormal concentrations or more particularly genetically determined variants of the hormone-binding molecules. The most clearly defined, albeit rare, group is of dysalbuminaemic variants (Lalloz *et al.*, 1985).

The physiological regulation of thyroid hormone secretion is conceptually important if only to interpret the biochemical findings in thyroid disease. The maintenance of normal free T_4 and free T_3 levels is achieved by a number of mechanisms but paramount is the secretion of pituitary TSH, a heterodimeric glycoprotein. The distribution of the secreted thyroid hormones between the various binding proteins and the free hormone compartment is the result of the protein concentrations and their affinity constants for T_4 and T_3. The level of TSH drive to thyroidal secretion is itself the consequence of an interplay of factors, primarily a positive drive exerted by the hypothalamus via thyrotrophin releasing hormone (TRH; which is a tripeptide pyroglutamyl-histidyl-prolineamide) and negative feedback by rising levels of especially free T_4 (rapidly almost wholly deiodinated to T_3 and, because in such molar excess over circulating T_3, exerting a quantitatively major influence) that inhibits TSH secretion and if in persistent excess, also TSH synthesis. Other minor influences can be discerned such as a circadian rhythm of small amplitude and possible inhibitory influences from the hypothalamus in the forms of dopamine and somatostatin. It is also likely that rapidly rising thyroid hormone levels can inhibit the hypothalamic drive via TRH. These hypothalamic influences are believed to be hormonal and mediated by factors such as TRH liberated into fenestrated capillaries of the median eminence of the medial basal hypothalamus, whence they travel down the portal vessels connecting this primary capillary plexus with the secondary plexus that is a series of similarly fenestrated sinusosids bathing the anterior pituitary cells.

As would be predicted from this description of the physiological regulation of thyroid hormone secretion, in disease states where there is impaired synthesis and/or hormone secretion, the interruption of the negative feedback loop leads to progressive disinhibition of TSH secretion which tends to rise exponentially as the thyroid hormone levels, particularly T_4, fall. Conversely, in states of primary thyroid over activity, whether as a result of autonomous adenoma, multinodular goitre or, most commonly, immunoglobulin-driven thyrotoxicosis (Graves' disease), TSH secretion will be suppressed. This suppression can now be simply and precisely measured with the latest generation of TSH assays that are capable of detecting levels of TSH well below the normal range. It is a common finding on treating thyrotoxicosis that the thyroid hormone levels may fall well down in the normal or even subnormal range yet TSH secretion will remain suppressed inappropriately for up to several weeks, indicating that the prolonged experience of thyroid hormone excess affects the synthesis and indeed the biosynthetic machinery for TSH as well as the more rapidly modulated changes in TSH secretion.

Mode of action of thyroid hormone

The pleiotropic nature of thyroid hormone effects has led to the exploration of many possible cellular sites of action. These include the cell surface, for example in mediating the transport of sugars into the cell (Segal & Ingbar, 1982) or the rapid phase of TSH suppression mediated by the hypothalamus (Belchetz *et al.*, 1978). In view of the major role on metabolism much attention has been paid to the process of oxidative phosphorylation and in particular to mitochondrial function (Sterling, 1979). It remains possible that these represent physiologically significant mechanisms, but the major focus of recent evidence has been on a primary nuclear site of action (Oppenheimer *et al.*, 1972). This has led to the identification of a group of thyroid hormone receptors that differ in their distribution between the thyroid responsive tissues of the body (Lazar, 1993). The course of cloning these receptors occurred by an unanticipated route and indicated a far wider series of homologies than expected, especially with steroid hormone receptors. Detailed consideration of the sequence of investigations lies outside the scope of this chapter. In brief, workers examining the role of oestrogen receptors in breast cancer examined possible homologies with the v-erb-A oncogene, which is encoded by the avian erythroblastosis virus. In turn this led to study of the normal cellular counterpart of the viral oncogene, known as C-erb-A proto-oncogene. The ligand for this was not another steroid, but was instead T_3 (Sap *et al.*, 1986; Weinberger *et al.*, 1986). There followed a recognition of a highly conserved pattern in the receptors of what has become known as the steroid/thyroid hormone nuclear receptor superfamily. More than 30 genes in this family have been cloned which also includes receptors for 1:25 $(OH)_2$ vitamin D_3 and retinoic acid derivations as well as a number for which the activating ligands have not been identified, referred to as 'orphan receptors'.

For further details the reader is referred to recent review articles but briefly all members of the family can be defined with five domains (Carson-Jurica *et al.*, 1990; Lazar, 1993). A/B at the N-terminal end is the hypervariable transactivation region, C the DNA binding region and D a hinge domain joining on to the C-terminal ligand binding domain. Two classes of thyroid hormone receptors have been cloned in humans α on chromosome 17 and β on chromosome 3. Alternate splicing of receptor gene transcripts yields various isoforms but the $β_2$ variant lacks ligand binding properties at the C-terminus hence is not a true thyroid hormone receptor. Important insights have emerged from studies of families with congenital resistance to thyroid hormone (Retetoff, 1993). The great majority of mutations have been localised in the ligand binding region of the β receptor.

Catecholamines metabolism and action

The measurement of circulating endogenous catecholamine levels and the biological response to graded infusions of noradrenaline and adrenaline suggest that in normal circumstances the great majority of noradrenaline is released as a neurotransmitter from nerve terminals (Cryer, 1980). Most noradrenaline is cleared by reuptake mechanisms into sympathetic postganglionic neurones. The spillover into the circulation is about 5% and the levels usually seen in the circulation are below those normally required for endocrine activity. In circumstances of extreme sympathetic activity, such as heavy physical exercise, the circulating concentration may rise sufficiently to have metabolic effects. The adrenal medulla contributes only about 2% of the circulating noradrenaline in normal circumstances which is clearly physiologically insignificant. Adrenaline is synthesised and secreted almost wholly from the adrenal medullae by virtue of the presence of the enzyme phenylethanolamine-N-methyl transferase (PNMT) that enables noradrenaline to be methylated by *S*-adenosylmethionine (Wurtman & Axelrod, 1966). This is a true hormone secreted in a dose-responsive manner to hypoglycaemia, exercise, surgery and a variety of medical disorders such as diabetic ketoacidosis and myocardial infarction. The levels reached are compatible with the effects seen after graded infusions which with progressive increases lead to tachycardia; then lipolysis, systolic hypertension; next hyperglycaemia, ketogenosis and glycolysis; and at the highest levels suppression of insulin secretion.

Catecholamine actions

These are mediated by cell surface adrenoreceptors containing seven trans-membrane domains with an extracellular hormone binding domain and a long intracellular tail (Bouloux, 1992). These are intimately related to intracellular second messenger mechanisms, particularly G protein coupled to adenyl cyclase, and thence generation of cyclic adenosine monophosphate (cAMP) production. The original classification into α and β receptors still holds although there are various subtypes functionally recognised: α_1, α_2, β_1 and β_2 receptors. The β_1 versions are particularly important in metabolic processes. They also play a major regulatory role in modulating the clearance of catecholamines by desensitisation in the presence of agonist (downregulation of receptor numbers) as β receptors have a role in metabolising catecholamines. This summary is a considerable oversimplification as vascular beds and tissues vary in their receptor types, densities and responses.

Hormone interactions

This complex area can only be touched briefly. The clinical similarity of thyrotoxic patients to conditions of sympathetic hyperactivity has led to the notion that there may be sensitisation of tissues to the normal levels of catecholamines seen in thyrotoxicosis. This in turn has led to the use of β-antagonists such as propranolol and nadolol as well as cardioselective antagonists such as atenolol as adjuncts to the treatment of thyrotoxicosis. The complex relationships between catecholamines and insulin, glucagon and the repair of hypoglycaemia have been alluded to. The secretion of many hormones in response to hypoglycaemia has been documented including adrenocorticotrophic hormone (ACTH), vasopressin and growth hormone. The immediate events restoring plasma glucose require adrenaline and glucagon, either alone will suffice but the absence of both may prove disastrous (Cryer, 1980). Growth hormone has complex actions metabolically, both in its own right and mediated by insulin-like growth factor 1 (IGF-1). Growth hormone has marked effects on metabolic rate (which is largely determined by skeletal muscle) and this in turn may, at least in part, be mediated by enhanced conversion of T_4 to T_3 (Jørgensen *et al.*, 1989). Growth hormone hypersecretion has marked effects on sweat and sebum production, as seen in acromegaly. The converse situation of growth hormone deficiency is associated with diminished sweat production and the impaired ability to control body temperature with liability to hyperpyrexia in the face of high environmental temperatures (Juul *et al.*, 1993). A final important hormonal interaction is seen in the adrenal gland where PNMT activity depends permissively on adequate cortisol production, the adrenaline response to hypoglycaemia being reduced in hypopituitarism (Rudman *et al.*, 1981).

Thyrotoxicosis

This term is used to express the clinical sequelae of excessive thyroid hormone secretion, rather than the purely biochemical description implied by hyperthyroidism. Confirmation of the diagnosis, nevertheless, does rely on hormone measurements in plasma. Usually this is quite simple, requiring no more than finding raised total thyroxine and suppressed TSH concentration (Franklyn, 1994). There are sufficiently frequent situations where there may be suppression of TSH in the absence of hyperthyroidism to reject the once popular concept of screening by a single 'first-line' measurement of TSH alone; examples include non-thyroidal illness, various drugs including corticosteroids and dopamine, and not infrequently in healthy elderly patients. Similarly, just measuring total T_4 levels is inadequate, particularly because of the frequency of raised TBG concentration in women who are pregnant or are taking a combined oral contraceptive pill. These distortions are not encountered in measurements of so-called free T_4 concentration as discussed earlier, but there are rare situations where these measurements may mislead. The measurement of serum T_3 concentration need not be routine but it is indicated to diagnose the situation of 'T_3 toxicosis' when T_4 (total and free) will be normal but TSH is suppressed.

The most common cause of thyrotoxicosis, Graves' disease, is straightforward to diagnose if there is ophthalmopathy (conjunctival oedema and inflammation, diplopia, proptosis) either singly or in combination, and a smoothly enlarged thyroid, often with a bruit. It should be noted that the findings of lid retraction or lid lag are not specifically features of Graves' disease and are attributed to the enhanced sensitivity of the levator palpebrae superioris fibres, which possess adrenergic innervation, to catecholamines in thyroid hormone excess of any cause. Other important causes include toxic multinodular goitre, or more rarely toxic adenoma (Plummer's disease), subacute thyroiditis (de Quervain's thyroiditis), postpartum thyroiditis and the toxic phase of Hashimoto's thyroiditis, which is often relatively short-lived being succeeded by hypothyroidism. It is important to recognise the possibility of iodine-induced hyperthyroidism which can be caused by iodine-containing radiographic contrast agents (less common nowadays), ingestion of large amounts of kelp and probably the most commonly seen form is following amiodarone therapy (Franklyn *et al.*, 1985). The effects of amiodarone are complex partly because of the high iodine content of the molecule which is released and probably because of conformational resemblance of the intact molecule and its metabolites to thyroid hormones and thus interaction with thyroid hormone receptors. Residual effects from amiodarone administration may persist for many months. High concentrations predominantly interfere with T_4 deiodination to T_3 and chronic use is frequently associated with high total and free T_4 but normal total and free T_3 and normal TSH in patients remaining euthyroid. It can also induce hypothyroidism with raised TSH but by the same mechanism a less than might be expected reduction in T_4. When amiodarone induces thyrotoxicosis both T_4 and T_3 are raised and TSH is suppressed. This is quite often seen when the drug has been discontinued and the levels begin to fall leaving mainly an increased iodine pool. Elderly patients often have nodular goitres and may be more prone to develop iodine-induced thyrotoxicosis.

In circumstances other than clinical Graves' disease it may be, albeit infrequently, helpful to perform a radioiodine (or technetium) scan. This will be helpful in confirming the size and position of either single or multiple nodules and the absence of uptake is found in states of iodine-induced thyrotoxicosis or destructive inflammatory processes leading to the release of stored preformed thyroid hormones from the colloid, as seen with either subacute or silent thyroiditis (a variant apparently commoner in the USA than in the UK or Europe) or the fairly frequent but normally evanescent and clinically insignificant hyperthyroid phase of postpartum thyroiditis (Ginsberg & Walfish, 1977; Fung *et al.*, 1988).

The clinical features of thyrotoxicosis are well known. The features of hypermetabolism include heat intolerance, excessive perspiration, tachycardia and large volume pulse, weight loss despite hyperphagia, agitation and hyperkinesis plus fine tremor, increased gut transit time, looseness of bowel action, diarrhoea or even steatorrhoea. In the elderly the features may be less conspicuous, mainly because the heart is more susceptible to the deleterious effects of even relatively minor degrees of hyperthyroidism with atrial fibrillation and cardiac failure predominating (Rønnov-Jessen & Kirkegaard, 1973). Rarely this may present as apathetic thyrotoxicosis where the patient may be suspected initially of being hypothyroid, being torpid, having ptosis rather than lid retraction and lacking thyroid enlargement or excessive sweating. These patients often present with cardiac cachexia, marked weight loss, atrial fibrillation and marked dependent oedema, scaphoid hollowing of the temples is frequently observed. While thyrotoxic heart disease is uncommon in the UK, in countries with less widely available healthcare it is not rare to find patients aged less than 40 years with heart failure as a result of long-standing untreated thyrotoxicosis (Woeber, 1992).

The conventional therapy of thyrotoxicosis may be with thionamide antithyroid drugs such as carbimazole and propylthiouracil, radioiodine therapy using ^{131}I and surgery. It is recommended that antithyroid medication is used to render the patient euthyroid before submitting a patient to surgery and indeed before the use of radioiodine in very thyrotoxic patients to reduce the risk of 'thyroid crisis' or 'storm' (see later). The use of β blockers (especially propranolol and nadolol) should be avoided in asthma or heart failure. These drugs are useful adjuncts in rapid symptomatic control of tachycardia, tremor, sweating and anxiety in the early stages of treatment. The former recommendation that surgery can be safely performed in thyrotoxic patients under β-blockade without prior treatment (Michie *et al.*, 1974) with antithyroid medication has largely fallen out of favour. All antithyroid drugs carry a low risk of serious side-effects (Burrell *et al.*, 1956) of which agranulocytosis is the most dangerous and it is advisable to provide patients starting on these agents with written advice to attend the nearest hospital casualty department requesting an immediate full blood count in the event of a sore throat which is the major feature of this complication. The patient should await the result and in the event of marked neutropaenia, less than 1×10^9/L, should immediately discontinue the treatment and contact the clinician dealing with the overall management of the thyrotoxicosis. While the incidence is reputed to be dose-dependent in the case of carbimazole and usually occurs in the first three months of initiating therapy this is not invariably the case.

The major role of surgery in treatment of thyrotoxicosis is in patients with severe disease and large, perhaps compressive goitres. While surgery is used less often and radioiodine more often, it remains a valuable approach in the minority of patients in whom medical control is difficult and only attainable with high-dose carbimazole. The choice of surgeon is critical and in experienced hands the complication rate is minimal. The response is of course immediate and gratifying and in the immediate few months after the operation hypothyroidism is often seen which is often transient and requires either no treatment or short-term treatment, say with liothyronine for 12 months before stopping this and assessing endogenous secretion after two months (Wilkin *et al.*, 1979). Hypocalcaemia is a frequent immediate postoperative finding and mild long-term hypocalcaemia is not uncommon but permanent symptomatic hypoparathyroidism with severe hypocalcaemia should be rare as should problems with the recurrent laryngeal nerves. Well-healed collar scars in natural skin creases often fade to virtual invisibility, but of course keloid can be unsightly and develops unpredictably except in Afro-Caribbean patients in whom it might be expected. Recurrent thyrotoxicosis is quite rare after adequate surgery but there is a rising tide of hypothyroidism which seems to be delayed by a decade or so before it begins to rise linearly with time. This rise in incidence of hypothyroidism parallels that seen after radioiodine therapy except that after the latter it begins to occur immediately after treatment reaching 50% by ten to 25 years (depending on the dose of ^{131}I used) (Franklyn, 1994). These figures underscore the necessity for an efficient and economical long-term follow-up of all patients treated for thyrotoxicosis. There is a growing vogue for using higher doses to hasten the time when thyroxine substitution therapy can be introduced as it is hoped that this will be complied with and so avoid the increasing risk of default from follow-up with time from ablative treatment. Radioiodine is cheap, simple to administer and remarkably safe without significantly increased risk of other neoplastic disorders including leukaemia. It should be avoided in pregnancy, which should be strictly prevented for four months after therapy, although the trend set in the USA of using radioiodine in young adults or even children is gaining popularity in the UK.

Thyroid crisis or storm

This frequently fatal complication is now exceedingly rare as it is widely recognised that surgery should be avoided in untreated thyrotoxic patients (Burch & Wartofsky, 1993). Other precipitants include myocardial infarction, stroke, infection and pulmonary embolism. The distinction from uncomplicated severe thyrotoxicosis is blurred but key features include cardiovascular decompensation, usually with rapid atrial fibrillation, central nervous features (ranging from severe agitation to psychosis and even coma), pyrexia, usually severe, and hepatic/gastrointestinal disturbance.

The cornerstones of therapy are first a large loading dose of antithyroid drug, classically propylthiouracil because of its alleged capacity to inhibit deiodination of T_4 to T_3, then after one hour, to permit the initiation of antithyroid drug action, large doses of iodide, given as the sodium salt if using the intravenous route (1 g) or else potassium iodide orally or by nasogastric tube. In fact, large doses of carbimazole are more easily administered using

80 mg and probably as effective as propylthiouracil because the doses required to inhibit deiodination probably far exceed those obtained therapeutically. The full panoply of supportive measures should be used simultaneously. These include propranolol in high dose (2–5 mg intravenously or 320–480 mg orally daily in four-hourly divided doses). Pyrexia should be lowered by external cooling and chlorpromazine has been recommended for this purpose as well as sedation. Active treatment of heart failure, underlying infection, rehydration and corticosteroids are generally required. The use of sodium ipodate is often recommended to inhibit thyroid hormone release. The author has personal experience of the benefits derived in this regard and also of improving the mental state by administration of lithium carbonate.

Phaeochromocytomas

These are rare tumours, probably responsible for no more than 0.1% of all cases of hypertension. Their fascination derives from their often dramatic and varied clinical features that challenge and sometimes defeat medical, surgical and anaesthetic skills. They vividly exemplify the physiological consequences of excessive catecholamine secretion, yet if successfully treated lead to a fully normal state including blood pressure in 75% of cases.

Phaeochromocytomas may present as small tumours of a few grams to large palpable tumours of over 1 kg; yet there may be severe symptoms with any size of phaeochromocytoma (Fonseca & Bouloux, 1993). The rule of 10% has been traditionally and reasonably accurately applied to phaeochromocytoma. Thus 10% occur outside the adrenal, 10% are malignant (of which the only reliable sign is the demonstration of synchronous or metachronous metastasis), 10% occur in children, 10% are bilateral (but more so in the several familial associated disorders), 10% are associated with hyperglycaemia and 10% with hypermetabolism. Extra-adrenal sites may be distant and occult, i.e. high in the neck, thoracic, within the heart, but most occur within the abdominal cavity. Here they are often associated with the paravertebral sympathetic chain and ganglia especially the organ of Zuckerkandl, around the origin of the inferior mesenteric artery but can be found widely for example in the wall of the bladder, prostate, testis, ovary, liver and kidneys.

Clinical features

These may be extremely varied often with crises that may prove lethal (Bravo & Gifford, 1993). Most patients are hypertensive, half only intermittently during paroxysms of catecholamine release, but of these who have persistent hypertension many exhibit fluctuations. Orthostatic hypotension is particularly associated with rare pure adrenaline secreting tumours (Baxter *et al.*,1992), but may succeed hypertensive episodes especially if there are associated crises such as gut infarction, hypovolaemia or lactic acidosis. Patients harbouring phaeochromocytomas usually complain of headaches, excessive sweating and palpitations. Other frequent symptoms include pallor, nausea and vomiting, tremor, weakness and exhaustion. Anxiety and nervousness may be marked even leading to 'angor animi': the conviction if impending doom, which is not always misplaced. Abdominal symptoms include constipation, which may not be solely related to catecholamine release as the tumours may contain many other products including enkephalins and somatostatin. About a fifth of patients flush. Cardiovascular problems range from brady to tachyarrhythmias and may be associated with myocardial infarction, heart failure, shock and myocarditis or even cardiomyopathy, both dilated and hypertrophic, are seen. Metabolic consequences may include diabetes, lactic acidosis, hypercalcaemia and ectopic ACTH secretion causing Cushing's syndrome with hypokalaemic alkalosis. Factors potentially releasing catecholamines from phaeochromocytomas include exertion, bending over, abdominal palpation, straining at parturition, or even defaecation, micturition (sometimes indicative of ectopic sites of tumours), induction of anaesthesia and administration of many drugs including glucagon, histamine, naloxone, metoclopramide, droperidol, tricyclic antidepressants, phenothiazines and β-blockers if not preceded by adequate α-blockade.

Investigation

The first question that arises is who to investigate. Suspicion may be raised by early age of onset of hypertension, severity, intermittency or provocation by β-blockage, induction of anaesthesia, labour or use of intravenous radiological contrast media. Hypertensive patients who are diabetic may have phaeochromocytomas, albeit rarely, more often than others. Patients at risk of familial phaeochromocytomas such as those with multiple endocrine neoplasia type 2 (MEN 2) need recurrent screening.

The classical screening using a 24 hour urine collection for vanillylmandelic acid (VMA) should be replaced by the more specific and sensitive measurement of metanephrines. Much more readily available in specialised centres is the measurement of urinary free catecholamines, most commonly using reversed phase high performance liquid chromatography (HPLC) with electrochemical detection. The urine needs to be acidified and several samples may need to be collected if intermittent secretion is not to be missed. Less commonly recourse is made to the measurement of plasma catecholamines which can be especially useful if blood is sampled during a hypertensive crisis. There may be some overlap between plasma noradrenaline in normal subjects and patients with phaeochromocytomas and so the use of suppressive tests has been suggested on the basis that suppression of central sympathetic activity with clonidine or ganglionic transmission with pentolinium should diminish the physiological secretion of noradrenaline but not from the autonomous production of phaeochromocytomas. Provocative tests are inherently hazardous and should be contemplated under α and β blockade; of the various agents used (including histamine, tyramine and naloxone), glucagon appears to be the safest. The value of these tests is when repeated basal values have proved normal but the index of clinical suspicion remains high (Bravo, 1994). Measuring the rate of fall in blood pressure following intravenous phentolamine in adrenergically unblocked patients with hypovolaemia has proved lethal and this test is obsolete.

Localisation of tumours

This can be attempted fairly easily if the condition is suspected, using computerised tomography (CT) scanning, initially of the adrenal glands alone (Reznek & Armstrong, 1994). To avoid pressor crises following the administration of intravenous contrast agents the patient should always receive α and β blockers. Further tissue characterisation is claimed for magnetic resonance imaging especially T_2 weighted images. In tumours which are difficult to locate multiple venous sampling from sites above and below the diaphragm and including the coronary sinus has proved helpful. The use of the tumour specific radionuclide metaiodobenzyl guanidine (mIBG) is helpful especially in identifying extra-adrenal paragangliomata and also metastases in the case of malignant tumours. It can also be used during the operation to confirm the removal of all labelled tissue.

Treatment

The key to safe surgery is adequate preparation which consists of using the irreversible α_1 and α_2 adrenergic blocking agent phenoxybenzamine orally in doses of 10–20 mg four times daily for one to two weeks, adding propranolol 40 mg three times daily after initial α blockade and expanding the often contracted plasma volume by blood transfusion as required (Ross *et al.*, 1967).

Preoperative management

Even with careful preparation with adrenergic blocking agents surgery is a hazardous matter with drugs, anaesthetics and physical handling of the tumour all potentially releasing catecholamines with swinging blood pressure and cardiac arrhythmias resulting. After tumour removal the rapid clearance of catecholamines may lead to profound hypotension that may be compounded by a relative reduction in plasma volume especially as the vascular bed expands and small vessels may be more than usually permeable to fluid. It is thus necessary to choose carefully premedicants (preferring diazepam and avoiding droperidol) and anaesthetic drugs. Pulse and blood pressure need to be continuously monitored and immediate access to intravenous sodium nitroprusside guaranteed so that hypertensive episodes can be controlled without delay. Tachyarrhythmias may need small intravenous doses of β blockers: traditionally propranolol but more recently esmolol. Magnesium sulphate may have a role in reducing the large swings in blood pressure.

Hypovolaemia requires prompt and adequate transfusion. The surgical technique requires a wide exposure and for this reason an abdominal incision is preferred so that the vascular pedicle (very short right adrenal vein draining directly into the inferior vena cava) can be approached with minimal handling of the tumour. The adrenal should be excised widely en bloc. With bilateral tumours or where bilaterality may be expected if only metachronously, surgery to both sides should be considered at one operation, hence further benefit of an anterior approach. Tumour extension may need removal from the renal vein or inferior vena cava. Although fewer than 20% of tumours are extra-adrenal, the variety of potential sites mandates accurate preoperative localisation because of the specialised approaches necessitated by intrathoracic (including pericardial and cardiac) or pelvic tumours. Phaeochromocytomas are notoriously dangerous in pregnancy and if diagnosed late, after preparation with phenoxybenzamine, elective caesarian section can precede abdominal exploration and tumour removal. Postoperative problems largely relate to the need to monitor plasma volume by measurement of central venous pressure and prompt replenishment. Although the often quoted figure for malignancy is 10%, this is probably an underestimate especially as metastatic disease may not become apparent until after surgery. The prognosis varies widely and amelioration appears to be conferred in many cases by chemotherapy using [131]I- mIBG (tracer doses of which are valuable for indicating tissue distribution; Brendel *et al.*, 1989).

Heritable conditions associated with phaeochromocytomas

Although the majority of phaeochromocytomas are sporadic, important groups are found in association with several neuroendocrine and neurocutaneous syndromes, reflecting the embryological origins of the tumour. These cases are frequently multicentric in origin with bilateral and extra-adrenal sites being encountered. The best known syndrome is multiple endocrine neoplasia type 2 (MEN 2a) which is caused by an autosomal dominant gene (ret-oncogene) localised to chromosome 10p (Mulligan *et al.*, 1993). It is linked to medullary carcinoma of the thyroid (MCT) which is the major clinical feature being expressed with increasing frequency from the age of about 5 years until by the age of 70 years about 60% of gene carriers have MCT. The occurrence of phaeochromocytomas is less and rare without pre-existing evidence of MCT. The precision of identifying gene carriers by genetic markers is greater than chemical screening by measuring simulated calcitonin release after intravenous pentagastrin. In those at risk annual measurement of 24 hour catecholamine excretion is recommended but prophylactic bilateral adrenalectomy is not indicated in contrast to total thyroidectomy on the basis of risk/benefit analysis. Hyperparathyroidism may also appear as part of the MEN 2a syndrome. Phaeochromocytoma may also occur in the rarer MEN 2b in which there are mucosal neuromas and constipation because of ganglioneuromatosis of the gut. The patients may look marfanoid and have lips thickened by the neurofibromas. Slit lamp examination may reveal medullated corneal fibres. Other conditions associated with higher than normal frequency of phaeochromocytomas include neurofibromatosis, von Hippel–Lindau disease, ataxia telangiectasia, tuberose sclerosis and multiple neoplasia triad syndrome (extra-adrenal paragangliomata, epithelioid leiomyosarcoma and pulmonary chordomas; Fonseca & Bouloux, 1993).

Conclusion

The endocrine system plays a major role in the physiological regulation of metabolic rate. Several hormones are involved particulary from the thyroid and adrenal medulla. The rarity of endocrine disorders leading to significant hypermetabolism is perhaps a testament to the effectiveness and reliability of the normal homeostatic mechanisms. The two major endocrine emergencies which threaten life and carry significant morbidity by virtue of inducing hypermetabolic states are thyroid crisis and phaeochromocytoma. The physiological basis to understanding these disorders, and the principles of diagnosis and management have been summarised.

References

Baxter, M. A., Hunter, P., Thompson, G. R. & London, D. R. (1992). Phaeochromocytomas as a cause of hypotension. *Clinical Endocrinology*, **37**, 304–6.

Belchetz, P. E., Gredley, G., Bird, D. & Himsworth, R. L. (1978). Regulation of thyrotrophin secretion by negative feedback of tri-iodothyronine on the hypothalamus. *Journal of Endocrinology*, **76**, 439–48.

Bouloux, P.-M. G. (1992). Phaeochromocytomas and related tumours. In *Clinical Endocrinolgy*, ed. A. Grossman. Oxford, Blackwell Scientific Publications. pp. 459–85.

Bravo, E. L. (1994). Evolving concepts in the pathophysiology, diagnosis and treatment of pheochromocytoma. *Endocrine Reviews*, **15**, 356–68.

Bravo, E. L. & Gifford, R. W. (1993). Pheochromocytoma. *Endocrinology and Metabolism Clinics of North America*, **22**, 329–41.

Brendel, A. J., Jeandot, R., Guyot, M., Lambert B. & Drouillard, J. (1989). Radionuclide therapy of phaeochromocytomas and neuroblastomas using iodine-131 metaiodobenzylguanidine (mIBG). *Clinical Nuclear Medicine*, **14**, 19–22.

Burch, H. D. & Wartofsky, L. (1993). Life-threatening thyrotoxicosis: thyroid storm. *Endocrinology and Metabolism Clinics of North America*, **22**, 263–77.

Burrell, C. D., Fraser, R. & Doniach, D. (1956). The low toxicity of carbimazole: a survey of 1046 patients. *British Medical Journal*, **1**, 1453–6.

Carson-Jurica, M. A., Schrader, W. T. & O'Malley, B. W. (1990). Steroid receptor family: structure and function. *Endocrine Reviews*, **11**, 201–20.

Chopra, I. J. Chopra, U., Smith, S. R., Reza, M. & Solomon, D. H. (1975). Reciprocal changes in serum concentrations of 3,3,5-triiodothyronine (reverse T_3) and 3,3,5-triiodothyronine (T_3) in systemic illnesses. *Journal of Clinical Endocrinology and Metabolism*, **41**, 1043–9.

Cryer, P. E. (1980). Physiology and pathophysiology of the human sympathoadrenal neuroendocrine system. *New England Journal of Medicine*, **303**, 436–44.

Fonseca, V. & Bouloux, P.-M. (1993). Phaeochromocytoma and paraganglioma. *Bailliere's Clinical Endocrinolgy and Metabolism*, **7**, 509–44.

Franklyn, J. A. (1994). The management of hyperthyroidism. *New England Journal of Medicine*, **330**, 1731–8.

Franklyn, J. A., Davis, J. R., Gammage, M. D., Little, W. A., Ramsden, D. B. & Sheppard, M. C. (1985). Amiodarone and thyroid hormone action. *Clinical Endocrinology*, **22**, 257–64.

Fung, H. Y. M., Kologula, M., Collison, K., John, R., Richards, C. J., Hall, R. & McGregor, A. M. (1988). Postpartum thyroid dysfunction in Mid-Glamorgan. *British Medical Journal*, **296**, 241–4.

Ginsberg, J. & Walfish, P. G. (1977). Post-partum transient thyrotoxicosis with painless thyroiditis. *Lancet*, **1**, 1125–8.

Gross, J., Pitt-Rivers, R. & Trotter, W. R. (1952). Effect of 3:5:3-L-triiodothyronine in myxoedema. *Lancet*, **1**, 1044–5.

Himsworth, R. L. (1992). Assessment of thyroid function. In: Grossman, A., editor. *Clinical Endocrinology*. Oxford, Blackwell Scientific Publications, pp. 264–273.

Jørgensen, J. O. L., Pedersen, S. A., Laurberg, P., Weeke, J., Skakkeback, N. E. & Christiansen, J. S. (1989). Effects of growth hormone therapy on thyroid function of growth hormone-deficient adults with and without concomitant thyroxine-substituted central hypothyroidism. *Journal of Clinical Endocrinology and Me-*

tabolism, **69**, 1127–32.

Juul, A., Behrenscheer, A., Tims T., Nielsen, B., Halkjaer-Kristensen, J. & Shak-kebaek, N. E. (1993). Impaired thermoregulation in adults with growth hormone deficiency during heat exposure and exercise. *Clinical Endocrinology*, **38**, 237–44.

Lalloz, M. R. A., Byfield, P. G. H. & Himsworth, R. L. (1985). A new and distinctive albumin variant with increased affinities for both triiodothyronines and causing hyperthyroxinaemia. *Clinical Endocrinology*, **22**, 521–9.

Larsen, P. R., Silva, J. E. & Kaplan, M. M. (1981). Relationships between circulating and intracellular thyroid hormones: physiological and clinical implications. *Endocrine Reviews*, **2**, 87.

Lazar, M. A. (1993). Thyroid hormone receptors: multiple forms, multiple possibilities. *Endocrine Reviews*, **14**, 184–93.

Magnus-Levy, A. (1985). Ueber den respiratorischen Gaswechsel unter dem Einfluss der Thyreoidea sowie unter verschiedenen pathologische Zuständen. *Berliner Klinishcen iner Wochenschrift*, **32**, 650–2.

Michie, W., Hamer-Hodges, D. W., Pegg, C. A. S., Orr, F. G. G. & Bewsher, P. D. (1974). Beta-blockade and partial thyroidectomy for thyrotoxicosis. *Lancet*, **1**, 1009–11.

Mulligen, L. M., Kwok, J. B. J., Healey, C. S., Elsdon, M. J., Eng, C., Gardner, E., Love, D. R., Mole, S. E., Moore, J. K., Papi, L., Ponder, M. A., Telenius, H., Tunnacliffe, A. & Ponder, B. A. J. (1993). Germline mutations of the RET proto-oncogene in multiple endocrine neoplasia Type 2A (MEN 2A). *Nature*, **363**, 458–60.

Nomura, S., Pittman, C. S., Chambers Jr. J. B., Buck, M. W. & Shimizu, T. (1975). Reduced peripheral conversion of thyroxine to triiodothyronine in patients with hepatic cirrhosis. *Journal of Clinical Investigation*, **56**, 643–52.

Oppenheimer, J. H., Koerner, D., Schwartz, H. L. & Surks, M. I. (1972). Specific nuclear triiodothyronine binding sites in rat liver and kidney. *Journal of Endocrinology and Metabolism*, **35**, 330–3.

Rapaport, B. & Ingbar, S. H. (1974). Production of triiodothyronine in normal human subjects and in patients with hyperthyroidism. *American Journal of Medicine*, **56**, 586–91.

Retetoff, S., Weiss, R. E. & Usala, S. J. (1993). The syndromes of resistance to thyroid hormone. *Endocrine Reviews*, **14**, 348–99.

Reznek, R. H. & Armstrong, P. (1994). The adrenal gland. *Clinical Endocrinology*, **40**, 561–76.

Rønnov-Jessen, V. & Kirkegaard, C. (1973). Hyperthyroidism–a disease of old age? *British Medical Journal*, **1**, 41–3.

Ross, E. J., Prichard, B. N. C., Kaufman, L., Robertson, I. A. G. & Harries, B. J. (1976). Preoperative and operative management of patients with phaeochromocytoma. *British Medical Journal*, **1**, 191–8.

Rudman, D., Moffitt, S. D., Fernhoff, P. M., Blackstone, R. D. & Faraj, B. A. (1981). Epinephrine deficiency in hypocorticotropic hypopituitary children. *Journal of Clinical Endocrinology and Metabolism*, **53**, 722–9.

Sap, J., Munoz, A., Damm, K., Goldberg, Y., Ghysdale, J., Lentz, A., Beug, H. & Vennstrom, B. (1986). The c-erbA protein is a high affinity receptor for thyroid hormone. *Nature*, **324**, 635–40.

Segal, J. & Ingbar, S. H. (1982). Specific binding sites for triiodothyronine in the plasma membrane of rat thymocytes: correlation with biochemical responses. *Journal of Clinical Investigation*, **70**, 919–26.

Slag, M. F., Morley, J. E., Elson, M. K., Crowson, T. W., Nuttall, F. Q. & Shafer, R. B. (1981). Hypothyroxinemia in critically ill patients as a predictor of high mortality. *Journal of the American Medical Association*, **245**, 43–5.

Sterling, K. (1979). Thyroid hormone action at the cell level. *New England Journal of Medicine*, **300**, 177–23.

Weinberger, C., Thompson, C. C., Ong, E. S., Lebo, R., Gruol, D. J. & Evans, R. M. (1986). The c-erbA gene encodes a thyroid hormone receptor. *Nature*, **324**, 641–6.

Wilkin, T. J., Gunn, A., Isles, T. E., Crooks, J. & Swanson Beck, J. (1979). Short-term triiodothyronine in prevention of temporary hypothyroidism after subtotal thyroidectomy for Graves' disease. *Lancet*, **2**, 63–6.

Woeber, K. A. (1992). Thyrotoxicosis and the heart. *New England Journal of Medicine*, **327**, 94–8.

Wurtman, R. J. & Axelford, H. (1966). Control of enzymatic synthesis of adrenaline in the adrenal medulla by adrenal cortical steroids. *Journal of Biological Chemistry*, **241**, 2301–5.

Index